PERICARDIAL DISEASE

Developments in Cardiovascular Medicine

VOLUME 108

For a list of titles see end of volume.

PERICARDIAL DISEASE

New Insights and Old Dilemmas

edited by

J. SOLER-SOLER

G. PERMANYER-MIRALDA

J. SAGRISTÀ-SAULEDA

Service of Cardiology, Hospital General Vall d'Hebron, Barcelona, Spain

Preface by Ralph Shabetai

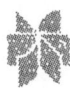

KLUWER ACADEMIC PUBLISHERS

DORDRECHT / BOSTON / LONDON

Library of Congress Cataloging-in-Publication Data

ISBN-13: 978-94-010-6702-7

Enfermedades del pericardio. English.
   Pericardial diseases : new insights and old dilemmas / edited by
J. Soler-Soler, G. Permanyer-Miralda, J. Sagristà-Sauleda.
      p.   cm. -- (Developments in cardiovascular medicine ; v. 108)
   Revised translation of: Enfermedades del pericardio.
   ISBN-13:978-94-010-6702-7   e-ISBN-13:978-94-009-0481-1
   DOI:10.1007/978-94-009-0481-1
   1. Peridardium--Diseases.   I. Soler Soler, J. II. Permanyer, G.
III. Sagristà-Sauleda, J., 1946- IV. Title. V. Series.
   [DNLM: 1. Pericardial Effusion. 2. Pericarditis.   W1 DE 977VME
v. 108 / WG 275 E56]
RC685.P5E54 1990
616.1'1--dc20
DNLM/DLC
for Library of Congress   89-24437
                                                              CIP

Published by Kluwer Academic Publishers,
P.O. Box 17, 3300 AA Dordrecht, The Netherlands.

Kluwer Academic Publishers incorporates
the publishing programmes of
D. Reidel, Martinus Nijhoff, Dr W. Junk and MTP Press.

Sold and distributed in the U.S.A. and Canada
by Kluwer Academic Publishers,
101 Philip Drive, Norwell, MA 02061, U.S.A.

In all other countries, sold and distributed
by Kluwer Academic Publishers,
P.O. Box 322, 3300 AH Dordrecht, The Netherlands.

This book is a revised version of an edition originally published in Spanish as: *Enfermedades del Pericardio*, Ediciones Doyma, SA, 1988
Translated by Dr. G. Permanyer-Miralda. Translation revised by Dr. R. Shabetai.

Printed on acid-free paper

There are no closed issues;
there are only men worn out by them.

S. Ramón y Cajal

Contents

List of contributors

J. Angel-Ferrer, M.D.
Service of Cardiology, Hospital General Vall d'Hebron, Barcelona, Spain.

Christopher P. Appleton, M.D.
Cardiology Section, Veterans Administration Medical Center, Tucson, Arizona, U.S.A.

J. Candell-Riera, M.D.
Service of Cardiology, Hospital General Vall d'Hebron, Barcelona, Spain.

Enrique Galve, M.D.
Service of Cardiology, Hospital General Vall d'Hebron, Barcelona, Spain.

H. García-del-Castillo, M.D.
Service of Cardiology, Hospital General Vall d'Hebron, Barcelona, Spain.

Liv K. Hatle, M.D.
Section of Cardiology, Regional Hospital, and Department of Medicine, University of Trondheim, Trondheim, Norway.

H. Sidney Klopfenstein, M.D., Ph.D.
Section of Cardiology, Department of Medicine, Bowman Grey School of Medicine, Wake Forest University, Winston-Salem, North Carolina, U.S.A.

M. Morlans, M.D.
Service of Nephrology, Hospital General Vall d'Hebron, Barcelona, Spain.

Marcos Murtra, M.D.
Service of Cardiac Surgery, Hospital General Vall d'Hebron, Barcelona, Spain.

J. Pascual Rodríguez, M.D.*
Primary care cardiologist, Madrid, Spain.

G. Permanyer-Miralda, M.D.
Service of Cardiology, Hospital General Vall d'Hebron, Barcelona, Spain.

Richard L. Popp, M.D.
Division of Cardiology, Stanford University School of Medicine, Stanford, California, U.S.A.

J. Sagristà-Sauleda, M.D.
Service of Cardiology, Hospital General Vall d'Hebron, Barcelona, Spain.

Ralph Shabetai, M.D.
University of California, San Diego, and Veterans Administration Medical Center, San Diego, California, U.S.A.

* deceased

J. Soler-Soler, M.D.
Service of Cardiology, Hospital General Vall d'Hebron, Barcelona, Spain.

David H. Spodick, M.D.
University of Massachusetts, Worcester, and Service of Cardiology, St. Vincent Hospital, Massachusetts, U.S.A.

Preface

In November 1986, I was invited to attend a symposium held in Barcelona on Diseases of the Pericardium. The course was directed by Dr. J. Soler-Soler, director of Cardiology at Hospital General Vall d'Hebron in Barcelona. During my brief but delightful visit to this institution, my appreciation of the depth and breadth of study into pericardial diseases, carried out by Dr. Soler and his group, grew into the conviction that these clinical investigators have accumulated a wealth of information concerning pericardial diseases, and that investigators and clinicians practicing in English speaking countries would greatly profit from ready access to the results of the clinical investigations into pericardial disease carried out in Barcelona.

The proceedings of the Barcelona conference were published in a beautifully executed volume in the Spanish language edited by Dr. Soler and produced by Ediciones Doyma. Because I believe that this work should be brought to the attention of the English speaking scientific and clinical communities, I encouraged Dr. Soler to have the book translated into English. I knew that this task could be accomplished and that the book would be translated into good English without change of its content. My confidence was based upon a translation of my own book, *The Pericardium*, into Spanish undertaken by Dr. Permanyer, who is a contributor and co-editor of the present volume.

The organization of the Service of Cardiology at the General Hospital Vall d'Hebron in Barcelona is such that clinical and research policies can be established by the chief of the Cardiology Service and the policies will be rigorously followed by the rest of the staff. The large number of patients followed for a decade and managed along predetermined lines constitute an invaluable source of clinical information and one, especially in this country, unlikely to be duplicated. I therefore consider it timely for this experience to become available in a monograph in the English language. Dr. Soler and his associates deserve great credit for establishing and maintaining prospective protocols (see Appendix) for the study of various pericardial diseases.

When I attended the symposium, I presented a paper on Clinical Aspects of Cardiac Tamponade and another on Constrictive Pericarditis and Restrictive Cardiomyophaty. Dr. Soler and his colleagues graciously asked me to include these in the English version. However, it seemed to me that this book should primarily present the clinical experience of Dr. Soler's group to English speaking readers, many of whom would be all too familiar with my own writings on this subject. Dr. Soler heads a group of clinical investigators that has not emphasized pathophysiology and animal experimentation; so, when Dr. Soler reluctantly accepted my wish not to be included as an author in the English book, his choice wisely fell on Dr. Sidney Klopfenstein for a discussion on cardiac tamponade and on Dr. Appleton, Dr. Popp and Dr. Hatle for a discussion of constrictive pericarditis and restrictive cardiomyo-

xi

J. Soler-Soler et al. (Eds.), Pericardial Disease, pp. xi–xvi.
© 1990 Kluwer Academic Publishers

phaty. These investigators have both made important new contributions to their subjects. I believe that readers of this volume will appreciate the wisdom of these choices. Dr. D. H. Spodick was also an invited guest from the United States at the Barcelona symposium, but for reasons similar to those regarding the chapters on cardiac tamponade and constrictive pericarditis, his contributions, like mine, are limited in this edition to the Round Table discussion (chapter 12).

It is not my intention to summarize, chapter by chapter, the contents of this book. I wish, however, to draw the reader's attention to the entity of transient constrictive pericarditis discussed by Dr. Angel, as this syndrome is not well known in this country. Likewise, it is becoming increasingly difficult in the United States to become experienced in the management of tuberculous pericarditis, and for this reason the contribution by Dr. Sagristà on this subject will be particularly useful. Likewise, few systematic studies of pericardial effusion in acute myocardial infarction have appeared in the English literature. For this reason, readers will find the contribution by Dr. Galve particularly interesting. Chronic effusive pericarditis characterized by massive effusion of unknown etiology is not encountered often, and presents a number of diagnostic and therapeutic difficulties which may be somewhat eased after reading the chapter by Dr. Soler. As practicing physicians, we are apt to think of pericardiectomy in the context of constrictive pericarditis, but Dr. Permanyer's discussion of other indications for pericardiectomy is highly relevant and his chapter constitutes a thought-provoking contribution to the present edition. The chapter by Dr. Murtra ends with a timely, if uncharacteristic, warning from a surgeon about the limitations of surgical treatment of pericardial disease.

Although the true functional significance of the pericardium remains enigmatic, the diseased pericardium can certainly make its presence felt. The pain of pericarditis sometimes simulates that of myocardial ischemia, but sometimes is pleuritic in nature. In either instance, more often than not, it is severe. Patients with relapsing acute pericarditis frequently use an adjective such as unbearable or excruciating to describe it. The pericardial friction rub, although capricious in behavior, is one of the most pathognomonic signs in clinical medicine. Likewise, the ECG manifestations of acute pericarditis are often florid.

Less common, but more dramatic are the manifestations of pericardial compression of the heart. The pericardium occupies a strategic position around the heart, such that compression by pericardial fluid under increased pressure, or constriction by pericardial scar, exerts dramatic effects on diastolic function which engender a remarkable degree of passive congestion.

The pathophysiology of constrictive pericarditis and cardiac tamponade has been considerably clarified by investigations over the last decade or so, employing a variety of new technological approaches. While appreciating the value of these recent contributions, it is salutary to look back on the work of Richard Lower on cardiac tamponade and Norman Chevers on constrictive pericarditis. In spite of all the limitations imposed by the lack of knowledge and technical amenities, both men recognized these two diseases as being major disorders of diastolic cardiac function. A distinguished English anatomist and physiologist, perhaps best known for his early studies on blood transfusion and intravenous drug infusion, Lower did much of his experimental work shortly after the death of William Harvey in 1657. In his famous "Treatise on the Heart", he wrote, "the fluid enclosed in the pericardium renders great service in lubricating the surfaces of the heart and in facilitating the movement: it likewise occasionally oppresses and floods the heart when it is in excess. For instance, when that envelope is full in *hydrops cordis*, and the walls of the organ are compressed on all sides by the surrounding fluid to such an extent that they are unable to dilate sufficiently to receive the blood, the heart beat diminishes greatly, until at length it is completely suppressed by too great an outflow of fluid, and syncope and death result." From his writings it is clear that he appreciated that impaired cardiac filling is the essential feature of tamponade. He also appreciated that, by a different mechanism, constrictive pericarditis can produce a similar result. He wrote, "Just as it injures the heart by accumulation of fluid within it, so when this is completely absent, it approaches so close to the heart, that at length, it adheres everywhere to this organ. Hence, as it is also joined to the diaphragm, it must combine and unite the heart's movement with that of the diaphragm." Then he goes on to describe the case of a thirty-year-old woman who complained of precordial discomfort and frequent fainting. He recorded his autopsy findings as follows: "when the body was opened, no abnormalities at all were visible among the abdominal viscera. While examining the other organs, however, we discovered a pathological condition of the heart, to which we may rightly attribute the cause of all her troubles. The thorax was opened and the lungs were healthy enough; the pericardium, however, had become closely attached all over to the whole surface of the heart, so that it could only with difficulty be separated from it. Further, this membrane had become thick, opaque and hard instead of being thin and transparent, as it should naturally have been. Hence, as there was no space for the free movement of the heart, and no fluids were moistening its surface, it is little wonder that she complained of all these ills." He then goes on to give what is probably the first description of pulsus paradoxus, proposing a theory popularized in more recent times by William Dock. Lower wrote, "Further, as the diaphragm is always attached to the pericardium in man, when the heart itself is also united to the pericardium, the diaphragm of necessity must have carried the heart down with it at every inspiration, and during that time, must have held up and suppressed its movement. So the observed intermission of the pulse succeeded regularly at every inspiration."

In 1842, the English physician Normal Chevers wrote concerning constrictive pericarditis, "The principal causes of dangerous symptoms in cases of the above appear to arise on the occurrence of gradual contraction of the layer of adhesive matter which has been deposited around the heart, com-

pressing its muscular tissue, and embarrassing its systolic and diastolic movements, *but more particularly the latter.* Under these circumstances, the circulation seems, after a time, in great measure to adapt itself to the en-
cumbered condition of the heart. The ventricles having become diminished in
capacity, make up for this loss by the rapidity of their contractions (hence the
small and rapid pulse). And thus the blood passes onward for a time, with
tolerable freedom; but the patients become incapable of continued muscular
exertion, and they are always liable to suffer from dropsy and other serous
effusions, upon the occurrence of very slight pulmonary obstructions... The
heart had, doubtless for a long time, continued to become more and more
compressed, weakened, and embarrassed by the gradual contraction of the
adventitious structure which surrounded it; distention of the great veins and
abdominal viscera had necessarily followed, and the resulting anasarca,
ascites and effusion of serum into the pleura, and air cells of the lung must
have had added still more to the obstruction with which the already almost
powerless heart had to contend." Modern medicine has emphasized the
pathophysiology of the compressive diseases of the heart, but from the preceding descriptions, it is apparent that the basic abnormality has been understood for a long time.

Removal of fluid from the pericardial space also has an interesting place in
medical history. Riolanus in 1653 suggested that pericardial effusion might
produce cardiac compression and suggested that trephining the sternum to
accomplish pericardiotomy might constitute the most effective treatment.
Franz Schuh (1804–1865), an Austrian physician, is credited with the first
closed pericardiocentesis which he performed on a twenty-four-year-old
woman who at autopsy five months subsequently was found to have a mediastinal neoplasm.

When I wrote my own book, *The Pericardium,* I stated that although
Francisco Romero was credited with the first open surgical drainage of
pericardial fluid, the original manuscript was lost. However, while attending
the Barcelona symposium, I learned from Dr. Pascual that he had, after years
of patient research, discovered the original published in Paris in 1815. The
story of Dr. Pascual's discovery is summarized in Appendix 3.

The function of the pericardium likewise has a long medical history.
Hippocrates described the structure as "a smooth membrane surrounding the
heart and containing a small amount of fluid resembling urine". Galen considered that function of the pericardium was to protect the heart, and thought
that "every structure has a function."

At the turn of the twentieth century, Barnard demonstrated that the pericardium can prevent acute over-distention of the heart. The importance or
lack thereof of pericardial constraint in normal physiology has often been
debated and written about in the ensuing ninety years. It is a relatively simple
matter to demonstrate that the pericardium significantly restrains left ventricular volume when the heart is subjected to an acute volume load such as rapid
infusion of a large volume of fluid, or the sudden appearance of severe mitral

regurgitation. It has been shown, both in experimental animals and in clinical studies, that sudden increase in preload shifts the left ventricular diastolic pressure-volume relation upwards, and sudden decrease in preload shifts the curve downward. If the left ventricle were to behave as an unrestrained body, alteration of preload would not displace the entire diastolic pressure-volume curve up and down its pressure axis, but would simply extend the original curve. In experimental animals, after the pericardium has been removed, alteration of preload does extend the curve rather than displacing it. This difference created by pericardiectomy on the effect of preload on the left ventricular diastolic pressure-volume relation furnishes clear evidence that the pericardium plays a major role in restraining acute cardiac dilatation. Indeed, when left and right atrial pressures are severely elevated by rapid fluid infusion, a substantial proportion of the pressure increase is borne by the pericardium, that is, pericardial pressure rises along with the atrial pressures, and the change in transmural atrial pressure is relatively small.

When the heart is subject to more gradual volume overload, such as occurs in heart failure, the pericardium adapts by hypertrophy and increased compliance. Thus, considerable cardiomegaly can occur without a significant increase in pericardial pressure or transmural atrial or ventricular diastolic pressure. However, acute exacerbations of heart failure, in which the already enlarged heart undergoes acute further enlargement, cause the heart to engage the pericardium. This engagement limits over-distention of the myocardium and must raise intrapericardial pressure. This phenomenon accounts for the observation that patients studied during acute exacerbation of heart failure often show equilibration of left and right ventricular diastolic pressure. This equilibration is a clear indication for the need for aggressive preload reduction; however, there is no evidence that pericardiectomy is of benefit in the treatment of heart failure.

For many years, pericardial pressure was measured in much the same way that intracardiac and vascular pressures are measured, using either fluid filled catheters attached to external pressure transducers, or transducer tipped catheters. In recent years, it has been proposed that this technique is suitable for measuring pericardial pressure only when there is pericardial effusion. It is posited that in normal physiology, the pericardium is in contact with the heart and therefore no true pericardial space exists, in spite of the presence of a small amount of pericardial fluid, conceived as a thin film between the layers. If it is true that there is no pericardial cavity, it is inappropriate to use techniques applicable to measurement of fluid pressure to the measurement of pericardial pressure. It then becomes necessary to assess the pericardial *contact force*, which may be several millimeters higher than conventionally measured pericardial liquid pressure. The originators of this manner of considering pericardial restraint offer several compelling analogies. One states that pressure in the knee joint of a standing subject measured by a catheter and Statham gauge would amount to only a few millimeters of mercury, whereas the condyles of the tibia obviously bear a much greater contact pressure. Likewise, if a heavy tent were to fall upon its occupant, and an interested observer were to put a catheter under the edge of the tent and attach it to a pressure transducer just outside the tent, the pressure recorded would be atmospheric, but the unfortunate occupant would not consider the weight of canvass pressing on his body as atmospheric. It is a more complicated matter to measure surface contact pressure than to measure liquid pressure. The proposed method is to insert a small flat unstressed balloon between the heart and pericardium, and to measure pericardial surface contact pressure, as the pressure within this balloon. This is clearly highly invasive and, for the most part, applicable only to experimental animals.

Of particular importance to the study of ventricular diastolic compliance is that pericardial contact pressure is close to right atrial pressure. Thus, if the balloon indeed yields a true estimate of pericardial pressure, then ventricular diastolic transmural pressure, a vital component of ventricular diastolic compliance, can be measured simply by subtracting right atrial from left ventricular diastolic pressure. When the pericardium contains fluid, the pressure within it can be measured by conventional technique and aside from hydrostatic differences is the same throughout the pericardial space. Pericardial surface contact pressure obeys no such rule of uniformity; inasmuch as regional differences in surface contact pressure can be demonstrated, and can be exaggerated by selective increase in the volume of specific cardiac chambers. Fortunately, clinicians are more frequently concerned with evaluating pericardial pressure in the presence of pericardial effusion; a circumstance that bypasses the current debate concerning the true nature of pericardial pressure.

William Osler emphasized that pericardial disease is often missed by clinicians simply because they fail to think of it. In today's terminology, successful diagnosis of pericardial disease requires a high index of suspicion. Spodick has pointed out that the pericardium can be involved in a myriad of systemic disorders. Sometimes this involvement is silent, but at other times seizes center stage from the hands of the underlying disease process, which may then escape early diagnosis. Dr. Soler and his collaborators, on the basis of their extensive clinical experience and the results of many years of patiently following prospective protocols, resolve some of these difficulties in diagnosis, provide a logical progression of investigative techniques and a logical basis for treatment. I believe that this volume will prove to be an invaluable source of clinical information on diseases of the pericardium.

San Diego, December 1989   RALPH SHABETAI

Introduction

This book is not a comprehensive monograph on pericardial disease. It rather is intended to be a review of several controversial aspects based on the experience of authors who mostly belong to the same working group.

In 1976 we attempted to put an end to the uneven fashion in which the diseases of the pericardium were approached in our Service. Accordingly, we elaborated a protocol for the diagnosis and management of pericardial disease which began to be operative in January 1977. From this time until December 1985 all patients who were admitted to the Cardiology Service were strictly evaluated and managed along the guidelines of the protocol, and then prospectively followed up. Throughout these nine years the original design of the protocol did not undergo any change. From 1986 onwards, only some particular types of pericardial disease have been prospectively followed. It should not be surprising to the reader, therefore, that the numbers related to the overall series change in some chapters. The total number of patients may change from 256 to 309, depending on the moment when the series was analysed for any particular topic. The initial analysis of our series induced us to change some basic aspects of the original protocol, mainly the indications for pericardiocentesis and pericardial biopsy. Accordingly, the protocol was modified and its new version may be found at the end of the present book.

The patients with end stage renal disease and pericardial disease have been prospectively studied on the basis of a separate protocol, which was elaborated by the Nephrology Service of our Hospital and began to be systematically applied on February 1978. The revised version (1986) of this protocol is also included at the end of this book.

Most of the present book, which is devoted to the Cinderella of heart disease, has a basically clinical emphasis, derived from our daily routine work. This is a deliberate approach, as for twelve years we have aimed to elaborate a rational systematization of the care of patients with pericardial disease based on clinical observation. This systematic work led us to confirm many already available clinical notions, to verify that old dilemmas have not gone away and to envisage new aspects of pericardial disease. Thus, the reader should not be surprised to find that topics as basic as the physical or electrocardiographic findings of acute pericarditis are not discussed in the book. This may, therefore, be of little use to the reader looking for a comprehensive text on pericardial disease. On the other hand, the book offers a new outlook to the clinician interested in less often discussed topics on which there is controversy. We hope the book may also prove useful to the expert physician who is puzzled by unsolved prevailing dilemmas, and is not satisfied with the explanation in the literature. The book does not emphasize pericardial physiology, pathophysiology or pathology, which are dealt in other available excellent monographs. However, some of the chapters provide

1

J. Soler-Soler et al. (Eds.), Pericardial Disease, pp. 1–3.
© 1990 Kluwer Academic Publishers

information on these topics and should prove useful to clinical and basic investigators.

The book includes a comprehensive discussion of one of the most common problems in everyday practice, the etiologic diagnosis and treatment of acute pericardial disease. This chapter has been elaborated in a Round Table format. This type of presentation may be surprising. However, we felt that the dialogue between members of different working groups might be the optimal means to present differing views on debatable issues. This Round Table actually took place in a Symposium on pericardial disease held at Barcelona on November 1986. Its present version is not a mere transcription of what was said, but its contents have been edited and updated. Also, bibliographical information concerning recent controversial areas, not previously discussed, has been included (acquired immunodeficiency syndrome, adenosine deaminase activity, newer imaging techniques, etc.). Although this chapter is placed at the end of the book, we strongly recommend the reader interested in getting a global view of our experience in the management of pericardial disease to begin by reading it before the remaining chapters.

The contribution of Dr. Ralph Shabetai has been of paramount importance for the elaboration of the English version of the present book. He not only obliged us by agreeing to write the Preface, but he also revised in a thorough and meticulous fashion the initial English translation that one of us (G.P.-M.) made of the original Spanish text. Owing to his painstaking efforts, the present text can now be offered to the English reader couched in a language that we would never be able to match. In addition to this cooperation, we are grateful to Dr. Shabetai for his invaluable editorial advice, his thoughtful criticism of our studies and, last but not least, the privilege of his friendship.

Dr. D. H. Spodick has always been particularly important to us. He was our first mentor. He was the first person not belonging to our group who carefully analysed the preliminary results of our study protocol. His encouraging criticism was decisive in making us continue to pursue the investigations which culminated in the present book.

We are grateful to Drs. Klopfenstein, Appleton, Popp and Hatle. Although their professional relation with us is recent, they have honored us by contributing valuable chapters which round out the information contained in the present text.

The large body of information that we have collected throughout the last twelve years could not be the result of our diligence alone. Without the willing continued cooperation of all the members of the Cardiology Service, who always complied faithfully with the study protocols, the studies could not have been adequately completed. We wish to acknowledge here our sincere gratitude to all of them. The anonymous task of the nurses of our Service should not be left unmentioned. One simply cannot tell how many pericardial fluid or biopsy specimens would not have been delivered to the laboratory in proper condition without their enthusiasm.

The Spanish edition of this book and, accordingly, the present revised

English translation, would not have been possible without the generous help of Laboratorios J. Uriach & Cía, S.A. This purely Spanish firm, which invests a great proportion of its financial resources in research, is to us a model of dedication, reliability and productivity. Our admiration for them exceeds even our gratitude.

The quality of transmission of a written message depends on its material form, no matter how good the message itself may be. For the present English edition we have been fortunate to secure the highly professional services of Kluwer Academic Publishers, and we particularly acknowledge our debt to Ms. H. P. Liepman. The firm has played a major role in furnishing an attractive volume in which to present our work.

Finally, it would be unfair not to acknowledge the technical assistance and unflinching personal loyalty of our secretaries Maravillas Llorente and Rosalía Coronado. To a degree, this is also their book.

Barcelona, October 1989   J. SOLER-SOLER
                                  G. PERMANYER-MIRALDA
                                    J. SAGRISTÀ-SAULEDA

1. Echocardiographic diagnosis of pericardial effusion: a critical evaluation

H. GARCÍA-DEL-CASTILLO, M.D.

Echocardiography is the technique most commonly used for the diagnosis of pericardial effusion (1, 2). In addition to its accuracy, it is noninvasive and comparatively nonexpensive. The characteristic finding of echocardiography is the presence of an echo free space behind the heart, between the free left ventricular wall and the posterior pericardium (Fig. 1.1). When the effusion is

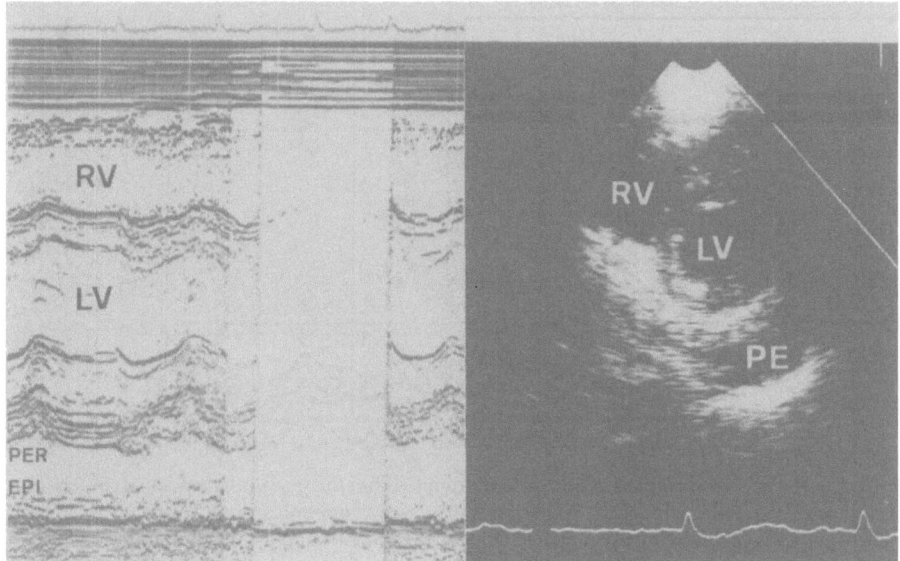

Fig. 1.1. M mode echocardiogram shows an echo free space between the epicardium (EPI) and the pericardium (PER) over the posterior cardiac wall indicating the presence of pericardial effusion. Two-dimensional echocardiogram in the short axis parasternal view shows an echo free space behind the left ventricular posterior wall, corresponding to pericardial effusion (PE). RV: right ventricle; LV: left ventricle.

J. Soler-Soler et al. (Eds.), Pericardial Disease, pp. 5–16.
© 1990 Kluwer Academic Publishers

large enough there may also be a separation between the anterior pericardium and the anterior right ventricular wall.

Diagnostic criteria

Both M mode and two dimensional techniques are useful for the detection of pericardial effusion. However, the M mode is more sensitive for the detection of small amounts of fluid owing to its better axial resolution (3). Using this technique, Horowitz et al. (4) established their widely accepted echocardiographic criteria of pericardial effusion in 1974. They compared the relation between epicardium and posterior pericardium with the amount of fluid removed from the pericardial cavity in 41 patients undergoing cardiac surgery, and described six patterns which they designated from A to E. In pattern A, the epicardium and pericardium maintained close contact throughout

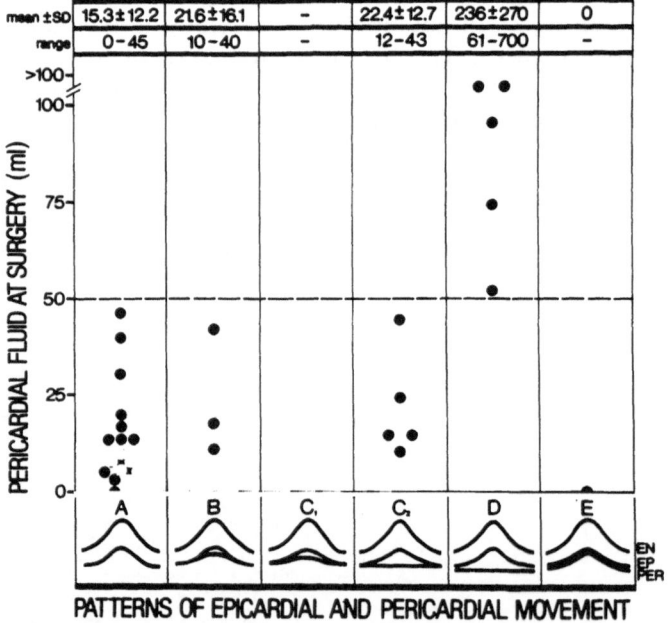

Fig. 1.2. Relation between the amount of fluid found within the pericardial cavity at surgery and the echocardiographic pattern of posterior wall pericardium-epicardium. The points in each column indicate the individual values. At the top of the figure the maximal, minimal and mean values and the standard deviation are shown, and at the bottom the echocardiographical patterns described by Horowitz et al. (4) is depicted. EN: endocardium; EP: epicardium; PER: pericardium. (From Galve E, García-del-Castillo H, Evangelista A, Batlle J, Permanyer-Miralda G, Soler-Soler J. Pericardial effusion in the course of myocardial infarction: incidence, natural history, and clinical relevance. Circulation 1986; 73: 294–299. Reproduced by permission of the American Heart Association, Inc.).

the cardiac cycle. In pattern B, the epicardium and pericardium were separated only in systole but remained in contact during diastole. In pattern C, the epicardium and pericardium remained separated during the systole and part of diastole. This pattern was divided into: C1 when the pericardium remained normally mobile, and C2 when it became immobile. In pattern D, the epicardium and pericardium remained separated during the whole cardiac cycle and the pericardium was immobile. Finally, in pattern E the pericardium and epicardium appeared as two closely separated parallel lines. Horowitz et al. (4) considered that the C2 and D patterns indicated the presence of effusion; this criterion has been subsequently accepted, although some authors (5) accept only pattern D as indicative of effusion. We have recently modified these criteria, in a study of pericardial effusion during acute myocardial infarction (6), to have our own criteria of effusion. We studied 33 patients with different types of heart disease on the day before cardiac surgery, and we interpreted the echocardiograms on the basis of Horowitz criteria. At operation the pericardium was carefully opened and a cannula was inserted to aspirate the fluid; the removed amount as measured and compared with the echocardiographic pattern (Fig. 1.2). Eighteen of the 32 patients with analyzable echocardiographic recordings had pattern A, three pattern B, five pattern C2, five pattern D and one pattern E; no instance of C1 pattern was found. The volumes of effusion found when the patterns were A, B or C2 had overlapped widely. None of the patients with any of these three patterns yielded more than 45 ml of pericardial fluid. When the echocardiogram showed pattern D the volume of effusion was consistently above 50 ml. Therefore, we consider that the only echocardiographic pattern that reliably indicated the presence of a sizeable pericardial effusion was pattern D. Pericardial fluid less than 50 ml in volume may show patterns A, B and C2, and should be considered as physiologic (7–9), as opposed to the opinion of Horowitz et al. (4) that 16 ml should be considered the upper normal limit.

Differential diagnosis

Not all echo free spaces behind the heart indicate pericardial effusion; several other structures which may result in similar images should be considered (Table 1.1). Two dimensional echocardiography is more reliable for this dif-

Table 1.1. Echocardiography in pericardial effusion. Differential diagnosis.

Left pleural effusion
Thoracic aorta
Venous coronary sinus
Aneurysmal left atrium
Pericardial tumors and cysts
Fibrous and calcific pericarditis
Epicardial fat

ferentiation than M mode, as it provides a real anatomical image of the heart and thus increases specificity.

The most difficult differential diagnosis is *left pleural effusion*, that often results in substantial amounts of fluid in the retrocardiac space. The lack of an anterior echo free space may help in the differentiation, as this is an uncommon occurrence in large pericardial effusion. However, the most useful finding is the position of the thoracic aorta as related to the heart (10). Normally, the aorta can be seen, in the different echocardiographic planes, to contact the posterior cardiac wall, approximately at the level of the atrioventricular groove. Pericardial effusion separates the thoracic aorta from the posterior cardiac wall, because the descending aorta is within the mediastinum but outside the pericardium. On the contrary, pleural effusion is located behind the thoracic aorta, which maintains contiguity with the posterior cardiac wall (Fig. 1.3).

Normal anatomical structures such as the *thoracic aorta* (11) or the *venous coronary sinus* (12) may be mistaken for small pericardial effusion in M mode presentation, but the two dimensional technique reliably establishes their true nature (Fig. 1.4).

An *aneurysmal left atrium* may also simulate pericardial effusion behind the left ventricle (13). The difference can be very difficult to establish with M mode, but it is readily appreciated with two dimensional technique, which may demonstrate that the echo free space behind the left ventricle communicates with the left atrium (Fig. 1.5).

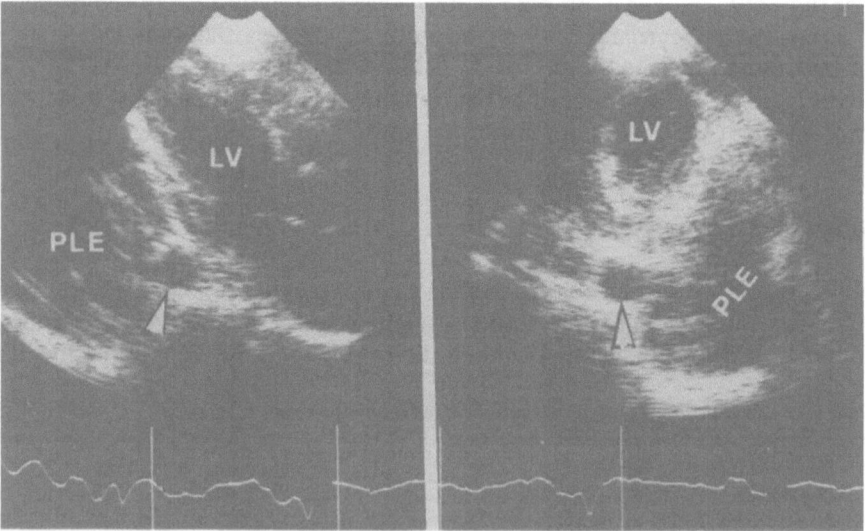

Fig. 1.3. Two-dimensional echocardiogram, parasternal long axis (left) and parasternal short axis (right) left ventricular views. The large fluid collection (PLE) behind the left ventricular posterior wall (LV) and the thoracic aorta (arrow head) is a pleural effusion. A small pericardial effusion can also be seen in front of the thoracic aorta.

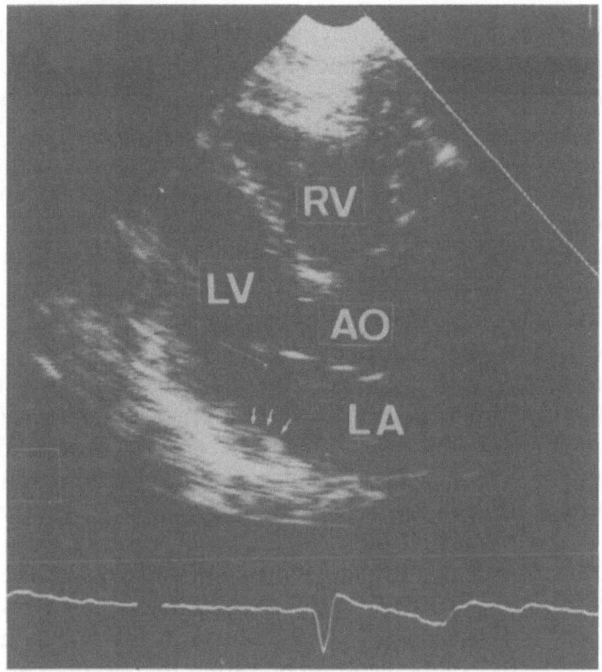

Fig. 1.4. Left parasternal long axis view showing the coronary sinus as an echo free space at the level of atrioventricular groove (arrows). AO: aorta; LA: left atrium; RV: right ventricle; LV: left ventricle.

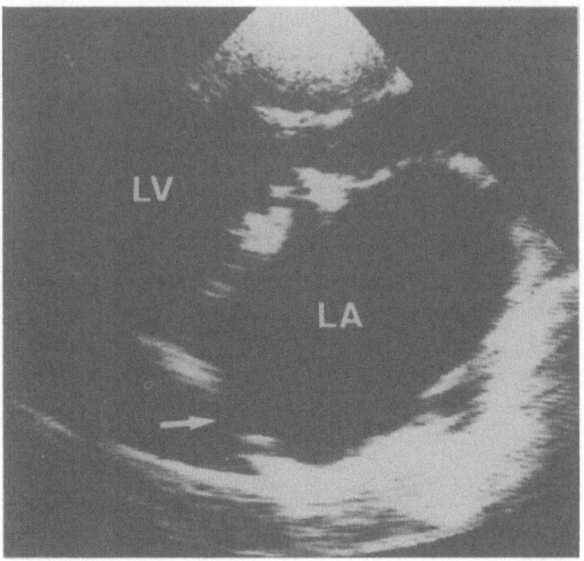

Fig. 1.5. Left parasternal long axis view showing an echo free space behind the posterior left ventricular wall communicating (arrow) with the left atrium. This is aneurysmal dilatation of the left atrium. LA: left atrium; LV: left ventricle.

Pericardial cysts and tumors may also simulate effusion, particularly with M mode. Figure 1.6 shows a cardiac angiosarcoma with a large anterior fluid collection and a small posterior pericardial effusion. At surgery a pericardial angiosarcoma communicating with the right atrium was found (14).

Fibrous or calcific pericarditis may be associated with a small pericardial effusion or fluid may be entirely absent, but the echocardiogram may simulate a moderately sized effusion (15). This possibility should be considered in cases with echocardiographic signs of effusion where pericardiocentesis is nonproductive (Fig. 1.7).

An anterior echo free space without a posterior echo free space is not considered evidence of pericardial effusion; it is attributed in most cases to *epicardial fat*, as has been confirmed by computed tomographic scans (16). Computed tomography has also shown that epicardial fat may be visualized not only as an anterior, but also a posterior echo free space. This space may be quite large, in which case it may be impossible to distinguish epicardial fat from pericardial effusion by echocardiography (17). On the other hand, Savage et al. (18) found that the prevalence of posterior echo free zones in 5652 individuals from the Framingham study was 6.5%. Particularly high prevalence was found in elderly individuals (higher than 10% in males and higher than 17% in females aged 70 years or more). These authors attributed such echo free spaces to subepicardial fat rather than to pericardial effusion.

Echocardiography is certainly not the ideal diagnostic tool for the accurate

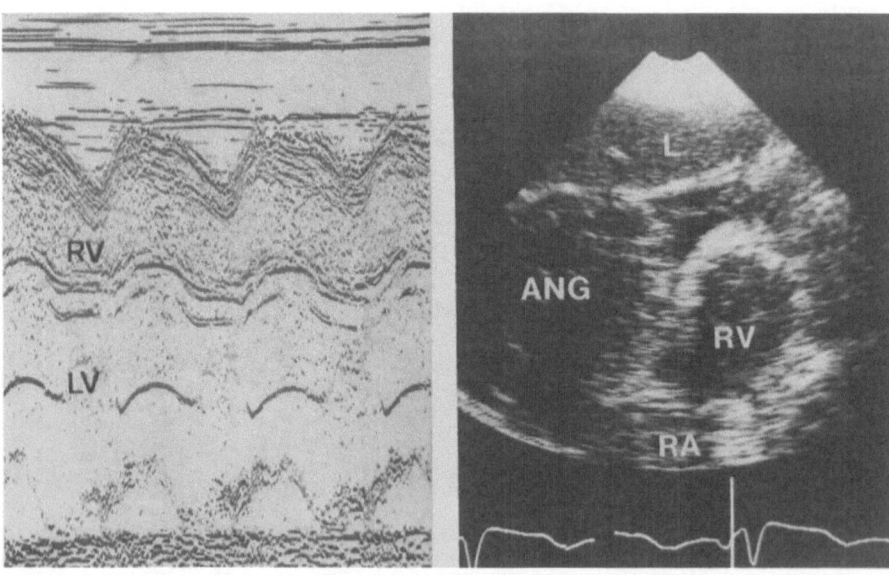

Fig. 1.6. Left panel: M mode echocardiogram showing a wide anterior echo free space. Right panel: subcostal view to show that the anterior clear space is caused by a large fluid filled mass. Cardiac angiosarcoma (ANG) was demonstrated at surgery. RA: right atrium; L: liver; RV: right ventricle.

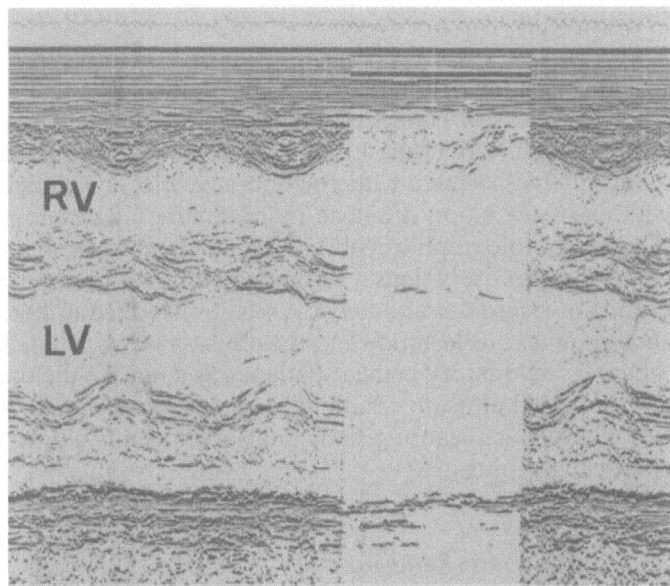

Fig. 1.7. M mode echocardiogram showing a wide posterior echo free space. One day after this recording was obtained, a pericardiocentesis was nonproductive. A few days later, surgery disclosed constrictive pericarditis with densely adherent pericardium without effusion. RV: right ventricle; LV: left ventricle.

identification of some of the above-mentioned situations. Newer noninvasive imaging techniques, such as computed tomography (16, 19–21) and nuclear magnetic resonance (22–24a) may provide more precise anatomic data. Furthermore, these techniques, particularly nuclear magnetic resonance, have even been claimed to give tissue and fluid characterizing information.

Specific situations

Pericardial effusion in acute myocardial infarction

Although the association of acute myocardial infarction and pericardial effusion is well known, only recently have the prevalence and significance of the latter been studied (6, 25–27). Pericardial effusion, usually small, is quite often found in patients with acute myocardial infarction (5.6%–37%). In our experience (6) it does not cause complications and is not a sequel of early postinfarction pericarditis or the level of anticoagulation, and has no influence on the mortality rate. These comments do not apply to hemopericardium secondary to cardiac rupture (28).

Pericardial effusion after cardiac surgery

Pericardial effusion after cardiac surgery can be detected in between 53% and 85% (29–31) of cases. The effusion usually develops between the second and tenth days after the operation, and is unrelated to the postcardiotomy syndrome. It is often associated with postoperative bleeding and, accordingly, patients with excessive blood drainage more commonly develop pericardial effusion. The echocardiographic evolution is charcteristic: the initial echo free space becomes progressively dense, so that it is difficult to differentiate from the neighboring myocardium and may even be overlooked if the echocardiographic study is limited to M mode and the effusion is loculated. Two-dimensional technique is mandatory in these patients, as it may be the only means of detecting a pericardial effusion resulting in cardiac tamponade (32); in addition, transesophageal echocardiography has been recently shown to be helpful in this particular setting (33).

Quantification of pericardial effusion

There are no definitive criteria for the echocardiographic quantification of pericardial effusion because of the lack of an alternative method to calculate the volume of fluid in the pericardial cavity to compare with the echocardiographic data. Pericardiocentesis is inadequate because removal of all the fluid is impossible in most cases. Aspiration during open chest surgery is accurate, but can be carried out only in a fraction of the patients.

Horowitz et al. (4) proposed a simple method for the quantification of pericardial effusion by M mode echocardiography. The distance between anterior and posterior pericardium at end-diastole is measured and cubed to estimate the volume of the pericardial cavity. The cardiac volume, estimated as the cube of the distance between anterior and posterior epicardium, is subtracted, and the difference corresponds to the volume of effusion. This method does not work well for small effusions and tends to underestimate larger effusions. Basically, the lack of precision of this technique is due to its being based on a small zone of anterior and posterior pericardium, neglecting others such as lateral recesses and the apex. Therefore, the calculation may be reasonably accurate if the fluid is evenly distributed in the pericardial sac, but in cases where it localises or loculates, the error may be considerable (Fig. 1.8). Martin et al. (34) used two dimensional technique to show that pericardial effusion is unevenly distributed particularly when it is small or very large. The distribution of moderate effusions tends to be more uniform, but not enough to allow accurate calculation of volume by the method of Horowitz et al. (4). Weitzman et al. (29) proposed a semiquantitative approach using M mode; effusion is considered small when the maximal diastolic separation between pericardium and epicardium is smaller than 10 mm, moderate if it is between 10 and 19 mm, and large when it is 20 mm or more.

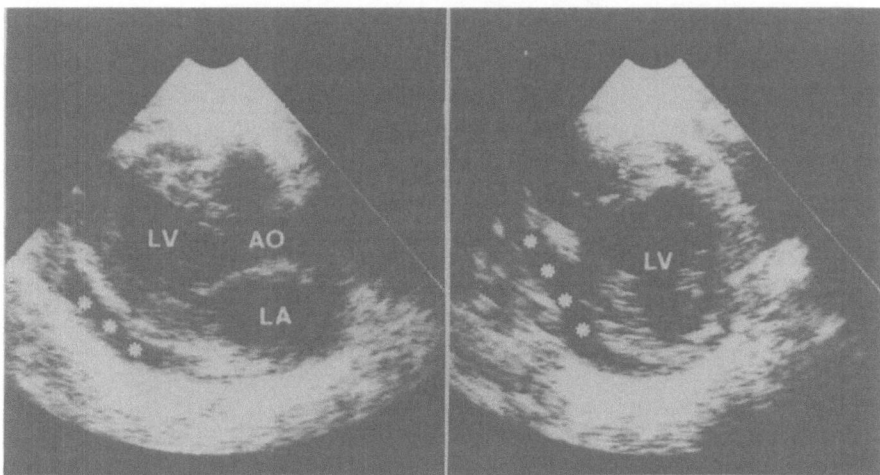

Fig. 1.8. Left panel, parasternal long axis view; right panel, short axis view at the ventricular level. An unevenly distributed pericardial effusion can be seen (asterisks), extending only through the posteroinferior area of the posterior sac. LA: left atrium; AO: aorta; LV: left ventricle.

A somewhat better quantification of effusion can be achieved using two dimensional technique. A simple quantification scheme could be the following: pericardial effusion present only behind the atrioventricular groove or extending slightly downwards without reaching the apex would be considered small. Those extending to the apex and to the lateral and posterior left ventricular wall and the anterior right ventricular wall would be considered large. Moderate effusions, probably the most difficult to quantify, would be in between the two extremes. Recently, nuclear magnetic resonance has been shown to be promising for the quantification of pericardial effusion (35).

Limitations of echocardiography

Although echocardiography provides a sensitive means to detect pericardial effusion, it may be missed particularly if one relies on M mode alone. When the recording technique is incorrect and the transducer is excessively angulated, the ultrasonic beam may not be directed through the pericardial effusion. This limitation does not exist with two dimensional technique, which allows study of the heart from different locations and in different sections. Localized effusion may be overlooked with the M mode study, but it is readily detected with two dimensional technique (Fig. 1.9).

The greatest diagnostic difficulty may arise when the pericardial effusion consists of blood, particularly when it contains clots (36, 37), as is frequently the case after cardiac surgery. M mode technique is insufficient for these cases, and two dimensional technique should always be used (32).

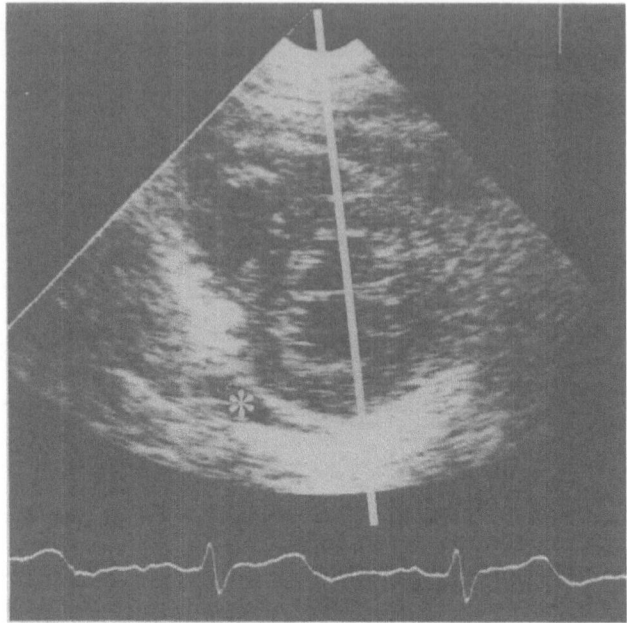

Fig. 1.9. Two dimensional echocardiogram showing a localized pericardial effusion (*) in the lateral zone of the posterior sac. The ultrasonic beam, in M mode, unless guided by 2D imaging, would miss the effusion. PE: pericardial effusion; RV: right ventricle; LV: left ventricle; IVS: interventricular septum.

Among the limitations of echocardiography for the diagnosis of pericardial effusion, false positive diagnosis due to the presence of epicardial fat should be included. Another shortcoming, common to all echocardiographic studies, is the inability to achieve satisfactory recording owing to a poor echocardiographic window. In spite of these limitations echocardiography performed with meticulous technique and with full awareness of the pitfalls of false positive and false negative diagnoses is one of the most sensitive and most specific tests available to the clinician.

References

1. Feigenbaum H, Waldhausen JA, Hyde LP. Ultrasound diagnosis of pericardial effusion. JAMA 1965; 191: 107–110.
2. Feigenbaum H, Faky A, Waldhausen JA. Use of reflected ultrasound in detecting pericardial effusion. Am J Cardiol 1967; 19: 84–90.
3. Feigenbaum H. Echocardiography. Philadelphia, Lea and Febiger, 1981; 490.
4. Horowitz MS, Schultz CS, Stinson EB, Harrison DC, Popp RL. Sensitivity and specificity of echocardiographic diagnosis of pericardial effusion. Circulation 1974; 50: 239-247.
5. Smith MD, Waters JS, Kwam OL, DeMaria AN. Evaluation of pericardial compressive disorders by echocardiography. Echocardiography 1985; 2: 67–86.
6. Galve E, García del Castillo H, Evangelista A, Batlle J, Permanyer Miralda G, Soler Soler

J. Pericardial effusion in the course of myocardial infarction: incidence, natural history and clinical relevance. Circulation 1986; 73: 294–299.

7. Sanmarco ME. Functional anatomy and developmental abnormalities of the pericardium and its diseases. Springfield, Charles C Thomas, 1971; 22–40.

8. Spodick DH. The pericardium: structure, function and disease spectrum. In: Spodick DH, ed. Pericardial diseases. Philadelphia, F.A. Davis Co. 1976; 1–10.

9. Roberts WC, Spray TL. Pericardial heart disease: a study of its causes, consequences and morphologic features. Cardiovasc Clin 1976: 7: 11–56.

10. Haaz WS, Mintz GS, Kotler MN, Parry W. Segal BL. Two-dimensional echocardiographic recognition of the descending thoracic aorta: value in differentiating pericardial from pleural effusion. Am J Cardiol 1980; 46: 739–743.

11. Mintz GS, Kotler MN, Segal BL, Parry WR. Two-dimensional echocardiographic recognition of the descending thoracic aorta. Am J Cardiol 1979; 44: 232–238.

12. Snider AR, Ports TA, Silverman NH. Venous anomalies of the coronary sinus: detection by M-mode, two-dimensional and contrast echocardiography. Circulation 1979; 60: 721–727.

13. Reeves WL, Ciotola T, Babb JD, Buonocore E, Leaman D. Prolapsed left atrium behind the left ventricular posterior wall: two-dimensional echocardiographic and angiographic features. Am J Cardiol 1981; 47: 708–712.

14. Mayor Molina G, García del Castillo H, Sagristà Sauleda J, Murtra Ferré M, Soler Soler J. Angiosarcoma de corazón. Hallazgos ecocardiográficos. Rev Esp Cardiol 1986; 39: 456–458.

15. Clark JG, Berberich SN, Zager JR. Echocardiographic findings of pericardial effusion mimicked by fibrocalcific pericardial disease. Echocardiography 1985; 2: 475–480.

16. Isner JM, Carter BL, Roberts WC, Bankoff MS. Subepicardial adipose tissue producing echocardiographic appearance of pericardial effusion. Documentation by computed tomography and necropsy. Am J Cardiol 1983; 51: 565–569.

17. Rifkin RD, Isner JM, Carter BL, Bankoff MS. Combined posteroanterior subepicardial fat simulating the echographic diagnosis of pericardial effusion. J Am Coll Cardiol 1984; 3: 1.333–1.339.

18. Savage DD, Garrison RJ, Brand F, Anderson SJ, Castelli WP, Kannel WB, Feinleib M. Prevalence and correlates of posterior extra echocardiographic spaces in a free-living population based sample (The Framingham study). Am J Cardiol 1983; 51: 1.207–1.212.

19. Moncada R, Baker M, Salinas M, Demos TC, Churchill R, Love L, Reynes C, Hale D, Cardoso M, Pifarré R, Gunnar RM. Diagnostic role of computed tomography in pericardial disease: congenital defects, thickening, neoplasms, and effusions. Am Heart J 1982; 103: 263–282.

20. Wong BYS, Lee KR, MacArthur RI. Diagnosis of pericardial effusion by computed tomography. Chest 1982; 81: 177–181.

21. Ansari A, Rholl AO. Pseudopericardial effusion: echocardiographic and computed tomographic correlations. Clin Cardiol 1986; 9: 551–555.

22. Stark DD, Higgins CB, Lanzer P, Lipton MJ, Schiller N, Crooks LE, Botvinick EB, Kaufman L. Magnetic resonance imaging of the pericardium: normal and pathologic findings. Radiology 1984; 150: 469–474.

23. Sechtem U, Tscholakoff D, Higgins CB. MRI of the abnormal pericardium. Am J Roentgenol 1986; 147: 245–252.

24. Meltzer RS, Vered Z, Neufeld HN (eds). Noninvasive cardiac imaging. Recent developments. Mount Kisco, Futura Publishing Company 1988, 289–351.

24a. Mulvagh SL, Rokey R, Vick W III, Johnston DL. Usefulness of nuclear magnetic resonance imaging for evaluation of pericardial effusions, and comparison with two-dimensional echocardiography. Am J Cardiol 1989; 64: 1002–1009.

25. Wunderick RG. Incidence of pericardial effusions in acute myocardial infarctions. Chest 1985; 85: 494–496.

26. Kaplan K, Davinson R, Parker M, Przybylek J, Light A, Bresnahan D, Ribner H, Talano

JV. Frequency of pericardial effusion as determined by M mode echocardiographic in acute myocardial infarction. Am J Cardiol 1985; 55: 335–337.

27. Pierard LA, Albert A, Henrard L, Lempereur P, Sprynger M, Carlier J, Kulbertus HE. Incidence and significance of pericardial effusion in acute myocardial infarction as determined by two-dimensional echocardiography. J Am Coll Cardiol 1986; 8: 517–520.

28. López Sendón J. Ruptura cardíaca subaguda. Tesis doctoral. Universidad Complutense de Madrid, 1985.

29. Weitzman LB, Tinker WP, Kronzon I, Cohen ML, Glassman E, Spencer FC. The incidence and natural history of pericardial effusion after cardiac surgery. An echocardiographic study. Circulation 1984; 69: 506–511.

30. Stevenson LW, Child JS, Laks H, Kern L. Incidence and significance of early pericardial effusions after cardiac surgery. Am J Cardiol 1984: 54: 848–851.

31. Ikäheimo MJ, Huikuri HV, Airaksinen KE, Korhonen UR, Linnaluoto MK, Tarkka MR, Takkunen JT. Pericardial effusion after cardiac surgery: incidence, relation to the type of surgery, antithrombotic therapy and early coronary bypass graft patency. Am Heart J 1988; 116: 97–102.

32. Kronzon I, Cohen ML, Wines HE. Cardiac tamponade by loculated pericardial hematoma: limitations of M mode echocardiography. J Am Coll Cardiol 1983; 3: 913–915.

33. Beppu S, Nakatani S, Tanaka N, Ikegami K, Kumon K, Nagata S, Myatake K, Nimura Y. Transesophageal echocardiographic diagnosis of localized pericardial coagula: a special cause of cardiac tamponade. Circulation 1988; 78: II-299 (abstr.).

34. Martin RP, Rakowski H, French J, Popp RL. Localization of pericardial effusion with wide angle phased array echocardiography. Am J Cardiol 1978; 42: 904–912.

35. Rokey R, Bolli R, Lewandowski D, Vick W, Roberts R, Johnston D. Detection and quantification of pericardial effusion using nuclear magnetic resonance imaging techniques. J Am Coll Cardiol 1988; 11 (suppl A): 158 A.

36. Kerber RE, Payvandi MN. Echocardiography in acute hemopericardium: production of false-negative echocardiograms by pericardial clots. Circulation 1977; 55–56 (supl III): III-24.

37. López Sendón J, García Fernández MA, Coma Canella I, Silvestre J, de Miguel E, Martín Jadraque L. Identification of blood in the pericardial cavity in dogs by two-dimensional echocardiography. Am J Cardiol 1984; 53: 1.194–1.197.

2. Tamponade and constriction: an appraisal of echocardiography and external pulse recordings

J. CANDELL-RIERA, M.D.

Cardiac tamponade and constriction are hemodynamic abnormalities which have traditionally been identified by cardiac catheterization; however, phono-cardiography, external pulse recordings and echocardiography play an important role in their clinical detection. External pulse recordings are not particularly useful for the diagnosis of tamponade, but the echocardiogram is the study of choice for the identification and quantification of pericardial effusion. On the other hand, several findings of Doppler echocardiography are indicative of the hemodynamic abnormalities of cardiac tamponade. In constrictive pericarditis, the phonocardiogram and external recording of the jugular venous pulse provide important information; in addition, Doppler echocardiography may provide some suggestive findings.

Cardiac tamponade

An important M mode echocardiographic finding of cardiac tamponade (Table 2.1) is an exaggerated variation in the ventricular diameters during the respiratory cycle (1), such that during inspiration right ventricular dimension increases while the left decreases, whereas during expiration the opposite takes place. In some severe cases the right ventricular diameter becomes smaller than 1 cm during expiration (Fig. 2.1). This finding supports the hypothesis that pulsus paradoxus is caused in part by a competitive filling of the two ventricles within a relatively rigid pericardial space (2). In a retrospective review of 22 patients with tamponade, Smith et al. (3) found this sign in 65% of patients. In Fig. 2.1, reciprocal changes in the ventricular diameters can be seen both in M mode and in two-dimensional recordings, with virtually complete collapse of the right ventricle during expiration. This is perhaps one of the more specific signs of cardiac tamponade; however, up to 10% of

J. Soler-Soler et al. (Eds.), Pericardial Disease, pp. 17–45.

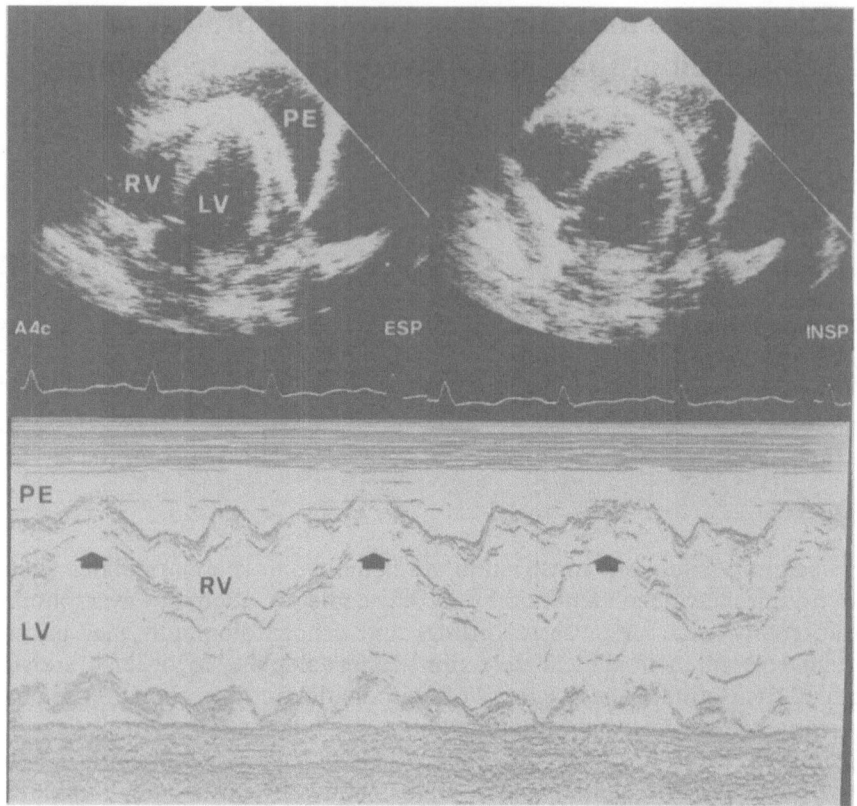

Fig. 2.1. M mode and two-dimensional echocardiographic recording of a patient with pericardial effusion (PE) and tamponade. There is a remarkable variation of ventricular diameters
during the respiratory cycle, both in the apical 4 chamber view (A4C) and in the M mode.
During expiration, the right ventricular (RV) end diastolic diameter is shorter than 1 cm and the
interventricular septum is virtually in contact with the right ventricular anterior wall (arrows).
ESP: expiration; INSP: inspiration; LV: left ventricle.

false positives have been reported (3). In patients with chronic obstructive
pulmonary disease wide variations of the ventricular diameters can also be
found during the respiratory cycle.

Two other characteristic signs are commonly found with two dimensional
echocardiography in patients with cardiac tamponade: end diastolic right
atrial collapse (4) and diastolic collapse of right ventricular free wall (5).
Figure 2.2 shows an end diastolic atrial collapse in the apical 4 chamber view;
a diastolic collapse of right ventricular anterior wall in the parasternal long
axis view can be seen in Fig. 2.3. These two findings should be carefully
looked for, particularly in apical and subcostal 4 chamber views, in all instances of pericardial effusion and whenever tamponade is suspected. Right
atrial collapse has been reported as one of the most sensitive and specific

Table 2.1. Cardiac tamponade. Echocardiographic findings.

M mode

Exaggerated reciprocal changes in ventricular diameters during the respiratory cycle (increase
   in right and decrease in left ventricular diameters during inspiration)*
Right ventricular diameter less than 1 cm at the end of expiration*
Swinging heart
Pericardial effusion behind the left atrium
Reduced EF mitral slope during inspiration
Early systolic notch of the right ventricular anterior wall
Interval mitral opening-X point longer than 0.05 sec.
Mitral pseudoprolapse
Abnormal motion (hypokynetic, paradoxical) of posterior left ventricular wall

Two-dimensional

End diastolic right atrial collapse*
Diastolic right ventricular collapse*
Swinging heart
End diastolic collapse of both atria
Diastolic left ventricular collapse
Absence of respiratory changes in the inferior vena cava diameter

Doppler

Wide respiratory variations in blood flow velocity through cardiac valves*
Absent respiratory variation in superior vena cava and hepatic vein flows

---

* Major findings.

signs in tamponade. Gillam et al. (4), in a series of 127 patients, found that
this sign had a 100% sensitivity and a 82% specificity. The beginning of this
collapse is coincident with atrial contraction, after the P wave of the electrocardiogram; it can be observed with greater accuracy when the M mode is
guided through the right atrial wall from the apical 4 chamber view (Fig. 2.4).
Probably, the mechanism of this sign is an increase of intrapericardial pressure above right atrial pressure at end diastole, when the ventricular volume is
largest. Accordingly, it might be absent or attenuated in cases with increased
right atrial pressure of other etiology, e.g., heart failure, tricuspid regurgitation
or severe pulmonary hypertension (6).

   Right atrial contraction may be seen after the P wave in patients with effusion without tamponade, and even without effusion. This movement may
complicate the evaluation of right atrial collapse, as an increased or vigorous
atrial contraction could be confused with right atrial collapse; the converse
might also happen. In a series of 25 patients with moderate to large pericardial effusion we were unable to demonstrate that the duration or amplitude of
right atrial collapse correlated with the level of intrapericardial pressure.
Quantification of right atrial motion was made in M mode guided from the
apical 4 chamber view (Fig. 2.4) and in the sagittal subcostal view of right
atrium and inferior vena cava (Fig. 2.5). This latter view, according to our
experience (7), permits detection of moderate and large pericardial effusions

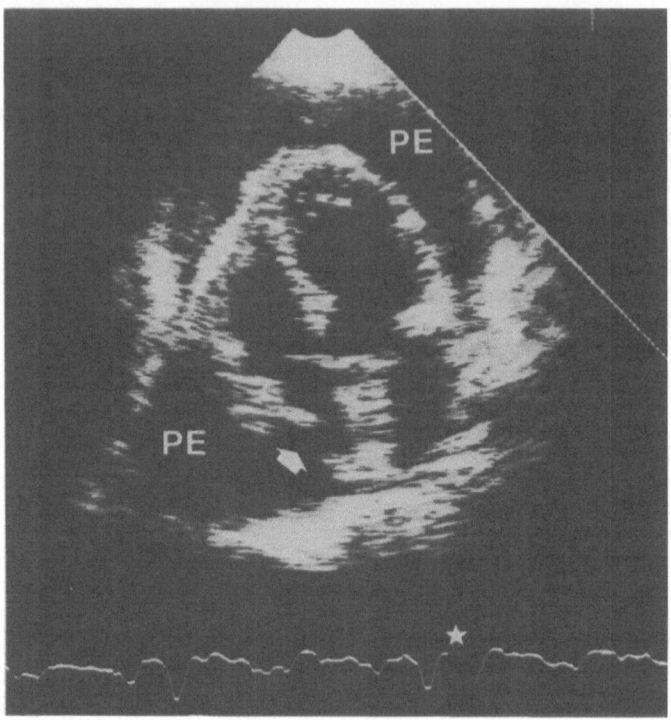

Fig. 2.2. Two-dimensional echocardiogram (apical 4 chamber view) of a patient with large pericardial effusion (PE) and cardiac tamponade. Right atrial collapse is apparent (arrow), persisting until early systole, as can be seen from the electrocardiogram (*).

between right atrial wall and the diaphragm. The lack of correlation between the magnitude of right atrial collapse and the level of intrapericardial pressure might be explained, at least in part, by frequent inability to cross the right atrium with the ultrasonic beam at right angles.

Experimental studies (8, 9) have shown that the sensitivity and specificity of right atrial and ventricular collapse improve with increasing severity of tamponade. Sensitivity and specificity are both consistently higher for right atrial than for right ventricular collapse. These signs indicate increased intrapericardial pressure even when pulsus paradoxus is not yet apparent (10–12). Abnormalities of intravascular volume may modify the relationship between right ventricular collapse and the severity of tamponade; thus, in hypovolemic states collapse may be observed with lower intrapericardial pressure (13, 14).

Several additional M mode and two dimensional echocardiographic findings (Table 2.1) have been reported in cases of cardiac tamponade (3, 15). The "swinging heart" (16, 17) may be observed in about a third of cases (3). Figure 2.6 shows the M mode echocardiogram of a patient with a huge pericardial effusion and oscillation of the heart every two cardiac cycles, which explains the electrical alternans. An echo free space behind the left atrium, in

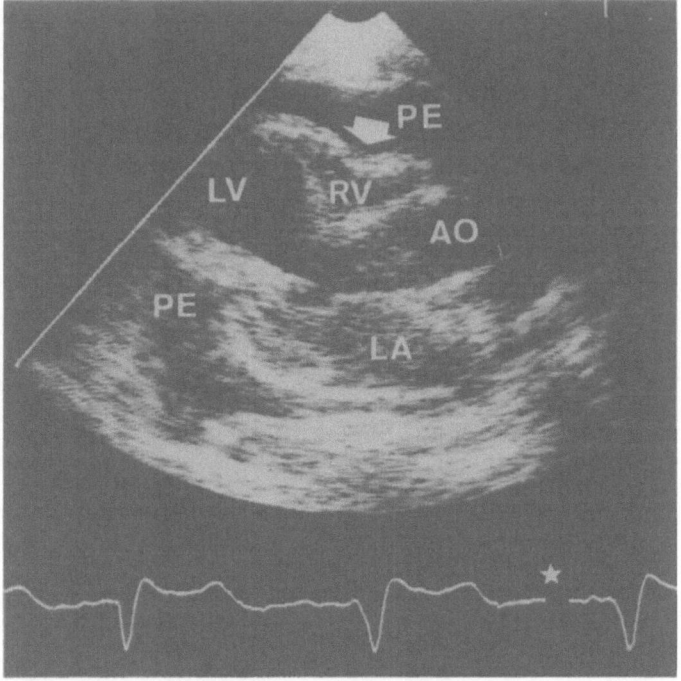

Fig. 2.3. Two-dimensional echocardiogram (parasternal long axis view) of a patient with peri-cardial effusion (PE) and cardiac tamponade. Collapse of right ventricular (RV) anterior wall (arrow) is apparent at end-diastole (*). AO: aorta. LA: left atrium; LV: left ventricle.

the oblique sinus (18, 19) is also present in about a third of cases (3). Mitral EF slope diminishes during inspiration (1), reflecting decreased left ventric-ular filling.

An early systolic notch (Fig. 2.7) in the anterior right ventricular wall has been described (20, 21), but the mechanism of this finding, which may be seen in one fourth of the patients (3), is poorly understood.

Engle et al. (22) reported that the interval between mitral opening and the X point (maximal posterior displacement of the right ventricular anterior wall) exceeded 0.05 seconds in the presence of tamponade.

Mitral "pseudoprolapse" (Fig. 2.7) has also been reported, consisting of a posterior holosystolic displacement and simulating the hammock image that can be seen in mitral prolapse. This apparent posterior displacement is really due to overall backwards displacement of the heart during systole (21, 23, 24). Abnormal motion of the posterior left ventricular wall has also been described (25) and an example is shown in Fig. 2.8.

Other reported findings depend upon two dimensional technique. In addition to the previously mentioned right atrial and ventricular collapses, end diastolic collapse of both atria (26), diastolic left ventricular collapse (27), and absence of the commonly found respiratory changes in the inferior

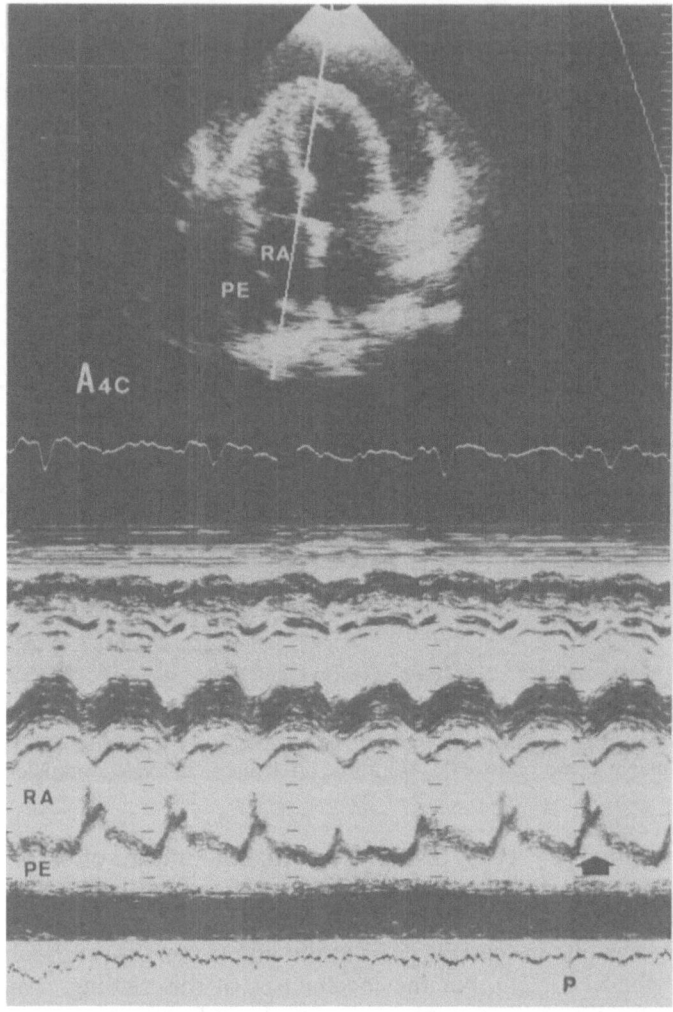

Fig. 2.4. Two-dimensional (apical 4 chamber view) and M mode echocardiogram (the ultra-sonic beam crosses the right atrial wall) in a patient with pericardial effusion, without clinical features of tamponade but with increased intrapericardial pressure. In the M mode recording it can be seen that the forward displacement (arrow) of the right atrial (RA) anterior wall begins after the P wave of the electrocardiogram. PE: pericardial effusion.

vena cava diameters (28) have also been reported. Figure 2.9 shows the respiratory variations in the diameter of inferior vena cava in the sagittal sub-costal view and the corresponding M mode recording in a healthy individual (left), in which the reduction of the vena cava size during inspiration is apparent. These variations are not found in instances with increased right atrial pressure, as shown in Fig. 2.9 (right). This sign usually accompanies right atrial collapse in cases of cardiac tamponade, but we have found it in

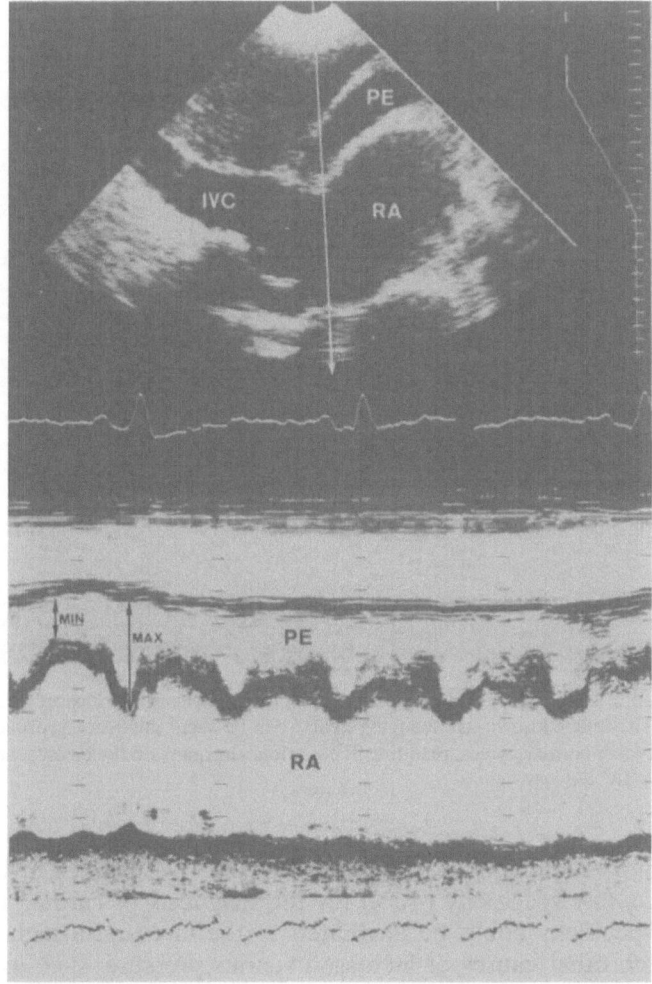

Fig. 2.5. Two-dimensional (sagittal subcostal view of right atrium and inferior vena cava) and M mode echocardiogram with the ultrasonic beam crossing the right atrial wall of a patient with pericardial effusion (PE) without clinical findings of tamponade. In the M mode recording the right atrial (RA) wall movement can be seen, showing a maximum posterior displacement (MAX) after the P wave of the electrocardiogram and the persistence of a separation between the atrial wall and the diaphragm for the remainder of the cardiac cycle (MIN). IVC: inferior vena cava. Copyrighted and reprinted with the permission of Clinical Cardiology Publishing Co.,/FACM, Inc., JBI Building, Box 832, Mahwah, New Jersey 07430, USA. (7).

instances of increased right atrial pressure of other etiology, such as in the patient in Fig. 2.9, who had mitral and tricuspid valve disease. In such cases there is no accompanying right atrial collapse. Himmelman et al. (29), in a retrospective series of 115 patients with moderate or severe pericardial effusion, found that the features suggesting "plethora" of inferior vena cava

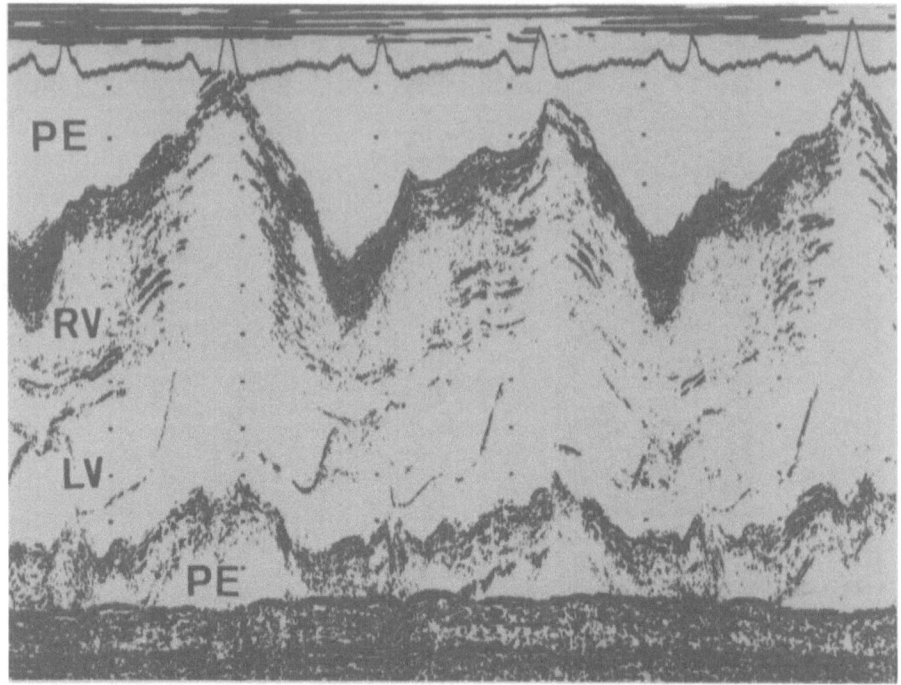

Fig. 2.6. M mode echocardiogram of a patient with large pericardial effusion (PE) and cardiac tamponade. The image known as "swinging heart" can be seen: the heart approaches the thoracic wall every two cardiac cycles, resulting in electrical alternans on the electrocardiogram. RV: right ventricle; LV: left ventricle.

(an inspiratory reduction in diameter of less than 50%) had a high sensitivity (97%) but a low specificity (40%) for the diagnosis of cardiac tamponade. This low specificity could be attributed to the fact that a high number of patients with other causes of increased venous pressure, such as congestive heart failure, were included in the series. On the other hand, the sensitivity of this sign would probably have been smaller if patients with low pressure tamponade (right atrial pressure lower than 12 mm Hg) (30) had been included in the series.

In some cases, transesophageal echocardiography may permit the diagnosis of special forms of cardiac compression, such as intrapericardial blood clots after cardiac surgery (31).

In cardiac tamponade, Doppler echocardiography may detect wide variations in the blood flow velocity through cardiac valves with the respiratory cycle and normalization after pericardiocentesis. In inspiration there is a marked reduction of flow through the left cardiac valves whereas flow increases through the right sided valves (32–33a). Figure 2.10 shows a reduced flow velocity in the left ventricular outflow tract during inspiration and normalization after pericardiocentesis. Exaggerated respiratory variations may

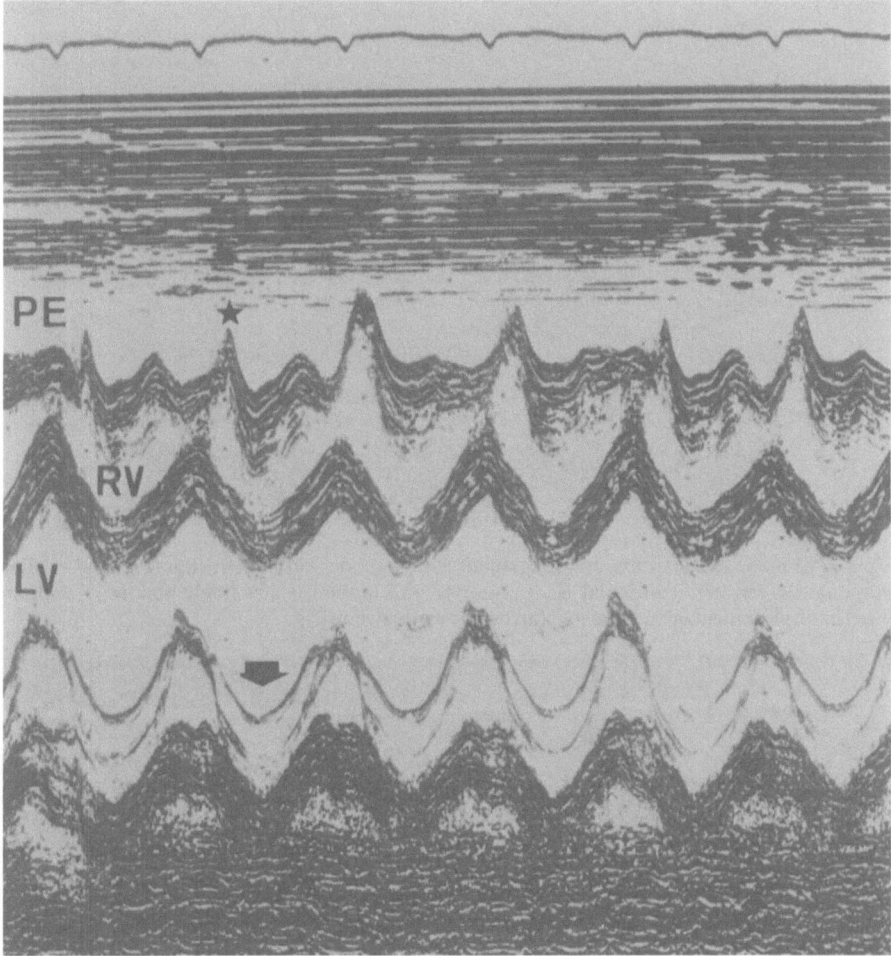

Fig. 2.7. M mode echocardiogram of a patient with pericardial effusion (PE) and cardiac tamponade, where a mitral pseudoprolapse (arrow) and an early systolic notch (*) in the right ventricular (RV) anterior wall can be seen. LV: left ventricle.

also be found, although in a lesser degree, in patients with large pericardial effusion and mild tamponade even in the absence of clinical findings of severe tamponade. Respiratory variations in flow velocity, particularly when confined to the right sided valves, should be evaluated with caution because they may be present in chronic lung disease and in normal individuals; in the latter, however, the magnitude of the changes is smaller. Flow oscillation related to the cardiac cycle in superior vena cava and hepatic veins during respiration may be less conspicuous in cardiac tamponade than in normal individuals. In normal subjects, systolic velocity always predominates over diastolic, and the predominance is increased during inspiration (Fig. 2.11). In cardiac tam-

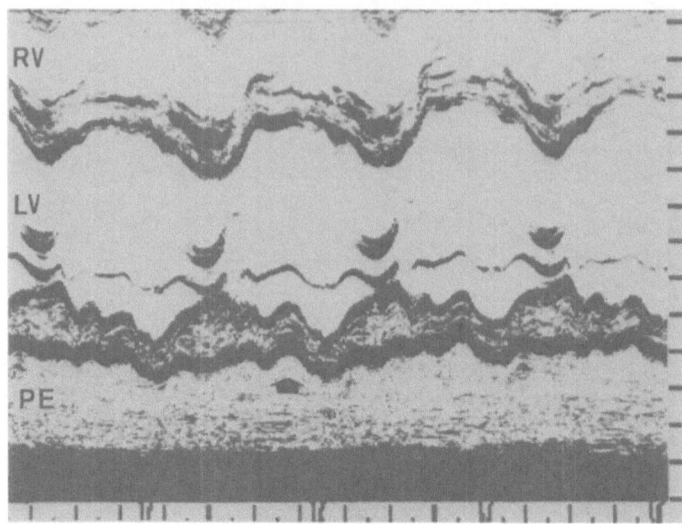

Fig. 2.8. M mode echocardiogram of a patient with large pericardial effusion (PE) and cardiac tamponade where left ventricular (LV) posterior wall motion is absolutely abnormal, with an anterior displacement in end diastole (arrow). RV: right ventricle.

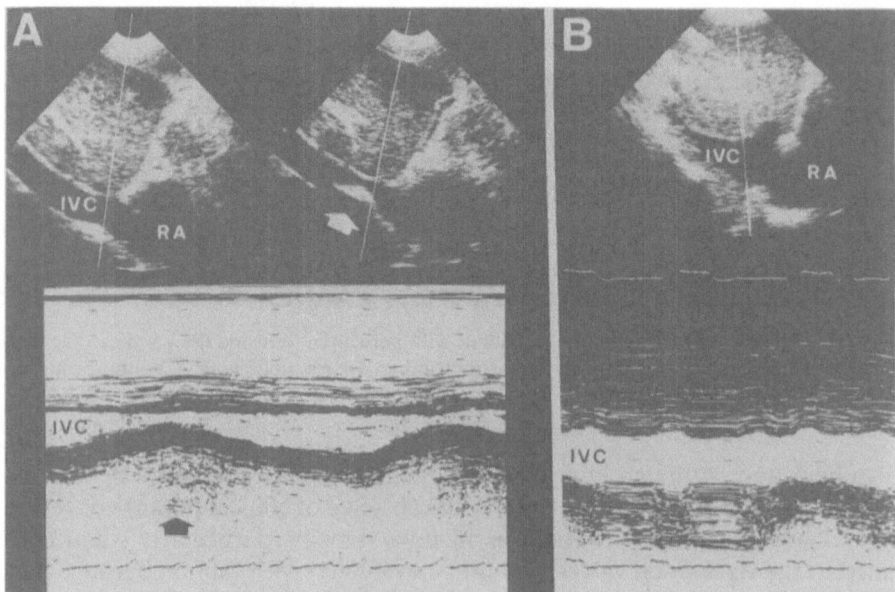

Fig. 2.9. Sagittal subcostal view of right atrium (RA) and inferior vena cava (IVC) of a healthy individual (A) and a patient with rheumatic mitral and tricuspid disease (B). In A, there is an apparent reduction in the diameter of inferior vena cava during inspiration, both in two dimensional and M mode echocardiograms (arrows). In B, IVC is dilated (23 mm) and shows a slight systolic expansion attributable to tricuspid regurgitation, but without changes in diameter during the respiratory cycle.

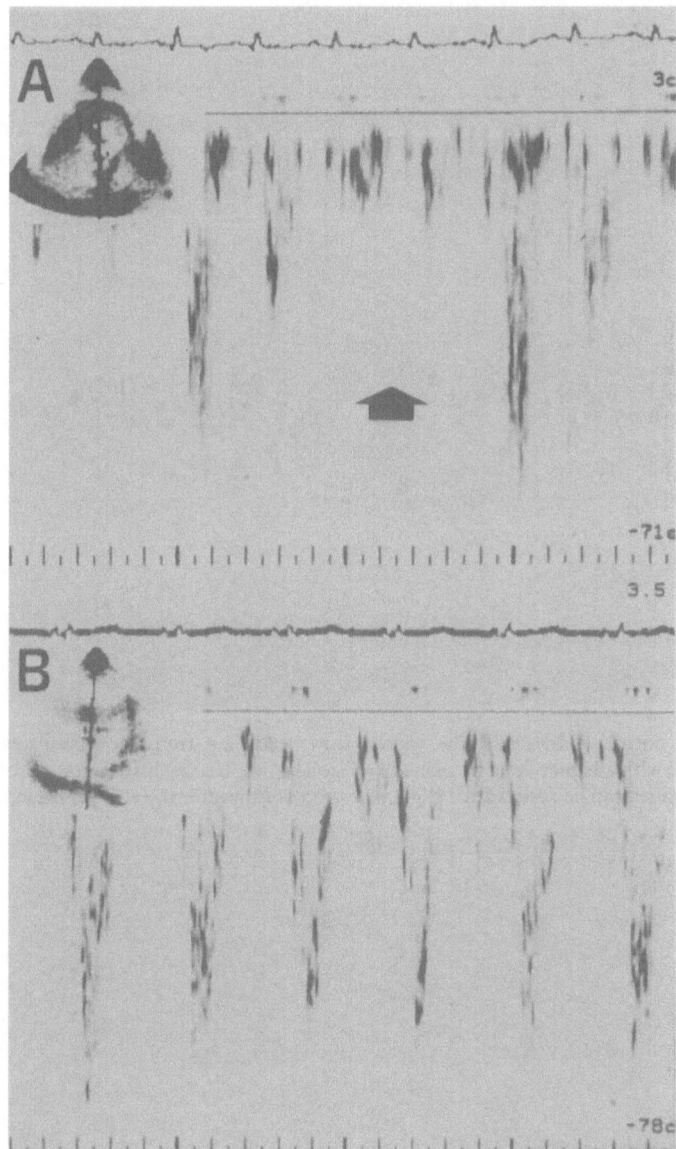

Fig. 2.10. *A*. Marked flow reduction (arrow) in the left ventricular outflow tract during inspiration, determined by pulsed Doppler in an apical 5 chamber view in a patient with cardiac tamponade. *B*. After pericardiocentesis (below) flow has returned to normal.

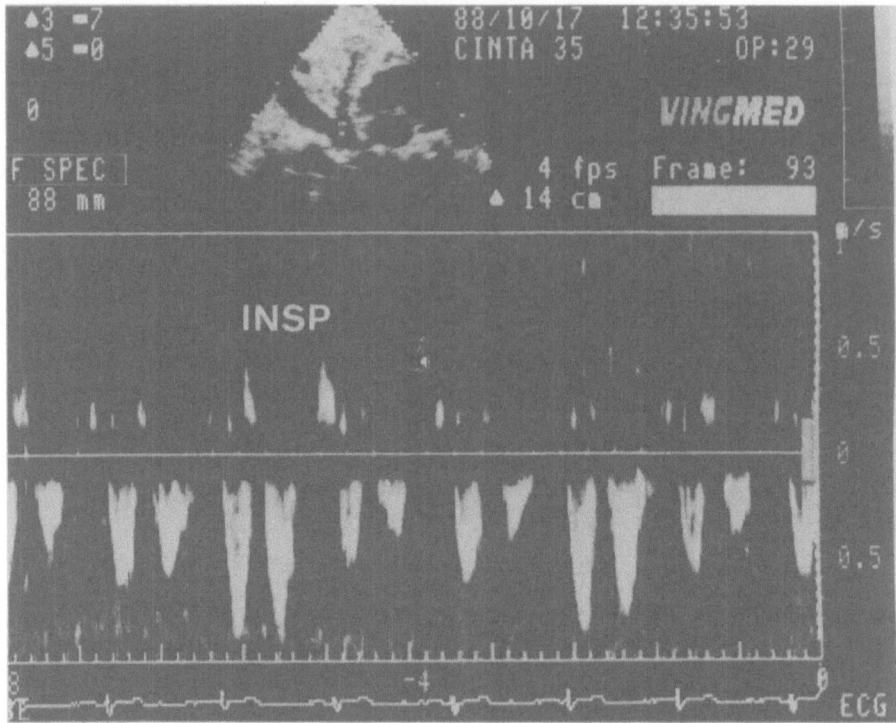

Fig. 2.11. In normal individuals, the venous flow recording from the hepatic vein shows a systolic wave with a higher velocity than the diastolic wave. During inspiration (insp) an increase in both velocities can be seen, with a slight inversion of flow after the atrial contraction.

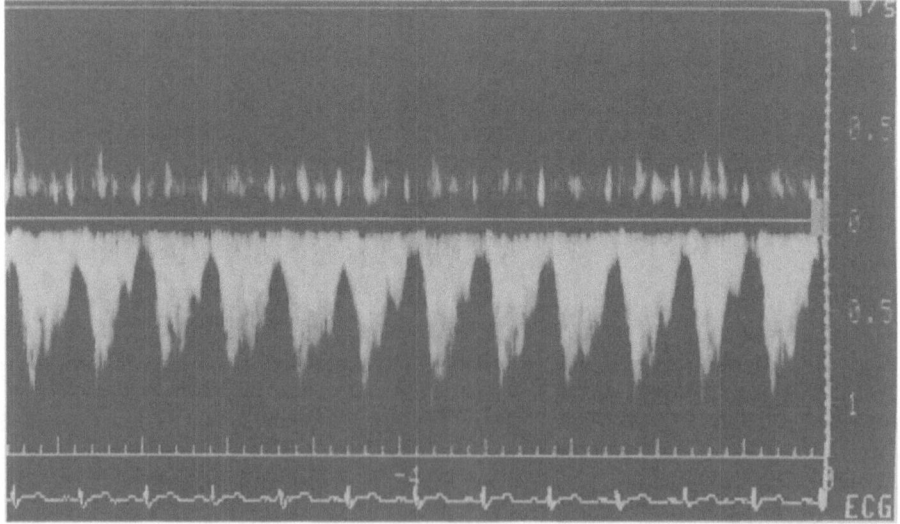

Fig. 2.12. Cardiac tamponade. The superior vena cava flow velocity measured by continuous wave Doppler from right supraclavicular area discloses a clear predominance of systolic over diastolic wave, and a virtual absence of variation of velocities with respiration.

ponade, the predominance of systolic flow is greatly enhanced and shows less marked variation during the respiratory cycle (Fig. 2.12). The diastolic flow wave may be absent.

To summarize, the basic role of echocardiography in cardiac tamponade is the detection of pericardial effusion; the identification of diastolic right atrial or ventricular collapse or both, particularly when associated with wide variations of ventricular diameters and transvalvular flows during the respiratory cycle, suggests that intrapericardial pressure is elevated and that cardiac compression is present, even in the absence of clinical signs of cardiac tamponade.

Cardiac constriction

Constrictive pericarditis

In contrast to cardiac tamponade, phonocardiography and external pulse recordings are highly useful in the diagnosis of cardiac constriction. An early

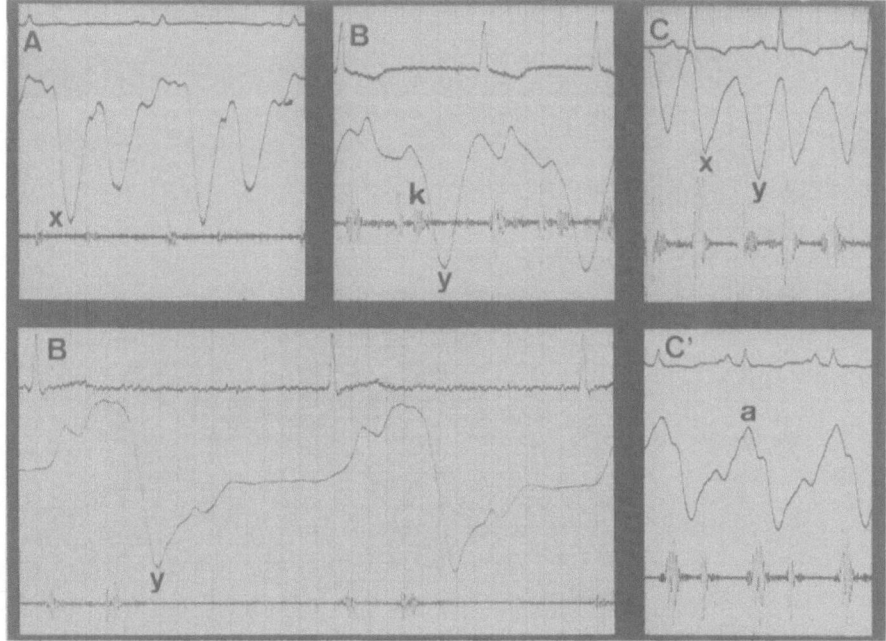

Fig. 2.13. Several types of jugular venous pulse in constrictive pericarditis. Type A (A): predominance of "x" trough, which is deeper than "y"; Type B (B): deep and brisk "y" trough with a slight delay after the early diastolic pericardial knock (B, upper panel) resulting in a dip-plateau morphology when diastole is very long (B, lower panel). Type C (C): "W" morphology with similar but very marked depth of both troughs. Type C' (C'): Predominant "a" wave in a case of subacute constrictive pericarditis.

diastolic pericardial knock, 0.07–0.13 seconds after the second heart sound, may be recorded in the phonocardiogram in 60–90% of patients with constrictive pericarditis (Fig. 2.13 and 2.14). The pericardial knock tends to increase in intensity during inspiration and to be closer to the second heart sound with greater severity of constriction (34). The morphology of the external recording of the jugular venous pulse may vary widely, as shown in Fig. 2.13. However, there is a brisk and deep "y" trough in more than 50% of cases. The nadir of "y" trough coincides with, or follows within a short delay, the early diastolic pericardial knock. Fishleder (34) described four types of jugular venous pulse, depending on whether the predominant wave was the "x" trough (type A), the "y" trough (type B, by far the most common), both "x" and "y" troughs (type C or "W" morphology), or the "a" wave (type C′). This latter morphology corresponds to the one reported by Kesteloot et al. (35) in cases of epicarditis with rapid development of epicardial constriction without calcification (Fig. 2.13). It is not uncommon to record a reverse apexcardiogram ("diastolic apical beat") in patients with sinus rhythm or atrial fibrillation (Fig. 2.14), which indicates the systolic retraction of the cardiac apex that may also be found at palpation.

The diagnosis of constrictive pericarditis cannot be made by echocardiog-

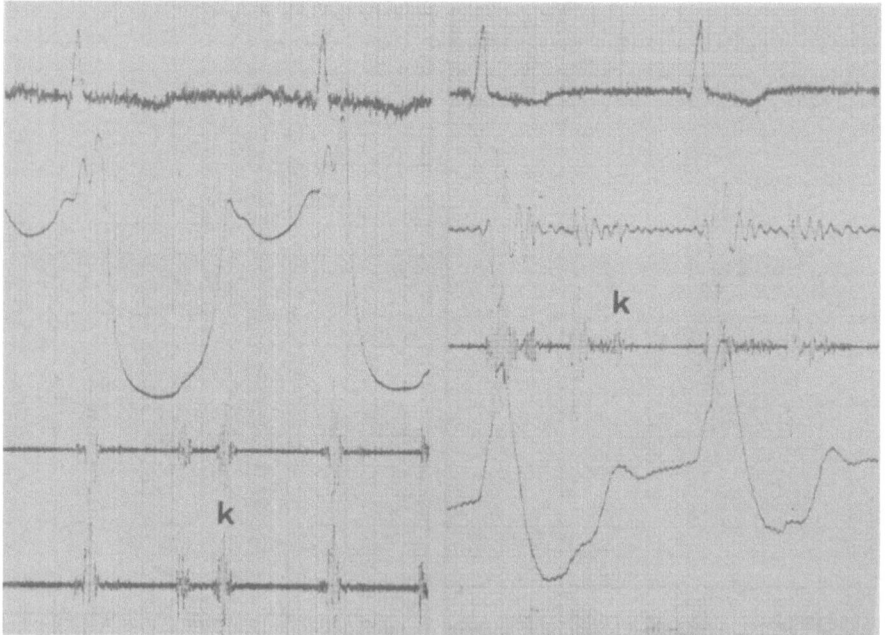

Fig. 2.14. Morphology of the apexcardiogram in two patients with chronic constrictive pericarditis. Both with sinus rhythm (left) and atrial fibrillation (right) there is a systolic retraction and a sudden expansion which coincides in its highest point with the early diastolic pericardial knock (k).

raphy alone; however, the echocardiogram may show abnormalities helpful in the diagnosis or in the follow up of pericardial diseases where constrictive pericarditis may develop.

Table 2.2 lists the echocardiographic findings that have been reported in constrictive pericarditis. We described the characteristic early diastolic notching of the ventricular septum (Fig. 2.15) in 1978 (36). This notch was identified in 92% of 25 patients evaluated in our Service (37) and was found to disappear or diminish after successful pericardiectomy (36). A notch of the ventricular septum coinciding with atrial systole (38) was considerably less common and in our series was present in only 20% of the patients (39). Our ability to recognize pericardial thickening by echocardiography was disappointing; we were able to document increased thickness of the pericardium in only about one third of the patients (38). The echocardiogram reflects the abnormal pattern of filling that develops as a result of constriction by the pericardium. Thus, following early diastolic filling, the posterior wall of the left ventricle remains flat (40), reflecting the absence of filling of the chamber in mid and late diastole. We documented this phenomenon in half of our series (37). We also observed abnormalities of systolic motion of the ventricular septum (41, 42). Systolic septal hypokinesis or flattening was seen in 46% and paradoxical motion in 20%. All these findings except the early diastolic notch of the ventricular septum lack sensitivity, but are reasonably specific. Early opening of the pulmonary valve (43, 44), which has been attributed to the increased right ventricular diastolic pressure, is not specific for constrictive pericarditis; we have even found this sign in normal individuals during inspiration (45).

M mode is more useful than two dimensional echocardiography, as its superior temporal resolution allows a more precise and objective definition of the sequence and timing of interventricular septal motion. However, other

Table 2.2. Constrictive pericarditis. Echocardiographic signs.

M mode
Early diastolic notch of the interventricular septum
Atrial systolic notch of the interventricular septum
Diastolic flattening of the posterior left ventricular wall
Increase in pericardial thickness
Abnormal motion (hypokinetic, paradoxical, flat in diastole) of interventricular septum

Two-dimensional
Small ventricles with dilated atria
Dense (double echo) immobile pericardium
Dilated inferior vena cava and suprahepatic vein
Inspiratory leftward bulging of interventricular and interatrial septum
Sudden cessation of diastolic ventricular filling

Doppler
Decrease in left ventricular early diastolic filling and increase in left ventricular isovolumic
    relaxation time at the onset of inspiration

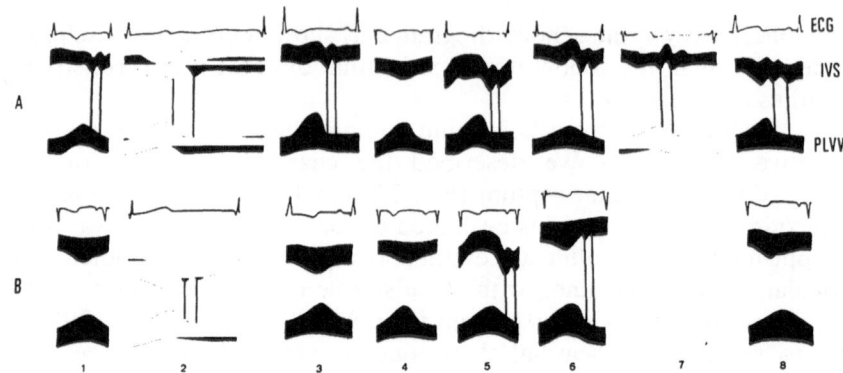

Fig. 2.15. Diagrammatic representation of interventricular septum (IVS) and posterior left ventricular wall (PLVW) motion in eight patients with chronic constrictive pericarditis, before (A) and after (B) pericardiectomy. Vertical lines indicate the onset and end of early diastolic notching of interventricular septum. (Reproduced from Candell-Riera J, García-del-Castillo H, Permanyer-Miralda G, Soler-Soler J. Echocardiographic features of the interventricular septum in chronic constrictive pericarditis. Circulation 1978; 57: 1154–1158. With authorization of the American Heart Association, Inc.).

signs of cardiac constriction have also been reported in two dimensional recordings (46, 47). Characteristically, the atria are enlarged in striking contrast to the small ventricular cavities. This combination is common to constrictive pericarditis and restrictive cardiomyopathy. The dense immobile pericardium is occasionally appreciated better on two dimensional images than by M mode. Sometimes the double echo is better seen on the two dimensional echocardiogram, but when present is often adequately recorded by M mode as well. Marked dilatation of the inferior vena cava is a characteristic finding of severe constriction. Subcostal views provide dramatic pictures of the greatly dilated hepatic veins. Inspiratory bulging of the ventricular septum toward the left ventricle may also be seen. Sudden cessation of diastolic ventricular filling may be highly apparent, specially in the apical view. We have found this dynamic abnormality particularly useful in patients with a poor parasternal acoustic window in whom an adequate M mode recording was not possible.

In our experience (36), the most consistent finding in constrictive pericarditis is the abnormal motion or early diastolic notch of the interventricular septum. Its onset coincides with the pericardial knock, and its maximal anterior displacement with the nadir of the "y" trough of the jugular venous pulse (Fig. 2.15). Thus, the early diastolic notch occurs during the early rapid ventricular filling period. In patients with sinus rhythm, septal bulging towards the left ventricle can also be seen immediately after the P wave of the electrocardiogram, coincident with the "a" wave of the jugular pulse recording (Fig. 2.16). Atrial fibrillation is present in about one half of the patients with constrictive pericarditis, reducing the prevalence of this sign. According to Tei et al. (38), the most likely cause of these abnormal movements of the

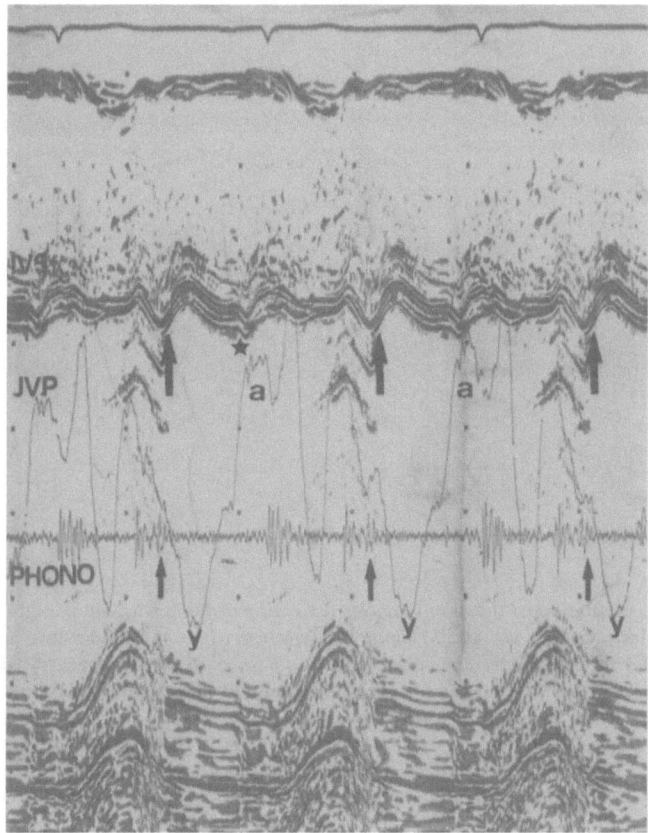

Fig. 2.16. Simultaneous recording of the M mode echocardiogram at ventricular level, jugular venous pulse (JVP) and phonocardiogram (PHONO) in a patient with cardiac constriction. Atrial systolic notch (*) of the interventricular (IVS) septum can be seen after the P wave of the electrocardiogram and coincident with the "a" wave of jugular venous pulse. There is also an early diastolic notch, beginning (large arrow) at the time of early diastolic pericardial knock (small arrow); its maximum forward displacement is simultaneous with the nadir of the "y" trough of the jugular venous pulse recording.

interventricular septum is the changing transseptal pressure gradients associated with atrial contraction and early rapid ventricular filling, as shown in Fig. 2.17.

Unfortunately, none of these signs is specific for constrictive pericarditis. An early diastolic notch may be observed in left ventricular volume overload, atrial septal defect (48), following ventricular premature beats, and in restrictive cardiomyopathy (49). We have found the atrial systolic notch in patients with left bundle branch block, pulmonary stenosis, cardiac tamponade, chronic obstructive pulmonary disease, restrictive cardiomyopathy and even in normal individuals (39).

To evaluate the usefulness of these signs for the differential diagnosis

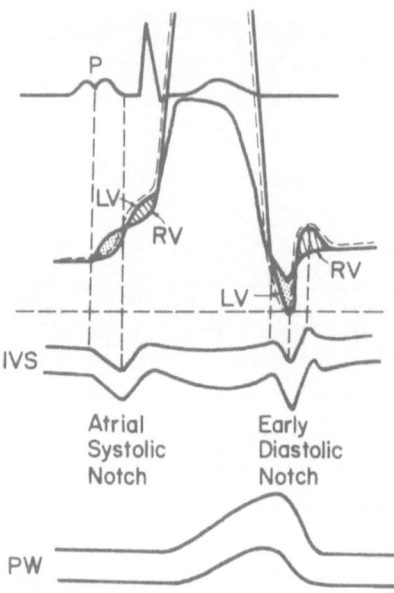

Fig. 2.17. Representation of the simultaneous recording of the intracavitary right (RV) and left (LV) ventricular pressures and the M mode echocardiogram at ventricular level in cardiac constriction. Atrial systolic notch takes place after the P wave of the electrocardiogram, at a time when RV pressure slightly exceeds LV pressure. Early diastolic septal notch takes place at the sudden end of the phase of rapid ventricular filling, when LV pressure is higher than RV pressure, thus resulting in a sudden forward septal displacement. IVS: interventricular septum; PW: posterior wall. (Reproduced, with permission, from Tei C, Child JS, Tanaka H, Shah PM. Atrial systolic notch on the interventricular septal echogram: an echocardiographic sign of constrictive pericarditis. J Am Coll Cardiol 1983; 1: 907–912).

between restrictive and constrictive syndromes, we reviewed (39) the echocardiograms of 25 patients with constrictive pericardits, and compared them with 14 with amyloidosis, 22 with idiopathic hemochromatosis, 10 with idiopathic restrictive cardiomyopathy, 4 hypereosinophilic syndromes and one endomyocardial fibrosis. An early diastolic notch was present in two of the cases of restrictive cardiomyopathy and in 23 (92%) with constrictive pericarditis. We found an atrial systolic notch in one patient with amyloidosis, in two with hemochromatosis and in one with hypereosinophilic syndrome (Table 2.3). Figure 2.18 illustrates the limitations of M mode echocardiography for the differential diagnosis between constrictive pericarditis and other types of heart diseases that may also be associated with early diastolic notch. The upper part of the figure shows the echocardiogram of a patient with constrictive pericarditis (A) where, in addition to a very apparent septal early diastolic notch, a definite increase of pericardial echoes (the pericardium was calcified) and apparent flattening of the posterior left ventricular wall are shown. The echocardiograms in the lower part of the figure are, from left to right, of a patient with idiopathic restrictive cardiomyopathy (B), in

Table 2.3. Cardiac constriction vs restriction (ECHO)

	Septal motion	
	Early diast. notch	Atrial syst. notch
25 constrictive pericarditis	23 (92%)	5 (20%)
14 amyloidosis	–	1
22 idiopathic hemochromatosis	–	2
10 idiopathic restrictive cardiomyopathy	2	–
4 hypereosinophilic syndrome	–	1
1 endomyocardial fibrosis	–	–

Diast.: diastolic; syst.: systolic.

which early diastolic septal notch was also found, a patient with cardiac amyloidosis with marked restriction to ventricular filling (C), and a patient with dilated cardiomyopathy (D). As shown in the figure, an early diastolic septal notch is not a specific finding of constrictive pericarditis. In the differential diagnosis of the restrictive and constrictive syndromes, M mode echocardiography may permit the differentiation of infiltrative cardiomyopathies from constrictive pericarditis; in the former there is a marked increase of myocardial mass and often impaired left ventricular systolic function (50, 51).

It has been pointed out that Doppler echocardiography may help to distinguish constrictive pericarditis from restrictive cardiomyopathy by analysis of tricuspid, mitral (52, 53) and central venous (54) flow profiles. In restrictive cardiomyopathy, flow velocity through the mitral valve is characterized by a prominent early diastolic filling wave, reduction in the atrial filling wave and the presence of diastolic regurgitation. This pattern is not altered by respiration, whereas in constrictive pericarditis a decrease in early diastolic filling, as well as an increase in left isovolumic relaxation time, can be seen at the onset of inspiration.

It has been suggested in a preliminary study (54) that the diastolic flow of superior vena cava and hepatic veins is higher than systolic flow in restrictive cardiomyopathy, whereas in constrictive pericarditis systolic flow might be predominant, with an increase in the first beat during inspiration and a characteristic expiratory reduction of diastolic flow. However, we think that the value of these signs still needs to be validated in large numbers of patients, as we have found diastolic flow velocity higher than systolic in eight patients with constrictive pericarditis (Fig. 2.19). This has also been the experience of other authors (55, 55a).

Pulsed transesophageal Doppler echocardiography has been used to record the pattern of flow velocities in the pulmonary veins (56). Pulmonary venous return is increased during expiration in patients with constrictive pericarditis.

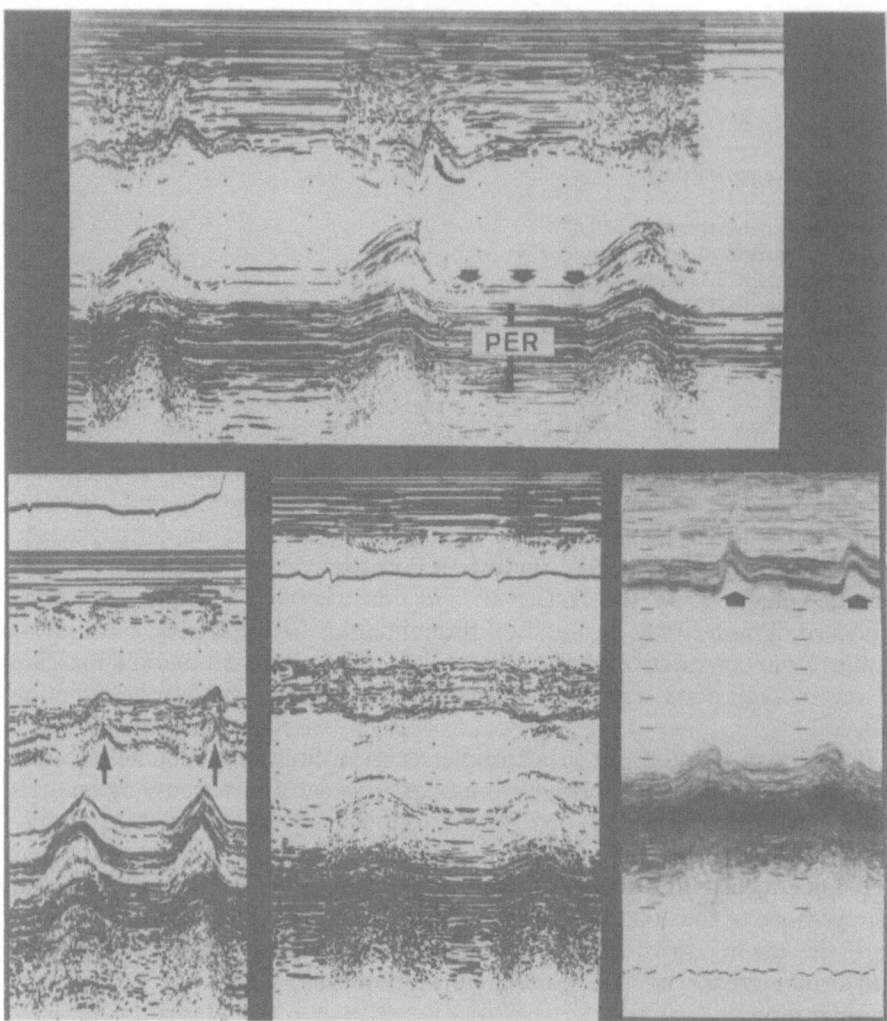

Fig. 2.18. Upper panel: Chronic calcific constrictive pericarditis. There is an early diastolic
notch (curved arrow) of the interventricular septum, a marked flattening (arrows) of the posterior left ventricular wall, and massive pericardial thickening (PER). Lower panel (*left*): Idiopathic restrictive cardiomyopathy. The abnormal early diastolic motion of interventricular
septum (arrows) is also seen in this case. *Middle panel*: Infiltrative cardiomyopathy (cardiac
amyloidosis) with a considerable increase in myocardial mass with diminished left ventricular
systolic function. *Right panel*: Dilated cardiomyopathy where, in addition to dilatation and
depressed left ventricular systolic function, a septal early diastolic notch can also be seen
(arrows).

Effusive-constrictive pericarditis

In contrast with chronic constrictive pericarditis, in which the parietal and visceral layers of the pericardium are fused, in subacute effusive-constrictive pericarditis effusion persists and cardiac compression results from both the pericardial effusion and the visceral pericardium. Hancock (57) reported 13 cases, nine idiopathic and four secondary to radiation, four of which went on to constriction without effusion after a few months. Effusive constrictive pericarditis may also be found in rheumatoid arthritis, uremia, neoplastic pericardial involvement, traumatic pericardial disease and tuberculous pericarditis. In the echocardiogram, signs of constriction, particularly abnormal motion of the interventricular septum can be seen in addition to pericardial effusion (Table 2.4). The jugular venous pulse of these patients is highly variable. It may have a morphology intermediate between the normal or that of tamponade, with a predominant "x" trough, and that of constriction, with a predominant "y" trough; or it may have a definitely constrictive configuration with a deep and brisk "y" trough. An early diastolic pericardial knock can often be recorded in the phonocardiogram, and, in our experience, early diastolic septal notching is frequently recorded. Doppler echocardiography may demonstrate transvalvular and venous flow profiles showing features of both tamponade and constriction, either one of which may predominate.

The presence of band-like echocardiographic images within the pericardial space has been reported in patients with tuberculous (58), neoplastic, uremic, infective and idiopathic pericarditis (59, 60). In a personal series (61) of 65 patients with moderate or large pericardial effusion followed up for two years we have found that intrapericardial band-like images are more common in patients with tuberculous pericarditis, and that patients with these tracts develop constrictive pericarditis more commonly. Figure 2.20 shows the two dimensional echocardiograms of a patient with tuberculous pericarditis and moderate pericardial effusion in whom, after one month, band-like images were detected within the pericardial cavity. At that time, signs of constriction were not present in the jugular pulse recording and the interventricular septal motion by M mode recording was normal. One month later, however, the phonocardiogram recorded pericardial knock, the external jugular pulse recording showed a deep "y" trough, and an early diastolic septal notch was present in the echocardiogram. Constrictive pericarditis was confirmed at subsequent pericardiectomy.

Transient constriction

In some patients with effusive acute idiopathic pericarditis we have documented the development of constriction, with subsequent spontaneous normalization (62, 63) (chapter 5). Phonocardiography, external venous pulse recording and echocardiography played a fundamental role in the recognition

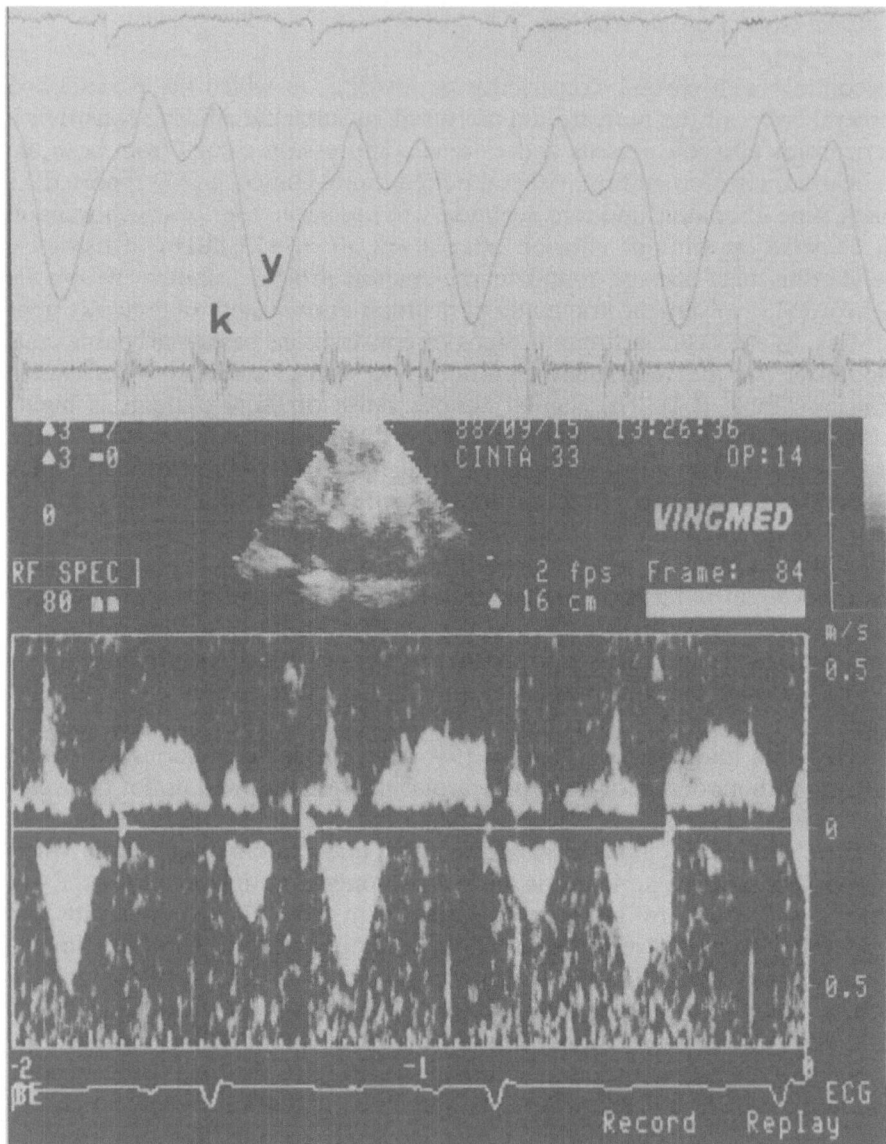

Fig. 2.19. Constrictive tuberculous pericarditis proven at surgery. Deep "y" trough in the jugular venous pulse and early diastolic pericardial knock (k) in the phonocardiogram. The hepatic vein flow, detected with pulsed Doppler, shows a similar morphology to that from jugular venous pulse, with a clearly more prominent diastolic wave and definite reversal of flow in late diastole.

Table 2.4. Differences between tamponade, constriction, and effusive-constrictive pericarditis.

	Tamponade	Effusive constr.	Chronic constr.
Echocardiogram			
pericardial effusion	+	±	−
early diastolic septal notch	−	±	+
Jugular venous pulse	X/Xy	Xy/XY/xY	XY/xY
Pericardial knock	−	±	+

X: absence of "y" trough; Xy: predominant "x" trough; XY: "x" and "y" troughs of similar amplitude; xY: predominant "y" trough.

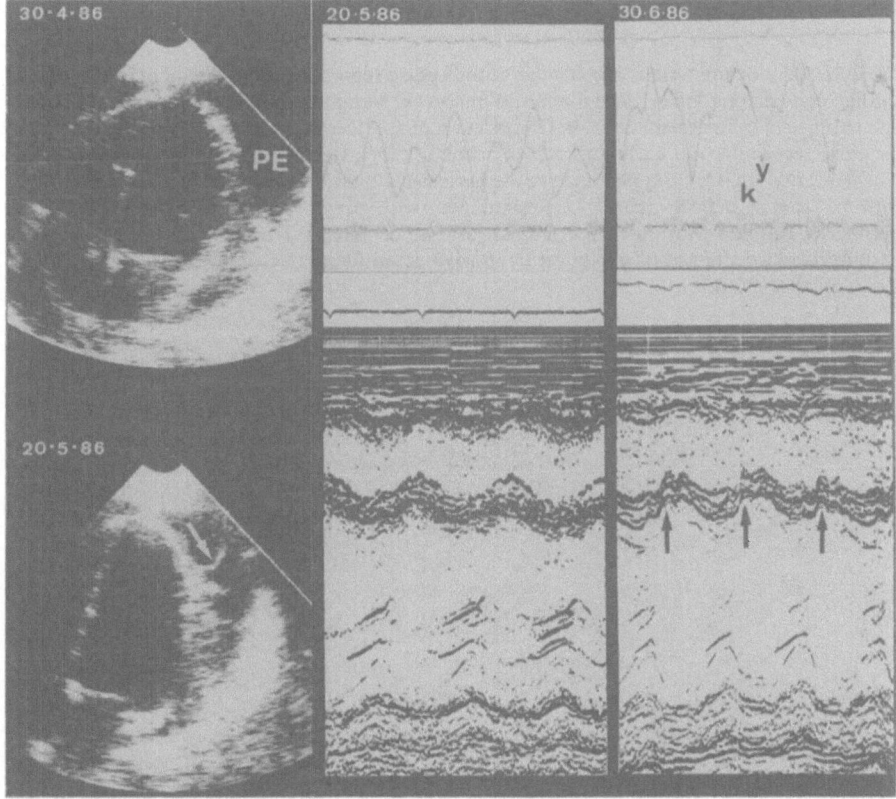

Fig. 2.20. Two-dimensional and M mode echocardiograms, phonocardiogram and jugular pulse recording in a patient with tuberculous pericarditis. *Left panel,* at admission (4.30.1986) there was a moderate pericardial effusion (PE). Twenty days later (5.20.1986) band-like images within the pericardial cavity were seen (arrow). At that time signs of constriction were not apparent in the M mode echocardiogram or in the external recordings (*middle panel*). *Right panel,* one month later (6.30.1986), a deep "y" trough was apparent in the jugular venous pulse, there was an early pericardial knock in the phonocardiogram (k), and an early diastolic septal notch (arrows) suggesting cardiac constriction could be seen in the echocardiogram. Constriction was demonstrated at surgery.

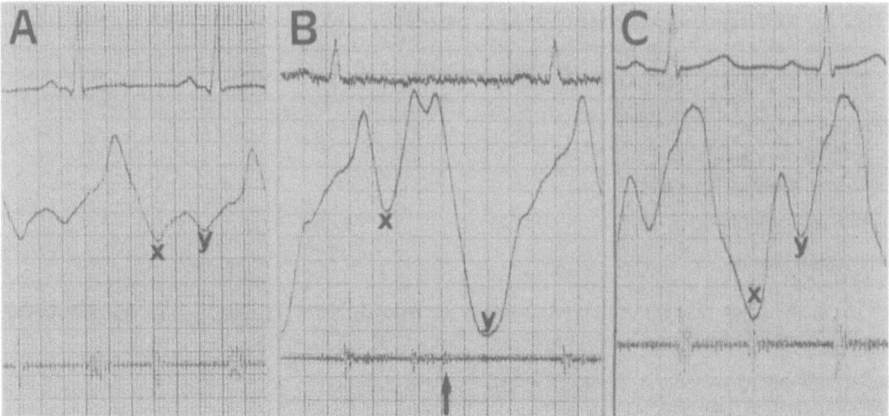

Fig. 2.21. Phonocardiograms and jugular venous pulse recordings from a patient with transient cardiac constricton. A: Pericardial effusion phase. "x" trough slightly more prominent than "y" and absence of pericardial knock. B: Constriction phase. Deep and brisk "y" trough in the jugular pulse recording with early diastolic pericardial knock (arrow) in the phonocardiogram. C: Normalization phase. Disappearance of the pericardial knock and normal jugular venous pulse with "x" trough deeper than "y". (Reproduced, with permission, from Sagristà-Sauleda J, Permanyer-Miralda G, Candell-Riera J, Angel J, Soler-Soler J. Transient cardiac constriction; an unrecognized pattern of evolution in effusive acute idiopathic pericarditis. Am J Cardiol 1987; 59: 961–966).

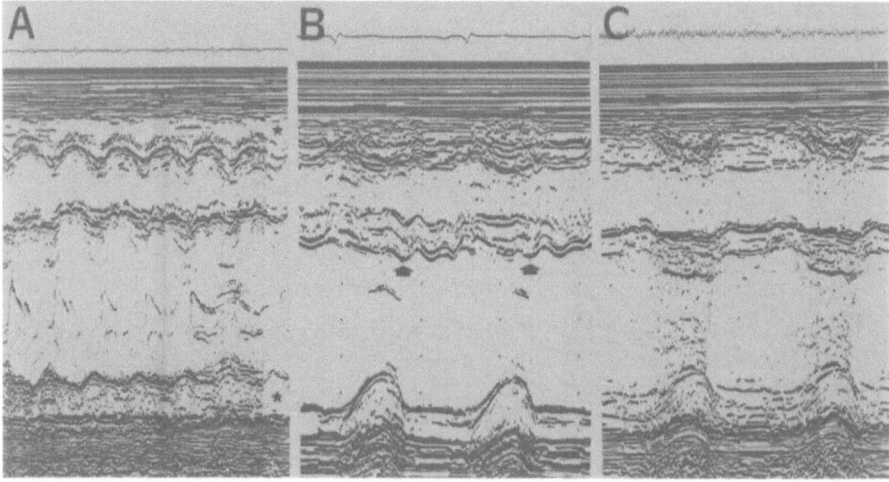

Fig. 2.22. M mode echocardiography recordings from the same patient of Fig. 2.21. A: Pericardial effusion (*) phase. B: Constriction phase. Presence of early diastolic septal notch (arrows) after the disappearance of effusion. C: Normalization phase: absence of pericardial fluid and normal motion of interventricular septum. (Reproduced, with permission, from Sagristà-Sauleda J, Permanyer-Miralda G, Candell-Riera J, Angel J, Soler-Soler J. Transient cardiac constriction: an unrecognized pattern of evolution in effusive acute idiopathic pericarditis. Am J Cardiol 1987; 59: 961–966).

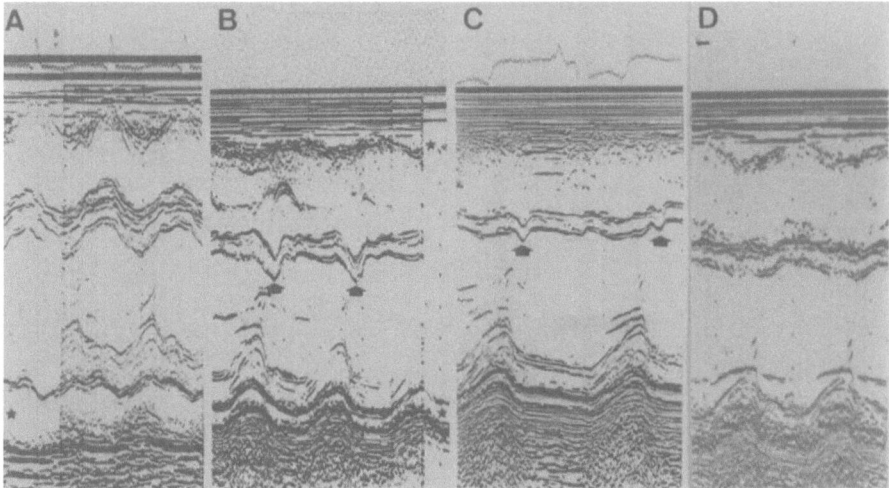

Fig. 2.23. M mode echocardiographic recordings in a patient with transient cardiac constriction. A: after the phase of pericardial effusion (*) a marked early diastolic septal notch developed (B, arrows), at a time when apparent separation between posterior pericardium and epicardium was still present (*). The septal motion progressively improved (C) until eventually it became normal (D). (Reproduced, with permission, from Sagristà-Sauleda J, Permanyer-Miralda G, Candell-Riera J, Angel J, Soler-Soler J. Transient cardiac constriction: an unrecognized pattern of evolute in effusive acute idiopathic pericarditis. Am J Cardiol 1987; 59: 961–966).

initial characterization of transient cardiac constriction. Figures 2.21 and 2.22 show how the jugular venous pulse, phonocardiogram and echocardiogram evolved in one of these patients. In the phase of pericardial effusion (A), the "x" and "y" troughs have a similar depth. Eighteen days later (B), a deep "y" trough and an early diastolic knock have appeared, while pericardial effusion has disappeared and an early diastolic septal notch has appeared. One month later (C), the pericardial knock has disappeared and both the jugular pulse and the echocardiogram have returned to normal. In some patients, the early diastolic septal notch suggestive of constriction appeared when a mild pericardial effusion still persisted (Fig. 2.23). The first echocardiogram (A) was obtained one month before the second (B), which shows both a septal notch and pericardial effusion. Two weeks later (C), the septal notch was less apparent and a double pericardial echo was present. Finally, return to the normal pattern was complete (D).

Occult constriction

In 1977, Bush et al. (64) reported the hemodynamic features of 19 patients who had a form of cardiac constriction which was only apparent after the rapid intravenous infusion (in 6–8 minutes) of 1000 ml of saline solution.

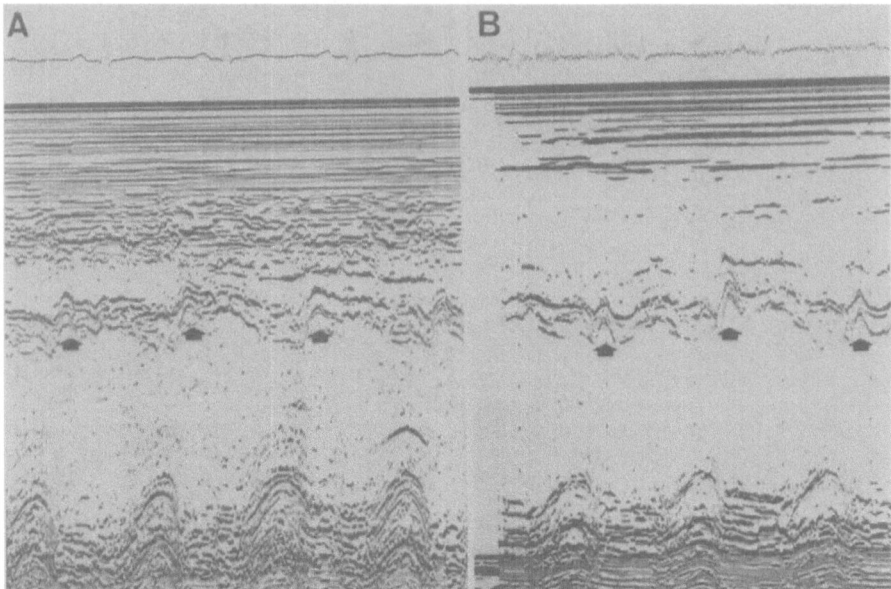

Fig. 2.24. M mode echocardiogram of a patient with occult constriction that was proven at catheterization. In baseline conditions (A) the recording was virtually normal except for a marked forward septal displacement in early diastole (arrows). After the infusion of 1000 ml of saline in 8 minutes (B), a definite early diastolic septal notch became apparent (arrows). (Reproduced, with permission, from Candell-Riera J, Permanyer-Miralda G. Constricción-restricción cardíaca. Utilidad de la ecocardiografía. Rev Latina Cardiol 1985; 6: 245–253).

With this method a characteristic constriction morphology in the right atrial and ventricular pressure curves was brought out, together with disappearance of the normal respiratory changes in the right atrial pressure and equilibration of intracardiac diastolic pressures. In some patients in whom no abnormality in septal diastolic motion could be recorded on the M mode echocardiogram under baseline conditions, or in whom abnormal early diastolic motion of intraventricular septum was questionable, we have been able to demonstrate, after rapid infusion of 1000 ml of saline, development or enhancement of the early diastolic septal notch (Fig. 2.24).

References

1. D'Cruz IA, Cohen HC, Prabhu R, Glick C. Diagnosis of cardiac tamponade by echocardiography: Changes in mitral valve motion and ventricular dimensions, with special reference to paradoxical pulse. Circulation 1975; 52: 460–465.
2. Cosío FG, Palacios Martínez J, Moro Serrano C, Sáenz de la Calzada C, Castro Alcaine C. Abnormal septal motion in cardiac tamponade with pulsus paradoxus. Echocardiographic and hemodynamic observations. Chest 1977; 71: 787–789.
3. Smith MD, Waters JS, Kwan OL, DeMaria AN. Evaluation of pericardial compressive disorders by echocardiography. Echocardiography 1985; 2: 67–86.

4. Gillam LD, Guyer DE, Gibson TC, King ME, Marshall JE, Weyman AE. Hydrodynamic compression of the right atrium: a new echocardiographic sign of cardiac tamponade. Circulation 1983; 68: 294–301.
5. Armstrong WF, Helper DJ, Schilt BF, Dillon JC, Feigenbaum H. Diastolic collapse of the right ventricle: Echocardiographic evidence of occult cardiac tamponade. (abstr.). Am J Cardiol 1982; 49: 1010.
6. Singh S, Wann S, Schuchard GH, Klopfenstein HS, Leimgruber PP, Keelan MH, Brooks HL. Right ventricular and right atrial collapse in patients with cardiac tamponade – a combined echocardiographic and hemodynamic study. Circulation 1984; 70: 966–971.
7. Candell-Riera J, García-del-Castillo H, Permanyer-Miralda G, Soler-Soler J. Pericardial effusion: Diagnostic value of the subcostal acoustic window (Inferior vena cava – right atrial projection). Clin Cardiol 1987; 10: 261–266.
8. Rifkin RD, Pandian NG, Funai JT, Wang SS, Sharma SC, Lojeski EW, Levine HJ. Sensitivity of right atrial collapse and right ventricular diastolic collapse in the diagnosis of graded cardiac tamponade. Am J Noninvas Cardiol 1987; 1: 73–80.
9. López-Sendón J, García-Fernández MA, Coma-Canella E, Sotillo J, Silvestre J. Mechanism of right atrial wall compression in pericardial effusion: An experimental echocardiographic study in dogs. J Cardiovasc Ultrason 1988; 7: 127-134.
10. Naggar CZ, Dillon WD, Butterly JR, Malacoff RF. Echocardiographic manifestations of tense pericardial effusion. J Am Coll Cardiol 1985; 6: 467–470.
11. Alfonso F, Rey M, Villacastín JP, De Rábago P. Echocardiographically revealed collapse of the right ventricle and prolonged inversion of both atria without clinical cardiac tamponade. Eur Heart J 1987; 8: 1141–1145.
12. Bain RJI, Gammage MD, Murray RG, Davies MKD. Right ventricular diastolic collapse in the absence of cardiac tamponade. J Cardiovasc Ultrason 1988; 7: 177–180.
13. Klopfenstein HS, Cogswell TL, Bernath GA, Wann LS, Tipton RK, Hoffmann RG, Brooks HL. Alterations in intravascular volume affect the relation between right ventricular diastolic collapse and the hemodynamic severity of cardiac tamponade. J Am Coll Cardiol 1985; 6: 1057–1063.
14. Cogswell TL, Bernath GA, Keelan MH, Wann LS, Klopfenstein HS. The shift in the relationship between intrapericardial fluid pressure and volume induced by acute left ventricular pressure overload during cardiac tamponade. Circulation 1986; 74: 173–180.
15. Shapiro MR, Cohen MW. Review: The echocardiogram in cardiac tamponade. J Cardiovasc Ultrason 1983; 2: 87–95.
16. Gabor GE, Winsberg F, Bloom HS. Electrical and mechanical alteration in pericardial effusion. Chest 1971; 59: 351–356.
17. Usher TW, Popp RL. Electrical alternans: mechanism in pericardial effusion. Am Heart J 1972; 83: 459–464.
18. Tajik AJ. Echocardiography in pericardial effusion. Am J Med 1977; 63: 29–40.
19. Greene DA, Kleid JJ, Naidu S. Unusual echocardiographic manifestation of pericardial effusion. Am J Cardiol 1977; 39: 112–115.
20. Vignola PA, Pohost GM, Curfman GD, Myers GS. Correlation of echocardiographic and clinical findings in patients with pericardial effusion. Am J Cardiol 1976; 37: 701–707.
21. Chandraratna PAN. Uses and limitations of echocardiography in the evaluation of pericardial disease. Echocardiography 1984; 1: 55–74.
22. Engel PJ, Hon H, Fowler NO, Plummer S. Echocardiographic study of right ventricular wall motion in cardiac tamponade. Am J Cardiol 1982; 50; 1018–1021.
23. Nanda NC, Gramiak R, Gross CM. Echocardiography of cardiac valves in pericardial effusion. Circulation 1976; 54: 500–504.
24. Levisman JA, Abbasi AS. Abnormal motion of the mitral valve with pericardial effusion: pseudoprolapse of the mitral valve. Am Heart J 1976; 91: 18–20.
25. Hsu TL, Chen CC, Hsiung MC, Yu TJ, Chiang BN. Paradoxic motion of the left ventricular free wall in cardiac tamponade. Am Heart J 1986; 111: 807–808.

26. Kronzon I, Cohen ML, Winer HE. Diastolic atrial compression: A sensitive echocardiographic sign of cardiac tamponade. J Am Coll Cardiol 1983; 2: 770–775.
27. Steele RL, Pérez JE. Left ventricular diastolic collapse provoking cardiac tamponade. Echocardiography 1986; 3: 149–150.
28. Lunde P, Rasmussen K. Respiratory changes of the inferior caval vein in cardiac tamponade: An echocardiographic study. J Cardiovasc Ultrason 1986; 5: 111–114.
29. Himelman RB, Kircher B, Rockey DC, Schiller NB. Inferior vena cava plethora with blunted respiratory response: a sensitive echocardiographic sign of cardiac tamponade. J Am Coll Cardiol 1988; 12: 1470–1477.
30. Fowler NO. Inferior vena cava plethora as an echocardiographic sign of cardiac tamponade. J Am Coll Cardiol 1988; 12: 1478–1479.
31. Beppu S, Nakatani S, Tanaka N, Ikegami K, Kumon K, Nagata S, Miyatake K, Nimura Y. Transesophageal echocardiographic diagnosis of localized pericardial coagula: A special cause of cardiac tamponade. Circulation 1988; 78: II-299 (abstr.).
32. Leeman DE, Levine MJ, Come PC. Doppler echocardiography in cardiac tamponade: Exaggerated respiratory variation in transvalvular blood flow velocity integrals. J Am Coll Cardiol 1988; 11: 572–578.
33. Appleton CP, Hatle LK, Popp RL. Cardiac tamponade and pericardial effusion: Respiratory variation in transvalvular flow velocities studied by Doppler echocardiography. J Am Coll Cardiol 1988; 11: 1020–1030.
33a. Burstow DJ, Oh JK, Bailey KR. Cardiac tamponade: characteristic Doppler observations. Mayo Clin Proc 1989; 64: 312–324.
34. Fishleder B. Exploración cardiovascular y fonomecanocardiografía clínica. México, La Prensa Médica Mexicana, 1978; p. 896–907.
35. Kesteloot H, Denef B. Value of reference tracings in diagnosis and assessment of constrictive epi- and pericarditis. Br Heart J 1970; 32: 675–682.
36. Candell-Riera J, García-del-Castillo H, Permanyer-Miralda G, Soler-Soler J. Echocardiographic features of the interventricular septum in chronic constrictive pericarditis. Circulation 1978; 57: 1154–1158.
37. Candell-Riera J, García-del-Castillo H, Permanyer-Miralda G, Soler-Soler J. El ecocardiograma en la pericarditis constrictiva crónica. Rev Esp Cardiol 1979; 32: 119–126.
38. Tei C, Child JS, Tanaka H, Shah PM. Atrial systolic notch on the interventricular septal echogram: An echocardiographic sign of constrictive pericarditis. J Am Coll Cardiol 1983; 1: 907–912.
39. Candell-Riera J, Gutiérrez-Palau L, García-del-Castillo H, Permanyer-Miralda G, Soler-Soler J. "Atrial systolic notch" and "Early diastolic notch" on the interventricular septal echogram in constrictive pericarditis. J Am Coll Cardiol 1985; 5: 1020–1021.
40. Voelkel AG, Pietro DA, Folland ED, Fisher ML, Parisi AF. Echocardiographic features of constrictive pericarditis. Circulation 1978; 58: 871–875.
41. Pool PE, Seagren SC, Abbasi AS, Charuzi Y, Kraus R. Echocardiographic manifestations of constrictive pericarditis. Abnormal septal motion. Chest 1975; 68: 684–688.
42. Gibson TC, Grossman W, McLaurin LP, Moos S, Craige E. An echocardiographic study of the interventricular septum in constrictive pericarditis. Br Heart J 1976; 38: 738–743.
43. Doi YL, Sugiura T, Spodick DH. Motion of pulmonic valve and constrictive pericarditis. Chest 1981; 80: 513–515.
44. Vandenbossche JL, Jacobs P, Decroly P, Primo G, Englert M. Significance of inspiratory premature opening of pulmonic valve in constrictive pericarditis. Am Heart J 1985; 110: 896–898.
45. Gutiérrez L, Bolaños F, Minguez A, Candell-Riera J. Mid-diastolic opening motion of pulmonary valve during inspiration in normal individuals. J Cardiovasc Ultrason 1986; 5: 163–166.
46. Lewis BS. Real time two dimensional echocardiography in constrictive pericarditis. Am J Cardiol 1982; 49: 1789–1793.

47. D'Cruz I, Dick A, Gross C, Hand C. Left ventricular-left atrial posterior wall contour: A new 2-D echo sign in pericardial constriction. Circulation 1988; 78: II-133 (abstr.).
48. Hoche JP. Interventricular septum in chronic constrictive pericarditis. (letter). Circulation 1979; 59: 846–847.
49. Acquatella H, Puigbó JJ, Suárez C, Mendoza J. Sudden early diastolic anterior movement of the septum in endomyocardial fibrosis. (letter). Circulation 1979; 59: 847–848.
50. Candell-Riera J, Lu L, Serés L, Batlle J, García-del-Castillo H, Soler-Soler J. Estudio ecocardiográfico en la amiloidosis y en la hemocromatosis idiopática. Rev Esp Cardiol 1983; 36: 411–416.
51. Candell-Riera J, Permanyer-Miralda G. Constricción-restricción cardiaca. Utilidad de la ecocardiografía. Rev Lat Cardiol 1985; 6: 245–253.
52. Hatle LK, Appleton CP, Popp RL. Differentiation of constrictive pericarditis and restrictive cardiomyopathy by Doppler echocardiography. Circulation 1989; 79: 357–370.
53. Appleton CP, Hatle LK, Popp RL. Demonstration of restrictive ventricular physiology by Doppler echocardiography. J Am Coll Cardiol 1988; 11: 757–768.
54. Appleton CP. Hatle LK, Popp RL. Central venous flow velocity patterns can differentiate constrictive pericarditis from restrictive cardiomyopathy. J Am Coll Cardiol 1987; 9: 119A (abstr.).
55. Suthar AL, Nanda NC. Doppler examination of superior vena cava, azygos vein, and hepatic veins. In: Nanda NC, ed.: Doppler echocardiography. New York, Igaku-Shoin, 1985, pp 136, 145.
55a. von Bibra H, Schober K, Jenni R, Busch R, Sebening H, Blomer H. Diagnosis of constrictive pericarditis by pulsed Doppler echocardiography of the hepatic vein. Am J Cardiol 1989; 63: 483–488.
56. Schiavone WA, Calafiore PA, Currie PJ, Lytle BW. Doppler echocardiographic demonstration of pulmonary venous flow velocity in three patients with constrictive pericarditis before and after pericardiectomy. Am J Cardiol 1989; 63: 145–147.
57. Hancock EW. Subacute effusive-constrictive pericarditis. Circulation 1971; 43: 183–192.
58. Chia BL, Choo M, Tan A, Ee B. Echocardiographic abnormalities in tuberculous pericardial effusion. Am Heart J 1984; 107: 1034–1035.
59. Martin RP, Bowden R, Filly K, Popp R. Intrapericardial abnormalities in patients with pericardial effusion. Circulation 1980; 61: 568–572.
60. Come PC, Miklozek, Riley MF, Carl LV, Morgan JP. Echocardiographic changes in rapidly developing pericardial constriction. Am Heart J 1985; 109: 1385–1387.
61. Alió J, Candell J, Monge L, García H, Sagristá J, Soler J. Imágenes intrapericárdicas y constricción cardiaca. Rev Esp Cardiol 1988; 41 (Supl 1): 55 (abstr.).
62. Permanyer-Miralda G, Candell-Riera J, Sagristá-Sauleda J, Soler-Soler J. Constricción cardiaca transitoria: una forma peculiar de evolución de la pericarditis aguda exudativa. Rev Lat Cardiol 1983: 4: 187–192.
63. Sagristá-Sauleda J, Permanyer-Miralda G, Candell-Riera J, Angel J, Soler-Soler J. Transient cardiac constriction: An unrecognized pattern of evolution in effusive acute idiopathic pericarditis. Am J Cardiol 1987; 59: 961–966.
64. Bush CA, Stang JM, Wooley CF, Kilman JW. Occult constrictive pericardial disease. Diagnosis by rapid volume expansion and correction by pericardiectomy. Circulation 1977; 56: 924–930.

3. Cardiac tamponade: current pathophysiological and diagnostic views

H. SIDNEY KLOPFENSTEIN, M.D., Ph.D.

This chapter will be devoted primarily to a discussion of the hemodynamic changes that occur in acute cardiac tamponade in conscious individuals and to an evaluation of newer noninvasive diagnostic methods and their limitations. Our understanding of newer noninvasive diagnostic methods and their limitations. Our understanind of the fundamental hemodynamic changes which occur during cardiac tamponade was obtained in large part from acute studies in anesthetized preparations and from clinical observations (1–3). Carefully controlled clinical studies are extremely valuable but are extraordinary difficult to perform and, of course, the measurements that can be made are limited. Relatively little information is available during acute cardiac tamponade from conscious animals who have recovered from surgery and almost no information exists concerning chronic tamponade in such preparations. There are some differences in the hemodynamic response to acute cardiac tamponade in conscious preparations from those seen in anesthetized or convalescent models. In conscious animals, for example, mean arterial blood pressure does not change significantly until late in tamponade when it abruptly decreases (4). A continuous decline in arterial blod pressure as intrapericardial pressure rises is characteristic of acute progressive tamponade in the presence of anesthesia or during convalescence from surgery. Furthermore, greater degrees of tamponade (higher intrapericardial pressures) are tolerated by healthy well hydrated conscious animals.

J. Soler-Soler et al. (Eds.), Pericardial Disease, pp. 47–58.
© 1990 Kluwer Academic Publishers

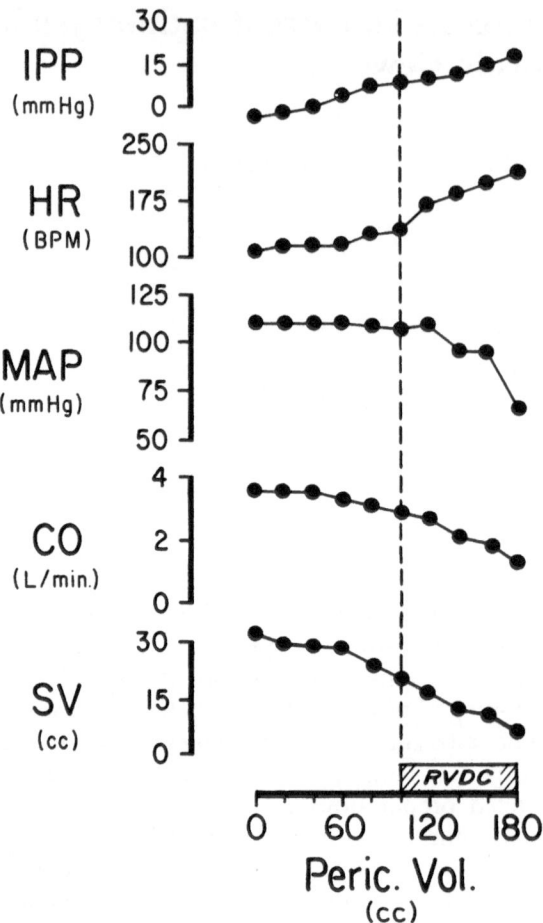

Fig. 3.1. Representative experiment illustrating the hemodynamic changes characteristically seen during experimental cardiac tamponade in a conscious euvolemic canine model. Pericardial volume (Peric. Vol.) was continuously increased at a rate of 10 ml/min. Mean intrapericardial pressure (IPP), heart rate (HR), mean aortic blood pressure (MAP), cardiac output (CO), and two-dimensional echocardiograms were recorded at 2 min intervals. Right ventricular diastolic collapse (RVDC) was first observed at a pericardial volume of 100 ml and persisted to the end point of the experiment (MAP <70% of control). CO and stroke volume (SV) declined consistently as tamponade progressed. MAP, however, was well maintained at the time RVDC was first observed and fell rapidly late in the course of cardiac tamponade. (From Leimgruber PP, Klopfenstein HS, Wann LS, Brooks HL. The hemodynamic derangement associated with right ventricular diastolic collapse in cardiac tamponade: an experimental echocardiographic study. Circulation 1983; 68: 612–620. Reprinted by permission of the American Heart Association, Inc.).

Pathophysiology

Definition

Cardiac tamponade is a unique hemodynamic derangement caused by the accumulation of pericardial fluid under pressure. It is not an all or nothing occurrence but is a continuum with severity likely dependent on several factors including atrial filling pressures, the intrapericardial pressure, and the compliance of the walls of the heart.

Hemodynamic progression

Figure 3.1 illustrates the typical changes that are produced in a conscious animal by the continuous infusion of warm saline into the pericardial space at a rate which will cause hemodynamic decompensation in 20 to 25 minutes. As intrapericardial pressures rises, cardiac output declines, and heart rate, left and right atrial blood pressures, and peripheral vascular resistance increase. Arterial blood pressure is well maintained until late in tamponade when it abruptly declines. It has generally been believed that reduced effective cardiac filling pressures in diastole play a key role in causing the decrease in cardiac output which is evident from the earliest stages of tamponade. Other factors may be contributing to the problem as well. For example, if the compliant chambers of the heart function as Starling resistors during tamponade, diastolic filling of the ventricles would be independent of ventricular pressures when they were lower than intrapericardial pressure and would be limited by the lower instantaneous pressure differences present between the inlet to the atria and the intrapericardial pressure (5). This concept will be touched on later. In any event, cardiac filling during tamponade must be a remarkably slow process. As heart rate increases the amount of time per minute devoted to diastole (and therefore available for cardiac filling) decreases, further contributing to this progressive diastolic dysfunction. The sizes of all cardiac chambers decrease as tamponade worsens. It is generally assumed that the increase in heart rate that is seen during cardiac tamponade serves to help maintain cardiac output as effective cardiac filling pressures and thus stroke volume are forced to decline. However, in recent studies in conscious dogs exposed to progressive tamponade, both without (control) and during beta adrenergic blockade, cardiac output was the same in both situations (6). Since heart rate during beta adrenergic blockade was lower and changed very little, compared to tamponade during control conditions in these euvolemic animals, stroke volume was consistently higher. These observations suggest the possibility that even further reductions in heart rate, which would provide more time for cardiac filling during tamponade, might actually result in better maintenance of cardiac output if they could be obtained without compromising systolic function. Agents with these properties have been identified but this provocative hypothesis has not yet been tested. Certainly, clinical interventions that increase heart rate during tamponade should be avoided until this problem has been more thoroughly studied in conscious individuals. The role played by systolic dysfunction in the absence of coronary artery disease is controversial. All investigators have observed a progressive decrease in coronary artery blood flow as intrapericardial pressure increases and it has been suggested that this change results in myocardial ischemia and systolic dysfunction. The work actually performed by the heart decreases during tamponade, however, and studies in euvolemic conscious dogs have shown that despite a continuous decline, coronary artery blood flow was always adequate to support aerobic metabolism, and a normal coronary artery vasodilatory reserve was present, even at the time of hemodynamic decompensation (7). Calculated mid diastolic coronary vascular resistance did not change in these animals. The decline in coronary artery blood flow resulted entirely from a progressive decrease in the blood pressure difference favoring coronary blood flow as intrapericardial pressure increased. One could speculate that if this study were repeated in animals having significant fixed coronary artery lesions, regional myocardial ischemia may have influenced the hemodynamic progression of cardiac tamponade. So far, this information is not available in conscious animals but myocardial necrosis has been observed in studies using anesthetized preparations exposed to prolonged hypotension during tamponade.

The ability of the conscious animal to maintain arterial blood pressure until very late in tamponade despite a continuous decline in cardiac output must reflect an enhanced ability to increase total peripheral vascular resistance as intrapericardial pressure increases (8). This increase in total peripheral vascular resistance is unaffected by beta adrenergic blockade or angiotensin converting enzyme blockade but is blunted by alpha adrenergic blockade. Both plasma renin activity and angiotensin II levels increase only at the time of decompensated cardiac tamponade in conscious animals when mean arterial blood pressure has fallen by 30%. Arginine vasopressin levels also increase only at the time of decompensation in this model (9) but the hemodynamic picture is unchanged by V_1 arginine vasopressin receptor blockade. Thus, the increase in total peripheral vascular resistance during cardiac tamponade is primarily dependent on alpha adrenergic mechanisms, with a limited late contribution from the renin-angiotensin system. The opioid receptor blocker naloxone was administered to dogs at the time of hemodynamic decompensation in order to try to understand why the final decline in arterial blood pressure is so precipitous in conscious animals during cardiac tamponade (10). The resulting prompt increase in mean arterial blood pressure from 58 ± 6.6 mmHg (mean $\pm$ SD) to the levels present before tamponade, occurred with no change in cardiac output or intrapericardial pressure and was associated with a corresponding increase in total peripheral vascular resistance. Clearly, much greater increases in total peripheral vascular resistance are possible at the time of hemodynamic decompensation but they are prevented by an opioid dependent mechanism. Since cardiac output did not change despite an average increase in mean arterial blood pressure of over 30 mmHg, one may also conclude that systolic function was not limiting cardiac output during tamponade in these animals. The effect of receptor blockade on the distribution of the declining cardiac output during tamponade in conscious animals is also of interest (6). Aortic and mesenteric artery blood flow decrease progressively during tamponade regardless of the presence or absence of blockade. Coronary artery blood flow does not change significantly during alpha adrenergic blockade, suggesting that the continuous decline observed during cardiac tamponade in the absence of alpha blockade or in the presence of beta adrenergic or angiotensin converting enzyme blockade is at least in part mediated by alpha adrenergic mechanisms. Renal artery blood flow, in contrast, is well maintained in all situations, confirming the importance of autoregulation in this vascular bed during cardiac tamponade.

It is surprising that atrial natriuretic peptide levels do not change at all during tamponade in this euvolemic conscious canine model (11). One might expect that atrial distention and not simply atrial blood pressure would play a dominant role in stimulating atrial natriuretic peptide release from the atria, and yet when atrial size continuously decreases during progressive tamponade serum levels of atrial natriuretic peptide are stable rather than decreasing. Certainly other factors must be influential and atrial natriuretic peptide release from noncardiac tissue must be considered.

A word of caution concerning the interpretation of arterial blood gas information during tamponade is in order. Acute cardiac tamponade in otherwise normal individuals breathing room air results in a profound arterial respiratory alkalosis, whereas mixed venous (pulmonary arterial) pH, pCO_2, and calculated serum bicarbonate levels remain relatively unchanged (12). As intrapericardial pressure increases and cardiac output declines, the difference between arterial and mixed venous pCO_2 progressively increase. Furthermore, whereas arterial oxygenation actually improves as cardiac output declines, mixed venous oxygenation steadily worsens. Thus, in spontaneously breathing individuals, mixed venous blood gases are superior to arterial blood gases in assessing acid-base status and oxygenation, even early in tamponade when the decline in cardiac output is in the range of 20 to 40% and arterial blood pressure has not changed significantly.

Modifying factors

If cardiac filling (diastolic function) is of critical importance during cardiac tamponade, then the level of intravascular volume should influence the hemodynamic course. Although the therapeutic value of maneuvers that increase cardiac filling pressures in patients have been questioned, they have long been advocated in the acute treatment of tamponade, whereas hypovolemia seems

to hasten the hemodynamic deterioration. It is clearly possible to substantial-
ly increase cardiac output in healthy conscious dogs exposed to progressive
cardiac tamponade but surprisingly large volumes of fluid are required (13).
Clinical trials in patients have been disappointing (14). This may be in part
because increases in intravascular volume not only lead to increased venous
pressures but also lead to increases in total heart size and thus increases in
intrapericardial fluid pressure which offset the value of the intervention (15).
There also may be danger. During significant tamponade one would expect
that the bulk of infused fluid would be confined to the systemic veins because
of the dominant effect of increased intrapericardial pressure on the right side
of the heart. When the pericardial fluid is removed one would expect that the
left ventricle would be promptly exposed to this volume load as well. In individuals with sufficient left ventricular dysfunction, acute left ventricular failure could be expected to occur. There have been clinical reports of acute
pulmonary edema following relief of cardiac tamponade (16) but no animal
studies have been performed, as yet, to confirm that this mechanism can produce these findings.

Pulsus paradoxus is a respiratory fluctuation in peak arterial blood pressure of 10 mmHg or greater, and is a traditional clinical sign of cardiac tamponade. Unfortunately, it is not as sensitive and specific for tamponade as one
might wish. An important clinical study resulted in the important observation
that patients with tamponade who have pre-existing left ventricular dysfunction with elevated left ventricular diastolic pressures do not exhibit pulsus
paradoxus (17). This has also been found in patients with aortic insufficiency
to produce elevated left ventricular diastolic pressures. The reasons for the
absence of pulsus paradoxus in these situations is not understood; indeed,
after many years and much effort, a complete understanding of the mechan-
ism(s) responsible for pulsus paradoxus in cardiac tamponade remain elusive.

Recent noninvasive diagnostic methods

A word of caution

All new diagnostic methods should be approached with caution since with all
there are likely to be clinical situations in which they falsely indicate the
presence of disease, situations in which they do not detect existing disease,
and other limitations which will only become apparent as we gain experience
in their use.

Echocardiography

If a pericardial effusion accumulates slowly enough the pericardium has time
to grow to accommodate the increased pericardial volume so that very large

effusions may be present with no significant increase in intrapericardial pressure (18). Only effusions that develop more rapidly elevate intrapericardial pressure, compete with the heart for the limited space in the pericardial cavity, and result in cardiac tamponade. Echocardiography allows the noninvasive identification and semiquantitation of pericardial effusions. However, since knowing the size of the effusion alone does not allow one to determine if the effusion is hemodynamically important and since currently available treatments for cardiac tamponade are invasive and associated with significant risks, it would be helpful if noninvasive landmarks were available to identify the presence of tamponade and the approximate degree of hemodynamic compromise. Since clinical reports described atrial and right ventricular free wall collapse during cardiac tamponade (19, 20), euvolemic conscious dogs were studied to define the hemodynamic derangement associated with diastolic collapse of the right ventricular free wall (4). All animals showed right ventricular collapse during acute progressive tamponade, and its appearance was associated with a 20% reduction in cardiac output and occurred prior to changes in mean arterial blood pressure. The onset of right ventricular collapse occurred in early to mid-diastole and its duration and the extent of the right ventricle involved increased as intrapericardial pressure rose. Short-term partial pulmonary artery obstruction led to increased right ventricular pressures and a prompt reduction in right ventricular collapse suggesting that collapse was caused by pericardial pressure exceeding right ventricular pressure in early diastole. An animal having severe right ventricular hypertrophy did not show right ventricular collapse even when intrapericardial pressures were high enough to produce hemodynamic decompensation. These observations apply only to effusions which are not loculated.

These findings were confirmed and extended in a series of clinical and canine studies which demonstrated that in the absence of hypertrophy or elevated intracardiac pressures, the chambers of the heart collapse as intrapericardial pressure rises in an order determined by wall stiffness when relaxed and the pressure of the blood in the chamber at the time (21, 22). These wall motion abnormalities are generally easily seen on 2D echocardiography. Thus, one would expect to see the right atrial free wall begin to invert in late systole and early diastole when intrapericardial pressure is only slightly elevated. Then, when intrapericardial pressure had increased to a somewhat higher level the left atrial free wall would begin to show a similar abnormality. When intrapericardial pressures are high enough to cause a 15 to 20% reduction in cardiac output in euvolemic individuals, right ventricular free wall collapse in early diastole begins. At much higher pressures in most subjects, shifting of the interventricular septum occurs with the same timing as right ventricular collapse. Once present, the wall motion abnormalities progress in extent and duration if intrapericardial pressure continues to increase. We have observed localized left ventricular free wall collapse in diastole in two patients having severe cardiac tamponade and right heart enlargement (presumably due to pressure and volume overload) but we have not studied this in an organized way.

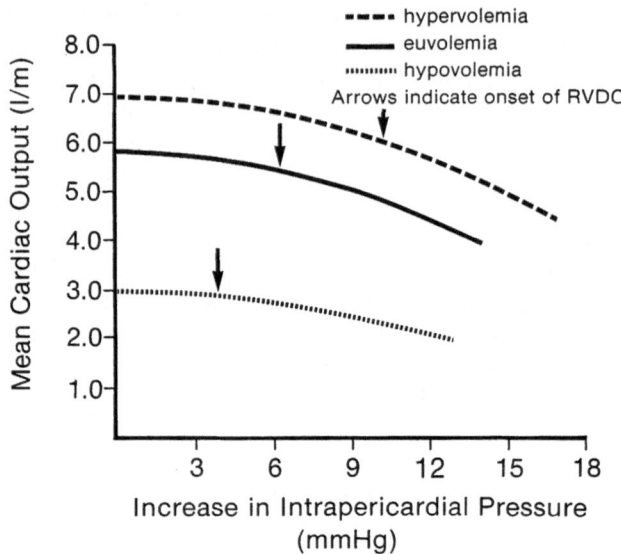

Fig. 3.2. Relation of mean cardiac output and increase in intrapericardial pressure during cardiac tamponade for each intravascular state. The curves all differ significantly from each other (p < 0.05 for any comparison). The cardiac output at the onset (arrows) of right ventricular diastolic collapse (RVDC) during euvolemia differs from that during hypovolemia (p < 0.001) and hypervolemia (p < 0.05). (From Klopfenstein HS, Cogswell TL, Bernath GA, Wann LS, Tipton RK, Hoffmann RG, Brooks HL, Janzer DJ, Peterson DM. Alterations in intravascular volume affect the relation between right ventricular diastolic collapse and the hemodynamic severity of cardiac tamponade. J Am Coll Cardiol 1985; 6: 1057–1063. Reprinted with permission from the American College of Cardiology).

Since the shape and position of the right ventricular free wall is related to the relative pressures within the pericardial space and the right ventricular chamber, one might expect the usefulness of right ventricular collapse to be influenced by intravascular volume and right heart filling pressures (Fig. 3.2). When compared to the euvolemic state in conscious dogs, the onset of right ventricular collapse in volume contraction occurs at a lower intrapericardial pressure (with a lower mean arterial blood pressure and cardiac output) while it occurs at a higher intrapericardial pressure (with a higher arterial blood pressure and cardiac output) in volume expanded states (13). It would be helpful to know what the relative value of right ventricular collapse is, compared to a more familiar traditional clinical sign of cardiac tamponade, such as pulsus paradoxus. It turns out that right ventricular collapse is more sensitive and specific than pulsus paradoxus in detecting increases in intrapericardial pressure during euvolemia and hypervolemia, but the two tests are equally valuable in hypovolemic states in these healthy animals (23, 24). A revealing recent clinical report (25) suggests that these echocardiographic signs may be more sensitive to the presence of cardiac tamponade in hypovolemic patients (so-called low pressure tamponade) than traditional invasive diagnostic methods and clinical signs. The relative value of pulsus paradoxus could not be evaluated in this report, however.

The clinical observation of right ventricular collapse with a small to moderate pericardial effusion in the setting of acute left ventricle failure led to canine studies which demonstrated that a rapid increase in left ventricular volume in the presence of an otherwise unimportant pericardial effusion may increase intrapericardial fluid pressure sufficiently to cause the alterations in right ventricular wall motion seen during cardiac tamponade (15). Therefore, if one is certain that acute enlargement of a cardiac chamber has occurred and the clinical reason for this change is reversible, we would suggest that therapy should be directed at treating the cause of chamber enlargement and not at pericardial fluid drainage, despite the presence of right ventricular chamber collapse.

Similarly, the clinical finding of right ventricular collapse in the presence of a small to moderate pericardial effusion and large pleural effusion led us to canine studies which showed that pleural effusions could indeed increase the pressure in an otherwise unimportant pericardial effusion enough to induce right ventricular collapse (26). Once again, the appropriate therapy is not a pericardial drainage procedure but rather removal of the pleural effusion. These two examples represent clinical situations in which right ventricular collapse is a false positive indication that pericardial fluid drainage is needed, even though the hemodynamics of cardiac tamponade are probably present.

In summary, a series of easily observed echocardiographic landmarks identifying various hemodynamic stages during progressive cardiac tamponade are now available. They can be extremely useful but if not applied with thought and caution, they may be misleading and dangerous. Cardiac tamponade may be lethal and current therapies are invasive and associated with significant risks. These noninvasive findings may be entirely absent, even when severe cardiac tamponade is present, if the walls of the heart are stiffened or intracavitary pressures are elevated. Further, as just discussed, the presence of right ventricular collapse, in particular, may not always indicate the need for pericardial fluid drainage. And finally, although the onset of wall motion abnormalities is clearly related to the hemodynamic state as intrapericardial pressure increases, this relationship is modulated by the current intravascular volume status of the individual. As suggested earlier, these landmarks in the progression of cardiac tamponade may result from the compliant chambers of the heart acting as Starling resistors. Since Starling resistors impose an upper limit to the rate of flow of fluid through them, the rate of cardiac filling during cardiac tamponade may be restricted below the rate one would expect based on conventional hemodynamic considerations.

Doppler

Several preliminary acute canine studies have found that during hemodynamically significant cardiac tamponade, an exaggerated respiratory variation in transvalvular blood flow velocities occurs (27, 28). Two recent clinical studies using standard transcutaneous Doppler techniques has confirmed these observations in spontaneous breathing patients having varying degrees of cardiac tamponade (29, 30). The direction of these changes is as one would expect – velocity increases with inspiration across the tricuspid and pulmonic valves and decreases across the mitral and aortic valves, with expiration having the opposite effect. It is the extent of this variation across individual valves which may eventually add to our ability to noninvasively identify patients having significant cardiac tamponade in need of an invasive drainage procedure. These exaggerated changes in transvalvular flow velocity are, of course, reflections of changes in intrathoracic pressure associated with respiration so one might expect that ventilator dependent patients may present a different pattern since inspiration in these people is associated with an increase in intrathoracic pressure rather than a decrease. Preliminary studies suggest that although the direction of the change in flow velocity is different at each valve in ventilator dependent patients from that found in spontaneous breathing patients, significant cardiac tamponade is still associated with an exaggeration of the normal variation in transvalvular flow velocities (31).

It is not yet clear how the degree of transvalvular flow velocity change in tamponade relates to the degree of hemodynamic compromise and the individuals state of hydration. Further studies will be needed to understand the limitations of this promising method as well as its relative value compared to better known findings such as pulsus paradoxus.

Conclusions

Cardiac tamponade is a unique hemodynamic progression which if not diagnosed and treated in a timely manner may cause death. Since the definitive therapies are invasive and require some time to prepare for once the diagnosis is made, early diagnosis is important. New noninvasive ultrasonic methods have emerged over the last 5 to 10 years which allow hemodynamically significant pericardial effusions to be identified early in the progression of cardiac tamponade. Although much has been learned about these methods and they already represent a valuable addition, much remains to be learned and they should be applied with caution in the context of each patients individual clinical situation.

The pathophysiology of cardiac tamponade is not completely understood. It would be especially helpful if more effective temporizing therapies were available for use, when needed, in patients awaiting pericardiocentesis or a surgical drainage procedure. It is hoped that further studies will improve our understanding of the hemodynamics of cardiac tamponade and lead to the development of such therapies.

References

1. Shabetai R. The pericardium. New York, Grune and Stratton, 1981.
2. Fowler NO. The pericardium in health and disease. Mount Kisco, Futura Publishing Co., 1985.
3. Reddy PS, Leon DF, Shaver JA. Pericardial disease. New York, Raven Press Books Ltd., 1982.
4. Leimgruber PP, Klopfenstein HS, Wann LS, Brooks HL: The hemodynamic derangement associated with right ventricular diastolic collapse in cardiac tamponade: An experimental echocardiographic study. Circulation 1983; 68: 612–620.
5. Brower RW, Noordergraaf A: Pressure-flow characteristics of collapsible tubes; a reconciliation of seemingly contradictory results. Ann Biomed Eng 1973; 1: 333–335.
6. Bernath GA, Cogswell TL, Hoffman RG, Klopfenstein HS: Influences on the distribution of blood flow during cardiac tamponade in the conscious dog. Circulation Research 1987; 60: 72–81.
7. Klopfenstein HS, Bernath GA, Cogswell TL, Boerboom LE: Coronary artery hemodynamics in conscious dog during cardiac tamponade. Circulation Research 1987; 60: 845–849.
8. Cogswell TL, Bernath GA, Raff H, Hoffman RG, Klopfenstein HS: Total peripheral resistance during cardiac tamponade: adrenergic and angiotensin roles. Am J Physiol 1986; 251: R916–R922.
9. Raff H, Cogswell TL, Bernath GA, Klopfenstein HS: Vasopressin and ACTH responses to acute cardiac tamponade in conscious dogs. Clin Res 1986; 34: 899A.
10. Mathias DW, Roberts J, Siegesmund D, Klopfenstein HS: Naloxone reverses hypotension during acute cardiac tamponade in conscious dogs. FASEB Journal 1988; 2: VI-A1693 (abstract).
11. Mathias DW, Bernath G, Cogswell T, Roberts J, Klopfenstein HS: Atrial natriuretic factor response to acute cardiac tamponade in conscious dogs. Clin Res 1987; 35: 303A.
12. Mathias DW, Clifford PS, Klopfenstein HS: Mixed venous blood gases are superior to arterial blood gases in assessing acid-base status and oxygenation during acute cardiac tamponade in dogs. J Clin Invest 1988; 82: 833–838.
13. Klopfenstein HS, Cogswell TL, Bernath GA, Wann LS, Tipton RK, Hoffman RG, Brooks HL: Alterations in intravascular volume affect the relation between right ventricular diastolic collapse and the hemodynamic severity of cardiac tamponade. J Am Coll Cardiol 1985; 6: 1057–1063.
14. Kerber RE, Gascho JA, Litchfield R, Wolfson P, Oh D, Pandian NG: Hemodynamic effects of volume expansion and nitroprusside compared with pericardiocentesis in patients with acute cardiac tamponade. N Engl J Med 1982; 307: 929–931.
15. Cogswell TL, Bernath GA, Keelan MH, Wann LS, Klopfenstein HS: The shift in the relationship between intrapericardial fluid pressure and volume induced by acute left ventricular pressure overload during cardiac tamponade. Circulation 1986; 74: 173–180.
16. VanDyke WH, Cure J, Chakko CS, Gheorchiade M: Pulmonary edema after pericardiocentesis for cardiac tamponade. N Engl J Med 1983; 309: 595–596.
17. Reddy PS, Curtiss EI, O'Toole JD, Shaver JA: Cardiac tamponade: hemodynamic observations in man. Circulation 1978; 58: 265–272.
18. Freeman GL, LeWinter MM: Pericardial adaptations during chronic cardiac dilatation in dogs. Circulation Res 1984; 54: 294–300.
19. Shiina A, Yaginuma T, Kondo K, Kawai N, Hosoda S: Echocardiographic evaluation of impending cardiac tamponade. J Cardiography 1979; 9: 555–563.
20. Gillam LD, Guyer DE, Gibson TC, King ME, Marshall JE, Weyman AE: Hydrodynamic compression of the right atrium: a new echocardiographic sign of cardiac tamponade. Circulation 1983; 68: 294–301.
21. Singh S, Wann LS, Schuchard GH, Klopfenstein HS, Leimgruber PP, Keelan MH, Brooks

HL: Right ventricular and right atrial collapse in patients with cardiac tamponade – a combined echocardiographic and hemodynamic study. Circulation 1984; 70: 966–971.

22. Singh S, Wann LS, Klopfenstein HS, Hartz A, Brooks HL: Usefulness of right ventricular diastolic collapse in diagnosing cardiac tamponade and comparison to pulsus paradoxus. Am J Cardiol 1986; 57: 652–656.

23. Klopfenstein HS, Schuchard GH, Wann LS, Palmer TE, Hartz AJ, Gross CM, Singh S, Brooks HL: The relative merits of pulsus paradoxus and right ventricular diastolic collapse in the early detection of cardiac tamponade: an experimental echocardiographic study. Circulation 1985; 71: 829–833.

24. Cogswell TL, Bernath GA, Wann LS, Hoffman RG, Brooks HL, Klopfenstein HS: Effects of intravascular volume state on the value of pulsus paradoxus and right ventricular diastolic collapse in predicting cardiac tamponade. 1985; 72: 1076–1080.

25. Labib S, Udelson J, Pandian NG: Echocardiography in low pressure tamponade. Am J Cardiol 1989; 63: 1156–1157.

26. Vaska KJ, Wann LS, Sagar K, Klopfenstein HS: Pleural effusion as a cause of right ventricular diastolic collapse and cardiac tamponade. J Am Coll Cardiol 1989; 13 (suppl A): 236 A.

27. Pandian NG, Rifkin RD, Wang SS: Flow velocity paradoxus – A Doppler echocardiographic sign of cardiac tamponade: exaggerated variation in pulmonary and aortic blood flow velocities. Circulation 1984; 70: II-381 (abstract).

28. Pandian NG, Wang SS, McInerney K, Caldeira M, Konstam M, Isner JM, Salem DN: Doppler echocardiography in cardiac tamponade: Abnormalities in tricuspid and mitral flow. J Am Coll Cardiol 1985; 5: 485 (abstract).

29. Leeman DE, Levine MJ, Come PC: Doppler echocardiography in cardiac tamponade: exaggerated respiratory variation in transvalvular blood flow velocity integrals. J Am Coll Cardiol 1988; 11: 572–578.

30. Appleton CP, Hatle LK, Popp RL: Cardiac tamponade and pericardial effusion: respiratory variation in transvalvular flow velocities studied by Doppler echocardiography. J Am Coll Cardiol 1988; 11: 1020–1030.

31. Pandian NG, Wang SS, Rifkin R, Sharma S, McInerney K, Caldeira M, Salem D: Effect of mechanical ventilation on the two-dimensional and Doppler echocardiographic signs of cardiac tamponade. Circulation 1985; 72: III-354 (abstract).

4. Differentiation of constrictive pericarditis and restrictive cardiomyopathy: general overview and new insights from two-dimensional and Doppler echocardiographic studies

CHRISTOPHER P. APPLETON, M.D., RICHARD L. POPP, M.D., AND LIV K. HATLE, M.D.

Introduction

Despite years of study and the description of numerous diagnostic tests, the differentiation of restrictive cardiomyopathy from constrictive pericarditis has remained difficult, even at experienced medical centers (1). This difficulty has been due, in part, to the inability to identify a basic difference in the underlying pathophysiology of the two diseases which could be easily identi-

59

J. Soler-Soler et al. (Eds.), Pericardial Disease, pp. 59–93.
© 1990 Kluwer Academic Publishers

fied and had a high degree of sensitivity and specificity. More recently, we have reported that Doppler echocardiography, through its ability to evaluate filling dynamics of all four cardiac chambers throughout the respiratory cycle, has provided new insights into the pathophysiology and differentiation of these conditions (2). In this chapter we will review these echo-Doppler findings in detail, and relate them to the clinical findings, pathophysiology and natural history of restrictive cardiomyopathy and constrictive pericarditis. Special emphasis will be placed on how ventricular diastolic properties and changes in intrathoracic pressures influence the observed findings in the two conditions. Unresolved issues and possible future directions for clinical research will also be discussed.

Definitions

For the purposes of this review restrictive cardiomyopathy is defined as a disorder of the heart muscle where the primary abnormality is a decrease in ventricular distensibility that is due to morphologic changes in either the endocardium or myocardium or both (3). This abnormality of diastolic function results in elevated filling pressures which are necessary to adequately distend the non-compliant ventricles and maintain cardiac output. Abnormalities of systolic function, if present, are usually mild and much less severe than the prominent diastolic abnormality.

Although some definitions of restrictive cardiomyopathy include only cases in which there is no definable etiology (3), infiltrative diseases (such as amyloidosis and hemochromatosis) that cause a marked decrease in ventricular distensibility will be included in this discussion. However, patients with marked abnormalities of diastolic function which are a result of ventricular dilatation or severe ventricular systolic dysfunction (such as dilated cardiomyopathy) are specifically excluded.

Constrictive pericarditis is defined as a condition in which the layers of the pericardium become scarred and fused, lose their compliance, and restrict ventricular and atrial distensibility in mid- or late diastole (4, 5). As with restrictive cardiomyopathy, the primary derangement is in the diastolic filling of the heart and any systolic dysfunction is mild or secondary to coexistent disease processes. Variants of constrictive pericarditis, such as constriction localized to a specific region of the heart, are rare and will not be discussed.

Etiology

A variety of conditions have been associated with restrictive cardiomyopathy and the development of constrictive pericarditis. These are discussed in several excellent reviews (3–5) and will not be discussed in detail here. However, of special mention is the recent description of both constrictive pericarditis (6) and more commonly a disorder which is similar to a restrictive cardiomyopathy in cardiac transplant recipients (7, 8). Recent studies suggests that during long term clinical follow-up up to 20% of these patients develop a hemodynamic picture consistent with "restrictive/constrictive" physiology (8). The etiology of this severe diastolic dysfunction is unknown, although chronic low-grade rejection, severe hypertension or a toxic effect of cyclosporin are possibilities. With the number of transplant recipients increasing worldwide, this group may be an increasingly important subset of patients with restrictive cardiomyopathy in the near future.

Pathophysiology

Abnormalities of diastolic function

Restrictive cardiomyopathy: The characteristic abnormality of restrictive cardiomyopathy, common to all etiologies, is a marked decrease in ventricular distensibility (3). This results in a shift of the ventricular diastolic pressure-volume relationship such that pressure is abnormally elevated for a normal end-distolic volume. Although not satisfactorily studied, it is generally assumed that the decrease in ventricular distensibility is the result of morphologic changes in the endocardium or myocardium. These changes usually include an increase in the amount of connective tissue and fibrosis, and in some cases infiltration by foreign substances such as amyloid. However, a few cases of restrictive cardiomyopathy have been reported without obvious changes in endo- or myocardial histology. In these instances the etiology of the marked decrease in ventricular distensibility remains unclear.

By definition, the restrictive process affects both ventricles, although the filling pressures are usually higher on the left side. This discordance in pressure is often cited as evidence for predominant left heart involvement, although this difference may simply reflect the normal relationship of the left heart being less compliant and having higher diastolic pressures than the right. In fact, the bi-ventricular involvement helps distinguish restrictive cardiomyopathy from other disorders which can be associated with a marked decrease in left ventricular distensibility, such as hypertensive heart disease, which can occasionally mimic it. In these cases diastolic right heart pressures and filling dynamics are normal or near normal.

Along with a decrease in distensibility, there is evidence that the rate of left ventricular relaxation is slowed in many patients with restrictive cardiomyopathy (9). This point has previously been underemphasized, but is important for understanding the filling dynamics and natural history of restrictive cardiomyopathy and how it differs from constrictive pericarditis. Recent studies have shown that if left atrial pressure does not change, a decrease in the rate of left ventricular relaxation will result in a reduction of the early diastolic transmitral pressure gradient (10) and consequently the rate of early diastolic ventricular filling (11). Just such a filling pattern has been reported in cardiac amyloidosis, where a decrease in early diastolic mitral flow velocity and increase in flow velocity at atrial contraction is seen in patients in the early stages of their disease (12, 13). A decreased rate of ventricular filling in early diastole is not typical of "pure" constrictive pericarditis and the marked difference in ventricular filling rates helps differentiate restrictive cardiomyopathy in its early stages from constrictive pericarditis (14–16). Unfortunately, in more advanced stages of restrictive cardiomyopathy, left atrial pressure is elevated and results in an increase in the rate of early diastolic filling, so that the differentiation of the two diseases by filling parameters alone is probably not reliable (2, 11).

Constrictive pericarditis: In contrast to restrictive cardiomyopathy, the primary abnormality of diastolic function in patients with constrictive pericarditis is not in the ventricular myocardium, but in the scarred, non-compliant pericardium which limits ventricular and atrial distensibility in mid- and late diastole (4, 5). In advanced cases total cardiac volume may even be reduced. However, unless co-existent disease processes are present, myocardial compliance and the rate of ventricular relaxation are normal. Therefore, early diastolic filling remains unimpeded throughout the natural history of the disease and the rate of left ventricular filling is normal in the early stages of the disease and then increased in later stages when atrial pressure is increased (15, 16).

The pressure-volume relationship of the cardiac chambers are also different in constrictive pericarditis from that in restrictive cardiomyopathy in that the major alteration is confined to mid- and late diastole when the pericardium exerts its constricting effect. In addition, both the atria and ventricles are affected in a similar fashion. This confinement of the heart inside a rigid shell results in an increase in mechanical coupling between the chambers so that a change in volume in one chamber affects both the pressure and volume in the other chambers.

Effect of respiration on intracardiac pressures and ventricular filling dynamics

The effect of respiration on intracardiac pressures is markedly different in constrictive pericarditis than in restrictive cardiomyopathy and is the key element which triggers the reciprocal ventricular filling which occurs in this condition.

In restrictive cardiomyopathy changes in intrathoracic pressure are transmitted normally to the cardiac chambers (2) so that changes in systolic and diastolic ventricular pressures with respiration are similar to changes in intrathoracic pressure in both direction and degree. Therefore, as shown in Figs. 4.1 and 4.2, the early diastolic pulmonary venous-left ventricular pressure gradient (estimated by the difference between pulmonary wedge and left ventricular pressure) and the left ventricular filling remain constant throughout the respiratory cycle.

In contrast, patients with constrictive pericarditis have less respiratory variation in intracardiac pressures than in intrathoracic pressures (2, 17–20); presumably because fluctuations in intrathoracic pressure are only partially transmitted through the scarred pericardium. As shown in Figs. 4.3 and 4.4, the reduced respiratory variation in left ventricular diastolic pressure results in a pulmonary venous-left ventricular pressure gradient, and consequently left ventricular filling, that changes continuously throughout the respiratory cycle. Because venous inflow pressure is elevated and the cardiac chambers are mechanically coupled inside the non-compliant pericardium, changes in filling on one side of the heart with respiration are associated with opposite changes on the other side. This respiratory driven, reciprocal ventricular filling is a cardinal feature of constrictive pericarditis and is the most important diagnostic hallmark that differentiates it from restrictive cardiomyopathy. The hemodynamic and Doppler findings associated with this reciprocal ventricular filling will be discussed in detail later in the chapter.

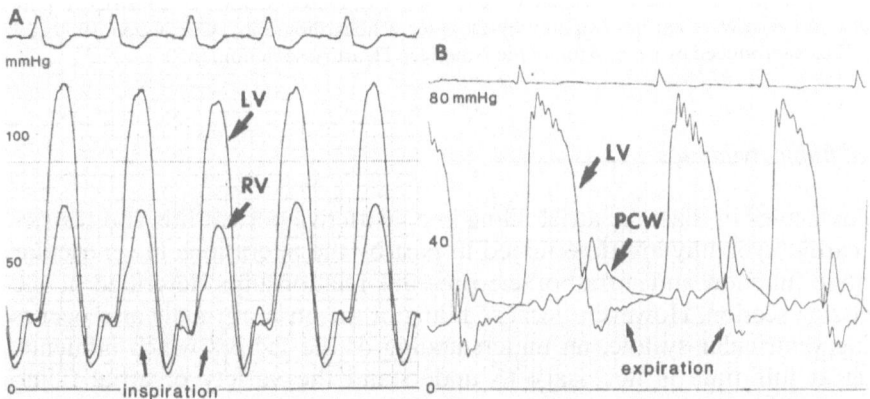

Fig. 4.1. Tracings of left ventricular (LV), pulmonary wedge (PCW), and right ventricular (RV) pressures recorded from patients with restrictive cardiomyopathy. Panel A: RV and LV diastolic pressures are markedly elevated and equalized but both systolic and diastolic pressures decrease with inspiration. Panel B: Simultaneous recording of LV and PCW pressures from a patient with restrictive cardiomyopathy who was in atrial fibrillation. LV diastolic and PCW pressures show a similar degree of change with respiration so that the early diastolic PCW-LV gradient remains nearly constant. (From: Hatle LK, Appleton CP, Popp RL. Differentiation of constrictive pericarditis and restrictive cardiomyopathy by Doppler echocardiography. Circulation 1989; 79: 350–370. Reproduced by permission of the American Heart Association, Inc.).

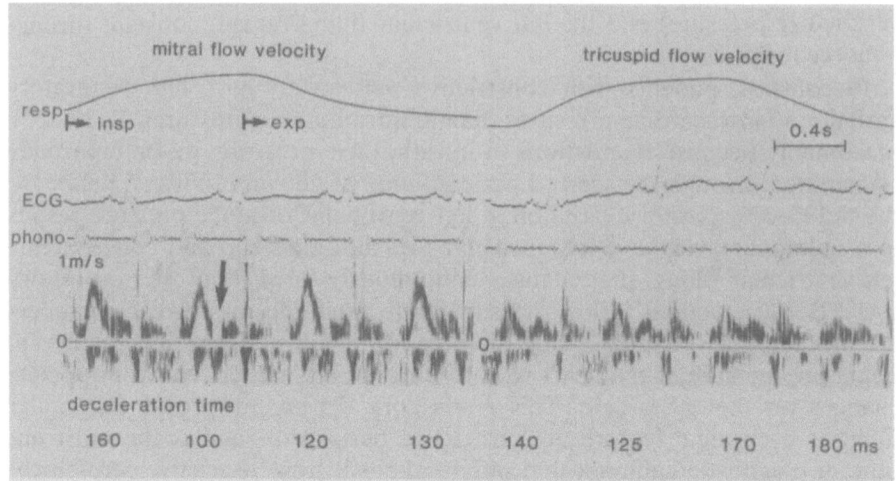

Fig. 4.2. Mitral and tricuspid flow velocity recorded with pulsed Doppler ultrasound and simultaneous ECG, phonocardiogram (phono) and respiration (resp) from a patient with restrictive cardiomyopathy. There is minimal respiratory variation in peak early mitral flow velocity with respiration and a relatively low flow velocity with atrial contraction. The mitral deceleration time is short, and shortens further (bottom values) during inspiration, with mid-diastolic reversal of flow (diastolic regurgitation, arrow) being seen at the same time. The early tricuspid flow velocity also shows marked inspiratory shortening of the deceleration time with only a moderate increase in peak velocity and there is no marked decrease in early velocity on the first beat of expiration. (From: Hatle LK, Appleton CP, Popp RL. Differentiation of constrictive pericarditis and restrictive cardiomyopathy by Doppler echocardiography. Circulation 1989; 79: 350–370. Reproduced by permission of the American Heart Association, Inc.).

Atrial filling dynamics

The dynamics of diastolic atrial filling in constrictive pericarditis and restrictive cardiomyopathy are determined in part by the alterations in ventricular diastolic function and intrathoracic pressure relationships described in the preceding section. However, because filling of the atria normally also occurs during ventricular systole, an understanding of the factors which influence filling at this time is necessary to understand the variety of atrial filling patterns which can be seen in the two diseases.

In normal individuals right atrial filling is bi-phasic, with the peak velocity of flow during systole being larger than that during diastole (21). This bi-phasic filling is composed of one "active" and one "passive" phase. The active phase occurs during ventricular systole, when atrial pressure falls rapidly (X descent) due to the combined effects of atrial relaxation and the apical descent of the tricuspid valve ring. By 2-D echocardiography this phase is characterized by a rapid elongation of the atrium. A smaller, passive filling phase of the atrium occurs during ventricular diastole when atrial pressure falls (Y descent) as a result of tricuspid valve opening. In this phase the atrium

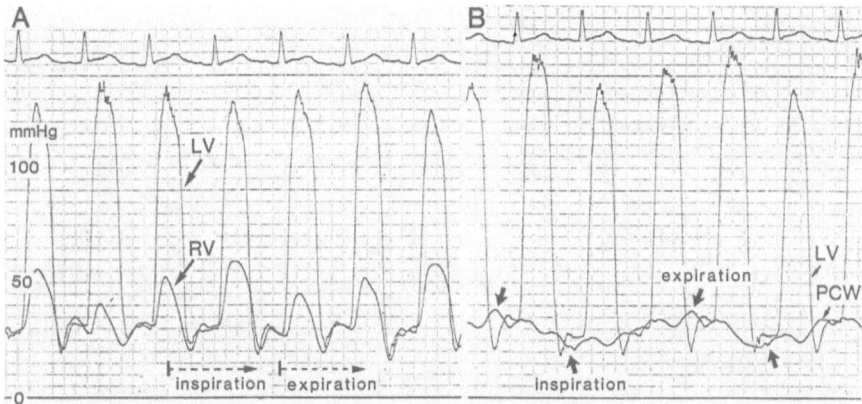

Fig. 4.3. Tracings of left ventricular (LV), pulmonary wedge (PCW) and right ventricular (RV) pressures recorded form a patient with constrictive pericarditis that demonstrate hemodynamic evidence of reciprocal ventricular filling. Panel A: RV systolic pressure is seen to increase on the second beat of inspiration while LV systolic and diastolic pressures are decreasing. Opposite changes are seen during expiration. Note also the marked respiratory changes in RV ejection time as estimated by the width of the RV systolic pressure recording. Panel B: Respiratory variation in diastolic LV pressure is seen to be less than PCW pressure, resulting in a decrease in the early diastolic PCW-LV pressure difference at the onset of inspiration (2nd and 4th arrows) and increased difference at the onset of expiration (1st and 3rd arrows). (From: Hatle LK, Appleton CP, Popp RL. Differentiation of constrictive pericarditis and restrictive cardiomyopathy by Doppler echocardiography. Circulation 1989; 79: 350–370. Reproduced by permission of the American Heart Association, Inc.).

is acting as a passive conduit for flow from the central veins to the relaxing ventricle. Minimal or reversed velocities occur in the central veins with atrial contraction (A wave) and at the end of ventricular systole (V wave). The similarity of the atrial filling pattern to the more widely recognized waves of the jugular venous pulse and right atrial pressure contour is shown in Fig. 4.5.

A decrease in atrial filling during systole may occur when right atrial or right ventricular systolic function is reduced and the rate and amount of active atrial expansion is slowed. In these cases atrial compliance is reduced and atrial pressures are usually elevated. Conversely, if the atrium or ventricle contracts vigorously, the amount of filling during systole may be increased. A decrease in the amount of diastolic atrial filling may occur when an impairment in ventricular relaxation is present and there is a reduced rate of ventricular pressure fall and early right ventricular filling. Increased diastolic filling may be seen when the ventricular relaxation is rapid and atrial pressure is increased. Flow reversals in the central veins are increased when atrial compliance is decreased and the pressure rise with either active or passive atrial filling is larger than normal.

Patients with restrictive cardiomyopathy may demonstrate a variety of atrial filling patterns depending on the stage of their disease. With mild dis-

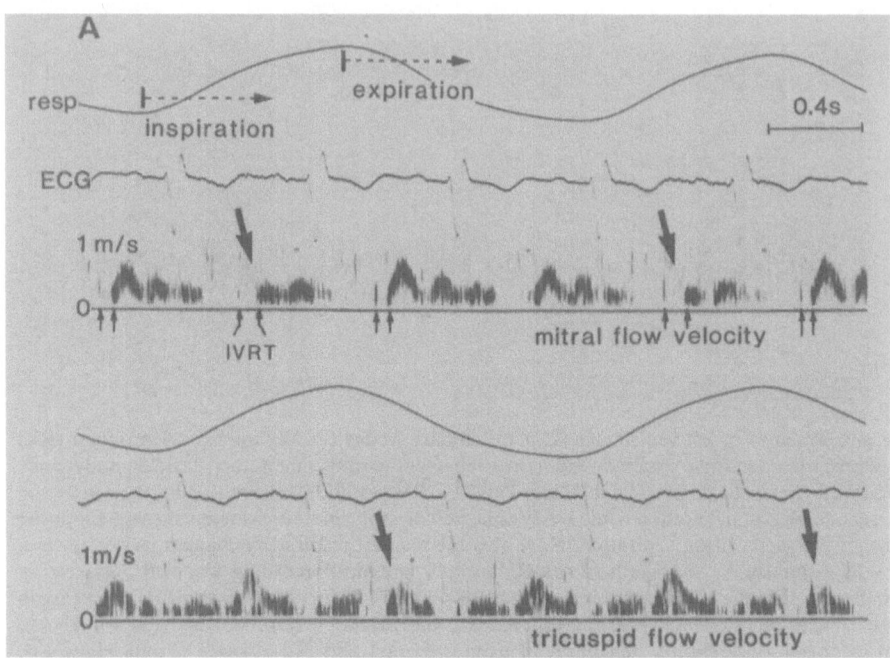

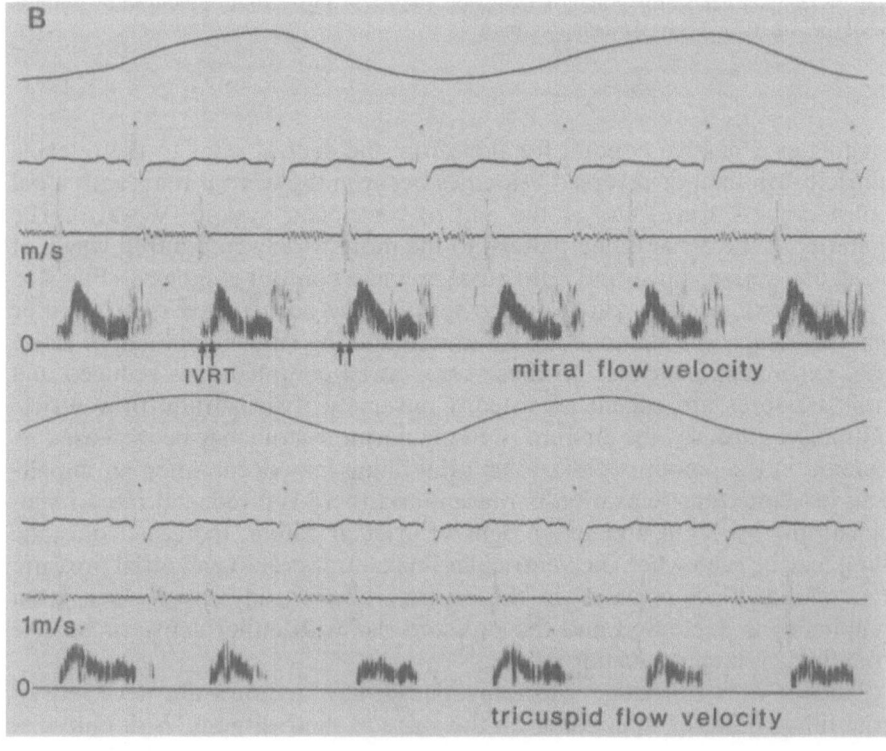

ease, ventricular relaxation may be impaired but atrial and ventricular systolic function may remain normal. In these cases atrial filling during systole is normal but passive filling during diastole is decreased (X>Y descent). With more advanced disease the atria are dilated and have an increase in pressure. In these cases atrial systolic function and compliance are usually reduced and atrial systolic filling is decreased while diastolic filling is increased (Y>X descent); a pattern opposite to that seen in the early stages of the disease. Intermediate stages may have filling which can be approximately equal during systole and diastole (X = Y descent), with prominent reversals of flow during atrial contraction.

In constrictive pericarditis the most common filling pattern seen is brisk biphasic filling (X = Y descent). This pattern may be seen because atrial function can be well maintained until the late stages of the disease, ventricular relaxation is unimpaired and central venous pressure is increased. However, predominance of either active or passive filling can occur if the atrium begins to fail or ventricular relaxation is impaired due to co-existent disease processes. These atrial filling patterns, and the effect of respiration on them, will be discussed further in the section on venous Doppler echocardiography.

Natural history

Restrictive cardiomyopathy

Recent data from echo-Doppler studies suggests that patients with restrictive cardiomyopathy progress through a sequence of alterations of cardiac function during the course of their disease (11–13). In the initial asymptomatic stages, ventricular relaxation may be impaired (slowed) but ventricular dis-

Fig. 4.4. Panel A shows mitral and tricuspid flow velocities recorded together with respiration (resp) in a patient with constrictive pericarditis. Note the marked decrease in early mitral flow velocity (beats 2 and 5, large black arrows) and the increase in left ventricular isovolumic relaxation time (IVRT, pairs of small arrows) on the first beat following the onset of inspiration compared to the other beats. The timing of aortic closure was verified by a simultaneous phonocardiogram not included in the figure. On the first beat following the onset of expiration (beats 3 and 6) and increase in mitral flow velocity and shortening of the IVRT is seen, when compared both to inspiration and to the intermediate beats. The tricuspid flow velocity shows reciprocal changes, with an increase on the first beat of inspiration (beats 2 and 5) and a decrease on the first beat of expiration (beats 3 and 6, arrows) compared with intermediate beats (1 and 4). The velocity recorded in systole in the tricuspid recording represents systolic flow in the right ventricular inflow tract and should not be confused with transvalvular flow. In panel B, recorded from the same patient one week after pericardiectomy, there is minimal respiratory variation in early mitral flow velocity and IVRT with respiration and the tricuspid flow velocity on the first beats following the onset of expiration (beats 2 and 5) is larger than the next expiratory beat (beats 3 and 6). (From: Hatle LK, Appleton CP, Popp RL. Differentiation of constrictive pericarditis and restrictive cardiomyopathy by Doppler echocardiography. Circulation 1989; 79: 350–370. Reproduced by permission of the American Heart Association, Inc.).

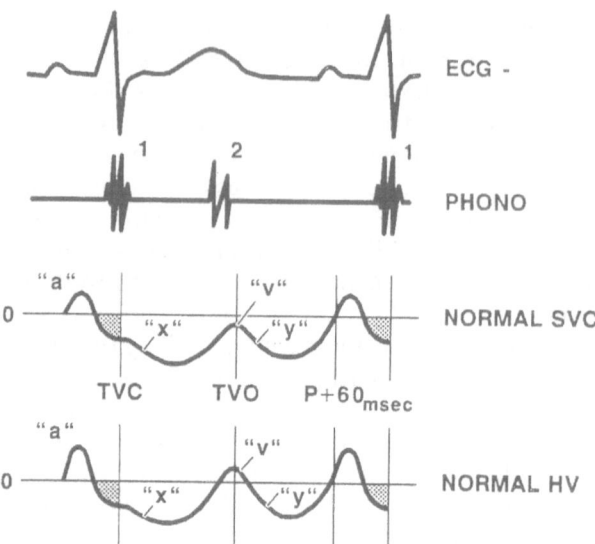

Fig. 4.5. Schematic diagram of flow velocity curves in the superior vena cava (SVC) and hepatic veins (HV) of normal adults. Flow below the zero reference line is toward the heart. Both curves demonstrate the biphasic nature of forward flow with the hepatic veins generally demonstrating slightly more prominent flow reversals at end systole and at the time of atrial contraction. The flow velocity contours accurately represent the waves seen in the jugular venous pulse and right atrial pressure recording and are labeled for analogy to these more familiar findings. phono = phonocardiogram; TVC and TVO = tricuspid closure and opening; A and V = waves; X and Y = descents. (Reproduced, with permission, from: Appleton CP, Hatle LK, Popp RL. Superior vena cava and hepatic vein Doppler echocardiography in healthy adults. J Am Coll Cardiol 1987; 10: 1032–1039).

tensibility only mildly decreased. At this stage patients are usually asymptomatic, but the impaired relaxation results in a decrease in the proportion of early diastolic ventricular filling and an increase in the proportion that occurs with atrial contraction (12–14). The atria may still be normal size, and, in fact, may appear hypercontractile; probably in part because the reduced volume of early ventricular filling results in less impedance to atrial emptying.

With progression of disease, ventricular distensibility decreases further and filling pressures increase. At this stage the effects of impaired ventricular relaxation on early diastolic filling are opposed by an elevated atrial pressure (10), so that the early diastolic transvalvular pressure gradient, ventricular filling rate and ventricular filling pattern return toward normal. We (11), and others (13), have termed this phenomenon "pseudonormalization" to indicate that although ventricular filling dynamics appear normal there are significant abnormalities of diastolic function present. With an increased ventricular diastolic pressure atrial emptying decreases and the atria begin to dilate. Patients begin to become symptomatic, usually with complaints of exertional dyspnea.

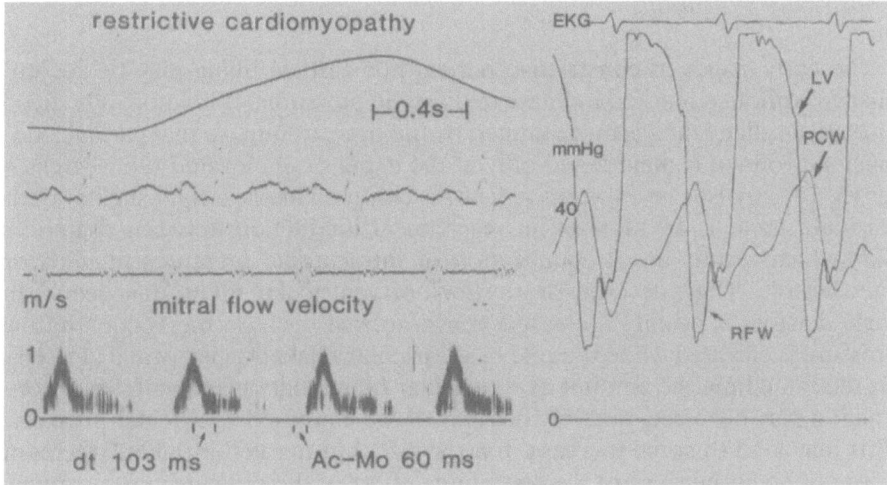

Fig. 4.6. Mitral flow velocity (left panel) and simultaneous LV and pulmonary wedge (PCW) pressure in a patient with restrictive cardiomyopathy. The short mitral deceleration time (dt, normal = 200 ms), short LV isovolumic relaxation time (Ac-Mo interval, nl = 80 ms) and minimal flow velocity at atrial contraction are typical of advanced restrictive cardiomyopathy and indicate the presence of high filling pressures, abrupt cessation of ventricular filling and poor atrial systolic function. However, note that there is no variation in mitral flow velocity throughout the respiratory cycle. The pressure recordings show that LV end diastolic pressure is markedly elevated and an increased rapid filling wave (RFW) is present. (Reproduced, with permission, from: Appleton CP, Hatle LK, Popp RL. Demonstration of restrictive ventricular physiology by Doppler echocardiography. J Am Coll Cardiol 1988; 11: 757–768).

In advanced cases of restrictive cardiomyopathy, ventricular distensibility is usually severely reduced, filling pressures are markedly elevated (and may be equalized), and the atria are often markedly dilated and show poor contractility (7, 12–13, 22). Despite impaired ventricular relaxation, the high venous pressures and severe decrease in distensibility result in more rapid than normal early diastolic filling which terminates abruptly because of an abnormally rapid rise in ventricular pressure (Fig. 4.6). Little or no filling occurs in late diastole and at atrial contraction, a pattern easily recognized with Doppler echocardiography (7) or at catheterization as a "dip and plateau" in ventricular diastolic pressure recordings. A mild to moderate decrease in left ventricular ejection fraction is also frequently seen at this advanced stage. Supraventricular arrhythmias and atrial fibrillation are common and the patients are often markedly dyspneic with only minimal exertion. A high central venous pressure, pleural effusions and peripheral edema are prominent clinical findings.

Constrictive pericarditis

In the early stages of constrictive pericarditis cardiac filling may be accomplished without a marked increase in diastolic pressures. With more advanced disease, cardiac filling is more limited by the pericardium, so that cardiac end-diastolic volume is maintained only at the expense of elevated filling pressures (5, 17–20). Because the entire heart is confined inside a rigid shell of pericardium, there is an increase in mechanical interaction between chambers (23) which results in an equalization of intracardiac pressures in mid- or late diastole. The rate (and proportion) of ventricular filling that occurs in early diastole is usually increased above normal because the venous inflow pressure is elevated while the rate of ventricular relaxation is normal (15–16). At the same time the amount of ventricular filling that occurs with atrial contraction may decrease, possibly because of the increased ventricular pressure. This may lead to some increase in atrial size, but marked atrial enlargement does not occur because of the restraining effect of the pericardium. Dyspnea, edema, ascites and hepatic dysfunction are common, but the dyspnea is often less prominent than in patients with restrictive cardiomyopathy.

In advanced cases, constrictive pericarditis may limit the diastolic volume of the heart so severely that stroke volume is fixed and tachycardia is necessary to maintain cardiac output. With further elevation of filling pressures atrial systolic function may deteriorate and atrial fibrillation occur. The rate of early diastolic filling remains increased above normal, with virtually no filling from mid-diastole on. Massive peripheral edema, ascites and cardiac cirrhosis and cachexia dominate the end-stage clinical picture (5, 18).

Diagnostic studies to differentiate constrictive pericarditis from restrictive cardiomyopathy

Clinical examination

Physical examination findings which favor constrictive pericarditis include pulsus paradoxus, a pericardial knock, collapsing X and Y descents in the jugular venous pulse and marked ascites which is out of proportion to the degree of peripheral edema. Typical findings in patients with restrictive cardiomyopathy include an apical third heart sound and an elevated central venous pressure which demonstrates a prominent Y descent. Venous engorgement, peripheral edema and Kussmaul's sign may be present in both disorders. Unfortunately, the clinical findings may be atypical or overlap in some individuals, and further diagnostic studies are usually required to establish the diagnosis with more certainty.

Pericardial knock. A pericardial "knock" is a frequent auscultatory finding in constrictive pericarditis. This high frequency, early diastolic sound usually occurs after the opening snap of mitral stenosis but before the third sound of left ventricular failure. Although the pathogenesis of this sound is still debated, the sound has been shown to occur at the abrupt cessation of rapid ventricular filling (24). Patients with restrictive cardiomyopathy commonly have a third heart sound which is of lower frequency and occurs at the time of peak mitral flow velocity (10). In our experience some patients with advanced restrictive cardiomyopathy have a very abrupt cessation of ventricular filling that is associated with a sound which is earlier, and of higher frequency than the typical third heart sound. This sound may mistakenly interpreted as a pericardial knock.

Pulsus paradoxus. The finding of pulsus paradoxus (> 10 mmHg inspiratory decrease in systolic blood pressure) strongly favors a diagnosis of constrictive pericarditis if other obvious causes of pulsus paradoxus (like obstructive pulmonary disease) can be excluded. This finding is a manifestation of the reciprocal ventricular filling that occurs with respiration in constrictive pericarditis but its reported incidence in clinical series has varied widely from approximately 10 to 60% (18, 24, 25). Pulsus paradoxus appears to be more prominent in subacute cases of constrictive pericarditis than in chronic cases. This may be related to the depth of respiration at the time of study, which is often greater in patients presenting subacutely, or to a greater sensitivity of Doppler techniques to detect the reciprocal filling dynamics. In these cases an increased respiratory effort may make a borderline abnormality more apparent (25). Although pulsus paradoxus has also been reported to occur in restrictive cardiomyopathy (5), we have not observed this finding in these patients unless coexistent disease were also present.

Jugular venous pulse. As described in the section on atrial filling dynamics, interpretation of the jugular venous pulse contour is facilitated by relating the observed findings to the clinical history, pathophysiology and natural history of each disorder. However, although certain patterns are more common in each of the disorders, the overlap is large enough to limit their diagnostic specificity without the results of other diagnostic studies (26). An inspiratory increase in the amplitude of A and V waves, the so called Kussmaul's sign, is seen in both conditions and does not aid the differentiation unless these reversals can be precisely timed to the respiratory cycle. The variety of patterns seen, and the difference in their response to inspiration, will be discussed in more detail in the section on venous Doppler echocardiography.

Echocardiography

M mode echocardiography

M mode echocardiographic patterns suggestive of pericardial thickening have been previously described (27). However, most investigators currently believe that echocardiographic techniques lack sufficient sensitivity and specificity to definitively make or exclude the diagnosis of pericardial thickening, and computerized tomography scanning has now become the diagnostic technique of choice for this evaluation in most medical centers (28).

A more important M mode finding in patients with constrictive pericarditis is evidence for the respiration related reciprocal right ventricle and left ventricle filling (2). This finding demonstrates the mechanical interaction between cardiac chambers in a fixed cardiac space and will only be seen if M mode recordings are made throughout the respiratory cycle. This finding is illustrated by a patient with effusive-constrictive pericarditis in Fig. 4.7, where an increase in right ventricular diameter during inspiration can be seen to be accompanied by a simultaneous decrease in the diameter of the left ventricle. In these cases the right ventricle and posterior left ventricle wall do not appear to move significantly in an anterior or posterior direction with respiration while the intraventricular septum shifts back and forth throughout the respiratory cycle. In patients with restrictive cardiomyopathy, and in normal subjects, an inspiratory increase in right heart volume does not impede filling of the left ventricle and the posterior left ventricular wall moves posteriorly with only a small change in left ventricle diameter.

Other M mode findings, such as abnormal intraventricular septal motion (29–33), digitized rates of early diastolic left ventricular diameter changes (15) and flat posterior wall motion (32–34) have been suggested as indicators of constrictive pericarditis. However, we believe these patterns do not have sufficient specificity to reliably differentiate the two diseases under all conditions. Ventricular septal motion reflects instantaneous differences in pressure

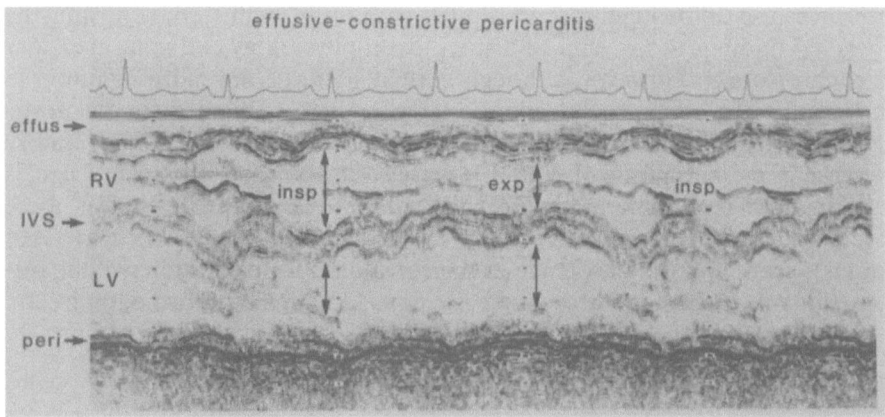

Fig. 4.7. Parasternal M mode recording of left and right ventricles demonstrating reciprocal ventricular filling in a patient with effusive-constrictive pericarditis who has a fixed cardiac volume. Note how the intraventricular septum (IVS) shifts back and forth with respiration while the RV free wall and posterior LV wall do not significantly move. This results in reciprocal changes in ventricular diameter with the right ventricle increasing in size during inspiration while LV diameter deceases (arrows). Opposite changes are seen during expiration. (effus = effusion, peri = pericardium).

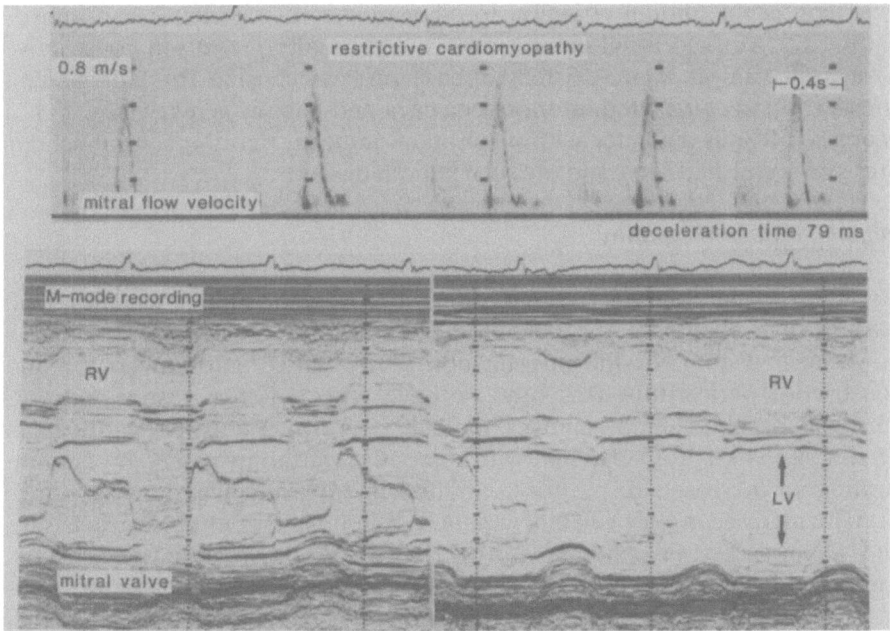

Fig. 4.8. Mitral flow velocity and parasternal M mode recordings of mitral valve and left ventricle in a patient with restrictive cardiomyopathy who is in atrial fibrillation. Note the extremely short mitral deceleration time indicating an abrupt cessation of LV filling in early diastole. M mode of left ventricle shows flat posterior wall motion (arrows) confirming that there is no significant flow occuring in mid- and late diastole. Despite the lack of late diastolic flow the mitral valve leaflets remain widely separated. (Reproduced, with permission, from: Appleton CP, Hatle LK, Popp RL. Demonstration of restrictive ventricular physiology by Doppler echocardiography. J Am Coll Cardiol 1988; 11: 757–768).

between the right and left ventricle (35) and would be expected to be affected by multiple factors other than those directly related to restrictive cardiomyopathy and constrictive pericardits. And as shown in Fig. 4.8, advanced cases of restrictive cardiomyopathy may have rates of early diastolic ventricular filling and flat posterior wall motion which are similar to those seen in constrictive pericarditis (2).

Two-dimensional (2-D) echocardiography

Two-dimensional echocardiographic findings which are characteristic of infiltrative cardiomyopathies such as amyloid heart disease have been described (12, 13, 22). These findings include small or normal left ventricle cavity size with markedly increased thickness of the ventricular walls, increased thickness of atrial septum, papillary muscles and cardiac valves, abnormal "texture" of the myocardium and marked bi-atrial enlargement. Of these findings, the marked atrial enlargement in the presence of normal size ventricles is the

most consistent finding common to all etiologies of restrictive cardiomyopathy (22). Marked atrial enlargement is not usually present in constrictive
pericarditis unless a pre-existent disease process causing the enlargement
coexists (2, 34). A dilated inferior vena cava and hepatic veins, which do not
decrease 50% in diameter with inspiration, indicate that the central venous
pressure is elevated (36), and are seen in both diseases.

Doppler echocardiography

Doppler echocardiography, with its ability to assess the filling dynamics of all
four cardiac chambers throughout the respiratory cycle, has provided a
powerful new tool for the investigation of restrictive cardiomyopathy and
constrictive pericarditis. Recently, we have reported that despite indistin-
guishable baseline hemodynamics, patients with constrictive pericarditis can
be differentiated from patients with restrictive cardiomyopathy by demonstrating an increased respiratory variation in transvalvular flow velocities
(2). The increase in flow velocity variation disappeared after pericardiectomy,
and was not seen in patients with restrictive cardiomyopathy or in normal
subjects. Furthermore, the Doppler findings were seen in constrictive pericarditis patients regardless of the presence of pulsus paradoxus, suggesting
that they are a more sensitive indicator of the presence of reciprocal ventricular filling than the traditional peripheral signs.

In Table 4.1 mean values for mitral and tricuspid flow velocity and related
variables during apnea, inspiration and expiration are given for 20 normal
subjects, 12 patients with restrictive cardiomyopathy and seven patients with
constrictive pericarditis. Changes in these variables with respiration, expressed as percent change from apnea, are shown for the groups in Fig. 4.9,
and for individual patients in Fig. 4.10. In patients with restrictive cardiomyopathy and in normal subjects, respiratory variation in left ventricle isovolumic relaxation time and peak early mitral flow velocity is minimal (mean
< 5%), with no individual showing greater than a 15% difference between
inspiratory and expiratory values. In contrast, patients with constrictive pericarditis show a marked respiratory variation in these variables (mean > 30%),
with all individuals showing a greater than 25% difference between inspiratory and expiratory values. Peak tricuspid flow velocity increased with inspiration in all three study groups. However, only patients with constrictive
pericarditis showed a marked decrease in tricuspid flow velocity on expiration.

Mitral flow velocity from a patient with constrictive pericarditis is shown in
Fig. 4.4 and illustrates the characteristic Doppler findings. On the first beat
after the onset of inspiration there is a decrease in early mitral flow velocity
and a lengthening of the left ventricle isovolumic relaxation time. Opposite
changes, with a marked increase in early mitral flow velocity and shortening
of the isovolumic relaxation time, are seen on the first beat of expiration.
Second and third inspiratory and expiratory beats (when present) show inter-

Table 4.1. Left ventricular isovolumic relaxation time, peak velocities of early mitral and tricuspid flow, and mitral and tricuspid deceleration times during apnea, expiration, and inspiration.

		Heart rate	IVRT (msec)	M_1 (cm/sec)	M_2 (cm/sec)	M_{dt} (msec)	T_1 (cm/sec)	T_2 (cm/sec)	T_{dt} (msec)
Normal ($n = 20$)	a	66 ± 11	69 ± 12	84 ± 18	61 ± 14	188 ± 28	56 ± 11	40 ± 5	218 ± 31
	e		72 ± 14	85 ± 18	59 ± 17	189 ± 26	56 ± 9	39 ± 6	219 ± 29
	i		74 ± 15	82 ± 17	58 ± 16	189 ± 27	64 ± 10	44 ± 6	220 ± 26
Restrictive cardiomyopathy ($n = 12$)	a	$90 \pm 18^*$	61 ± 13	89 ± 20	$32 \pm 12^*$	$123 \pm 32^*$	66 ± 16	$28 \pm 2^*$	$148 \pm 23^*$
	e		62 ± 13	89 ± 22	44 ± 18	$123 \pm 34^*$	65 ± 18	32 ± 9	$134 \pm 29^*$
	i		65 ± 12	86 ± 20	43 ± 19	112 ± 37	74 ± 14	33 ± 16	114 ± 30
Constrictive pericarditis ($n = 7$)	a	$94 \pm 7^*$	67 ± 14	79 ± 19	56 ± 34	156 ± 48	58 ± 17	27 ± 16	160 ± 44
	e		$56 \pm 14^*$	91 ± 19	60 ± 34	153 ± 43	50 ± 9	24 ± 17	$160 \pm 38^*$
	i		$84 \pm 19^*$	$60 \pm 10†$	55 ± 34	146 ± 34	74 ± 21	38 ± 14	$150 \pm 45^*$

IVRT, isovolumic relaxation time; M_1, T_1, mitral and tricuspid flow velocities in early diastole; M_2, T_2, mitral and tricuspid flow velocities at atrial contraction; M_{dt}, T_{dt}, mitral and tricuspid deceleration times; n, total number; a, apnea; e, expiration; i, inspiration. Values are mean ± SD.

* $p < 0.05$ versus normal.
† $p < 0.05$ versus restrictive cardiomyopathy.
‡ $p < 0.05$ versus restrictive cardiomyopathy and normal.

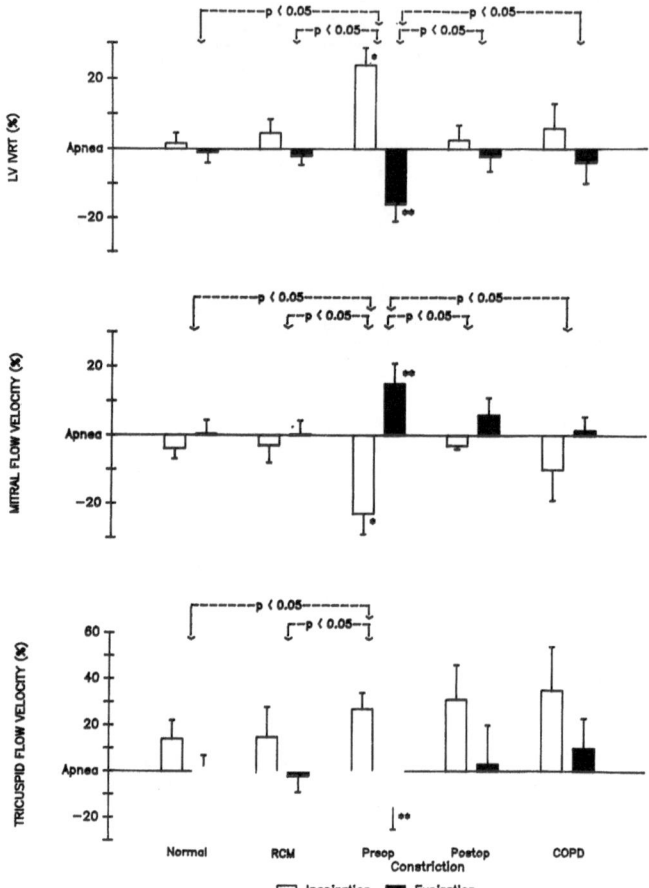

Fig. 4.9. Bar graphs illustrating the amplitude and direction of the mean percentage change from apnea in inspiratory and expiratory values for peak early mitral and tricuspid flow velocities and in LV isovolumic relaxation time (LV IVRT) in normal subjects (normal), patients with restrictive cardiomyopathy (RCM), patients with constrictive pericarditis (constriction) before (preop) and after pericardiectomy (postop) as well as in patients with chronic obstructive pulmonary disease (COPD) are shown. Bars represent mean ± SD; * = p <0.05 for inspiratory change only, constriction (preop) vs all other groups; ** p = <0.05 expiratory change only, constriction (preop) vs all other groups; dashed lines difference in total change from expiration to inspiration. (From: Hatle LK, Appleton CP, Popp RL. Differentiation of constrictive pericarditis and restrictive cardiomyopathy by Doppler echocardiography. Circulation 1989; 79: 350–370. Reproduced by permission of the American Heart Association, Inc.).

mediate values for these variables. Tricuspid flow velocity shows reciprocal changes, with the largest increase in velocity on the first beat of inspiration, and the largest decrease in velocity on the first beat after the onset of expiration. After pericardiectomy, the respiratory variation in mitral flow velocity is markedly decreased (Fig. 4.4). Patients with restrictive cardiomyopathy also have minimal, if any, change in mitral flow velocity with respiration, and

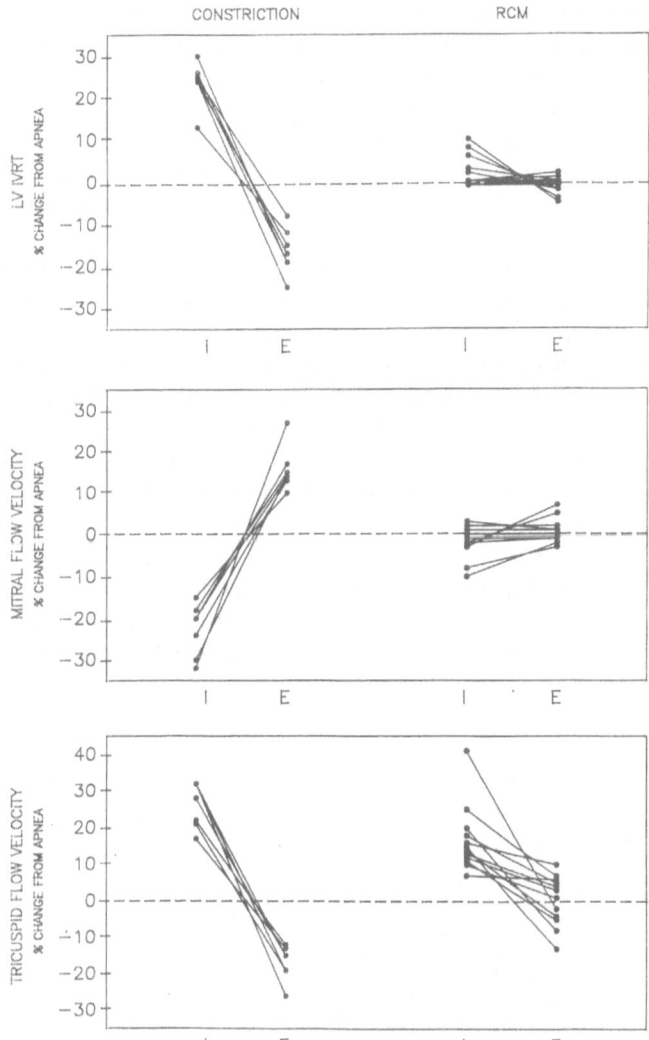

Fig. 4.10. Individual values are plotted for the respiratory variation (expressed as a percent change from apnea) in left ventricular isovolumic relaxation time (LV IVRT), peak early mitral flow velocity and peak early tricuspid flow velocity in all the patients with constrictive pericarditis (constriction, n = 7) and restrictive cardiomyopathy (RCM, n = 12). I = inspiration, E = expiration. (From: Hatle LK, Appleton CP, Popp RL. Differentiation of constrictive pericarditis and restrictive cardiomyopathy by Doppler echocardiography. Circulation 1989; 79: 350–370. Reproduced by permission of the American Heart Association, Inc.).

tricuspid velocity does not decrease to values below apnea at the onset of expiration (Fig. 4.2).

Increased respiratory variation in aortic and pulmonic flow velocities and ejection times, which parallel the changes in ventricular filling, are also seen in patients with constrictive pericarditis, but the differences from patients with restrictive cardiomyopathy and normal subjects were less marked than those seen across the mitral and tricuspid valves (2).

The hemodynamic events that correlate with the observed Doppler findings in constrictive pericarditis are shown in Fig. 4.3. Most strikingly, right and left ventricular systolic pressure change in opposite directions with respiration. An *increase* in right ventricular systolic pressure with inspiration is not normally seen in normal subjects and it indicates that a marked increase in stroke volume is occurring at this time. This increase in stroke volume is also seen as an increase in the width of the right ventricular pressure tracing, indicating that the ventricular ejection time also lengthens. In the same figure, simultaneous recording of pulmonary capillary wedge and left ventricular pressure shows that the respiratory variation in pulmonary capillary wedge pressure is larger than diastolic left ventricular pressure resulting in a decrease in the early diastolic pulmonary capillary wedge-left ventricular pressure difference at the onset of inspiration and an increased difference at the onset of expiration. These changes in pressure gradient parallel the changes in early mitral flow velocity that were described above. As shown in Fig. 4.1, patients with restrictive cardiomyopathy have respiratory changes in peak systolic pressures that parallel one another, and the pulmonary capillary wedge-left ventricular diastolic gradient remains nearly constant throughout

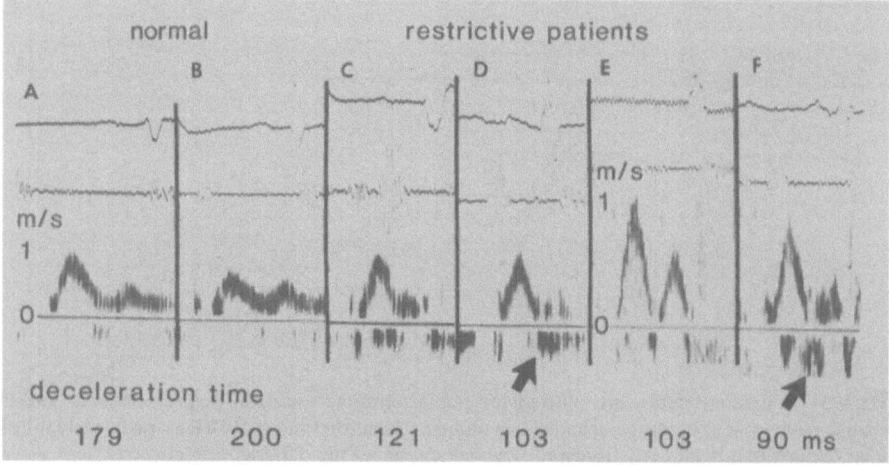

Fig. 4.11. Mitral flow velocity recordings from two normal subjects (panels A and B) and four patients with restrictive cardiomyopathy (panels C to F). Note the shortened deceleration time in the patients with restrictive cardiomyopathy indicating a more rapid than normal cessation of ventricular filling. In panel C, low velocity, and in panel D, reversal of flow (diastolic regurgitation, arrow) are seen with atrial contraction. In panels E and F, velocity with atrial contraction is normal, but in panel F there is mid-diastolic reversal of flow (arrow) representing diastolic mitral regurgitation. Patients with the worst atrial function have the lowest flow velocities at atrial contraction. (Reproduced, with permission, from: Appleton CP, Hatle LK, Popp RL. Demonstration of restrictive ventricular physiology by Doppler echocardiography. J Am Coll Cardiol 1988; 11: 757–768).

the respiratory cycle so that little variation in mitral flow velocity would be expected.

Although patients with restrictive cardiomyopathy have minimal variation in mitral flow velocity with respiration, characteristic Doppler findings are also seen in patients with advanced disease. These findings include an increase in the proportion of flow velocity in early diastole to that at atrial contraction, markedly shortened mitral and tricuspid deceleration times, further shortening of the tricuspid deceleration time with inspiration and diastolic mitral and tricuspid regurgitation (7). Figure 4.11 shows mitral flow velocity in four patients with restrictive cardiomyopathy which illustrate some of these Doppler findings. The variation in individual patients probably reflects slightly different stages of the disease process. In Fig. 4.12, a patient with Fabry's disease demonstrates an inspiratory shortening of the tricuspid deceleration time, which is shown to correlate with an abrupt increase in the rate of rise of diastolic right ventricular pressure. In Fig. 4.13, diastolic left

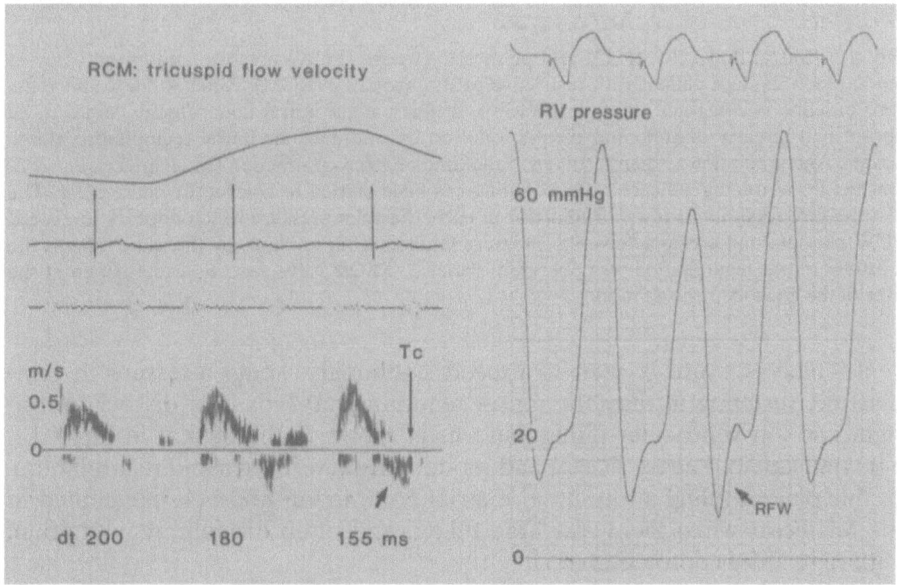

Fig. 4.12. Recordings of tricuspid flow velocity (left panel) and right ventricular (RV) pressure recording (right panel) in a patient with restrictive cardiomyopathy (RCM). Upward deflection on respiratory tracing (upper line in left panel) indicates inspiration (insp) and downward deflection expiration. With inspiration, peak tricuspid flow velocity increases, but there is abnormal shortening of the tricuspid deceleration time (dt), with reversal of flow in late diastole (arrow). RV systolic and diastolic pressure decrease normally with inspiration but show a corresponding more abrupt and larger increase in the rapid filling wave (RFW). These findings indicate that the RV is non-compliant so that an inspiratory increase in right heart filling results in an abnormal rise in RV pressure and consequently and abrupt cessation of ventricular filling. (Reproduced, with permission, from: Appleton CP, Hatle LK, Popp RL. Demonstration of restrictive ventricular physiology by Doppler echocardiography. J Am Coll Cardiol 1988; 11: 757–768).

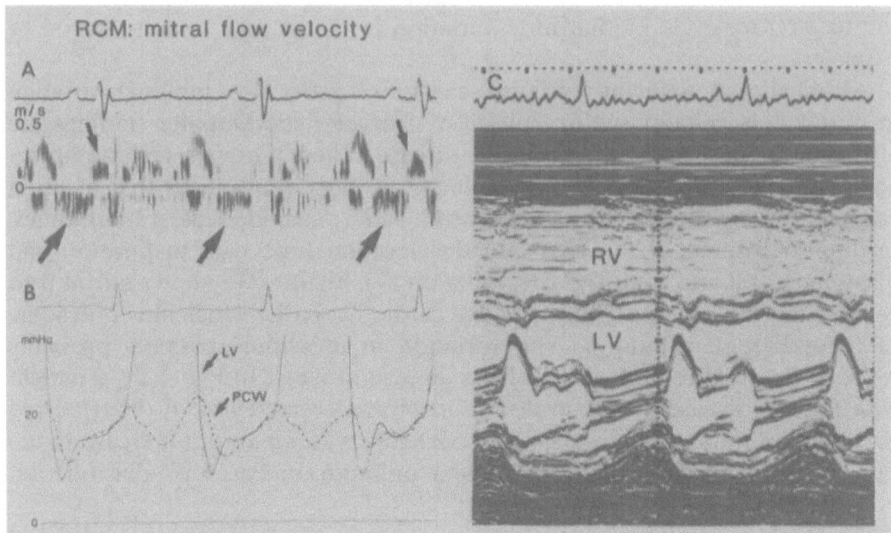

Fig. 4.13. Mitral flow velocity, LV and pulmonary wedge (PCW) pressure and mitral valve M mode recording in a patient with restrictive cardiomyopathy (RCM). Panel A: Flow above the zero baseline is antegrade through the valve. In this patient mitral flow velocity comes to an abrupt halt in early diastole and then is followed by mid-diastolic mitral regurgitation (large arrow). Antegrade flow is then resumed at the time of atrial contraction (small arrow). Panel B: Dashed PCW tracing indicates this recording has been shifted to correct for phase delay. The LV pressure recording shows a rapid rise in early diastolic pressure which appears to exceed PCW pressure and create a "reverse" pressure gradient at approximately the same time as the diastolic mitral regurgitation was observed. Panel C: Mitral valve remains widely open at the time of the diastolic regurgitation.

ventricular pressure is seen to exceed pulmonary wedge pressure in mid-diastole, resulting in diastolic mitral regurgitation. Finally, a dissociation in right and left ventricular filling patterns is shown in the patient in Fig. 4.14, who had amyloid heart disease and moderately severe tricuspid regurgitation. In this patient filling at the time of atrial contraction was well maintained in the left heart while there was little filling, and often diastolic regurgitation, with right atrial contraction.

A dissociation of right and left ventricular filling patterns can occur in restrictive cardiomyopathy because the limitation to filling is primarily into each ventricle, and there is relatively little ventricular interaction through the non-compliant septum (Fig. 4.15). Therefore, increases in ventricular filling may result in large rises in ventricular pressure which overshoot left atrial pressure and result in diastolic regurgitation. In contrast, in constrictive pericarditis the limitation to filling is imposed by the pericardium with all the chambers having similar pressure volume relationships. Therefore, an increase in filling on one side of the heart results in a more equal rise in ventricular and atrial pressure, and the compliant interventricular septum shifts and limits the simultaneous filling on the other side (Fig. 4.15).

Patients with constrictive pericarditis also have shortened mitral and tricuspid deceleration times which indicate the abrupt cessation of ventricular filling. In addition, a decrease in velocity at atrial contraction may occasionally be seen. Therefore, it should be emphasized that it is the increased respiratory variation in transvalvular flow velocities that is the most specific Doppler finding which differentiates restrictive cardiomyopathy from constrictive pericarditis.

Presystolic pulmonary valve opening has been described in patients with constrictive pericarditis (37). However, we have also observed this finding in patients with restrictive cardiomyopathy (2).

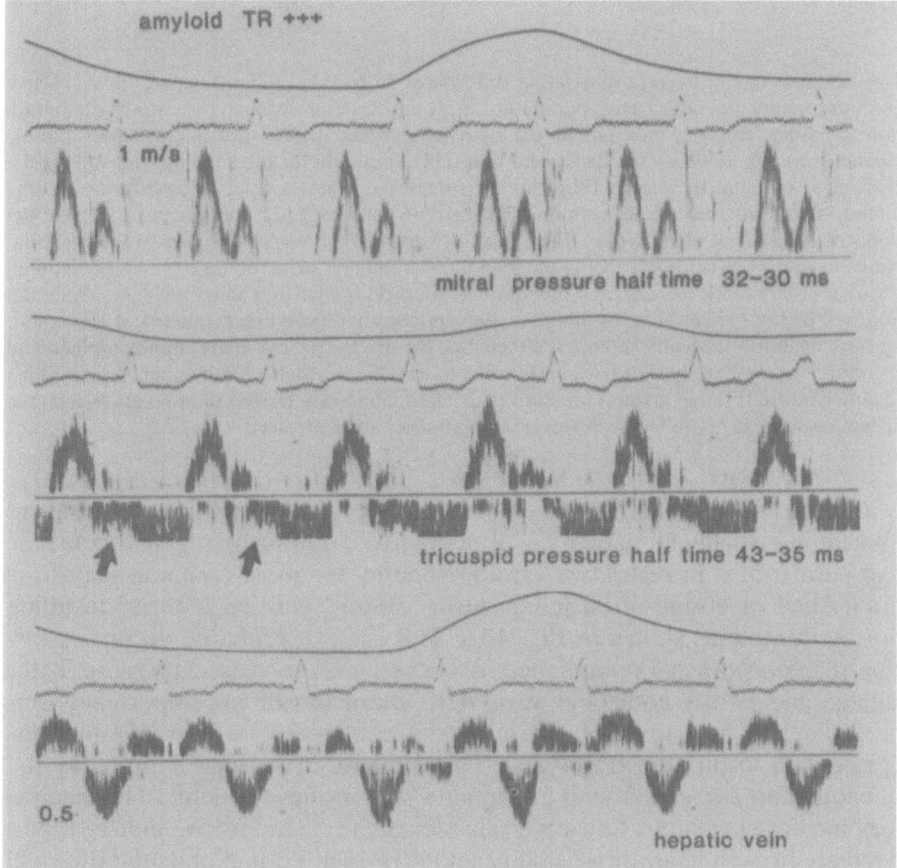

Fig. 4.14. Mitral, tricuspid and hepatic vein flow velocity recordings in a patient with amyloid heart disease and severe tricuspid regurgitation (TR). Mitral pressure half time is short (nl = 60 ms) indicating a more rapid than normal cessation of early diastolic LV filling. However, the normal velocity at atrial contraction indicates that left atrial systolic function is still present. Tricuspid pressure half time is also short (nl = 65 ms), but in this case atrial contraction is associated with diastolic tricuspid regurgitation (arrows). Hepatic vein recording shows only diastolic forward flow, with reversals both at the time of atrial contraction and during ventricular systole.

Constrictive Pericarditis   Restrictive Cardiomyopathy

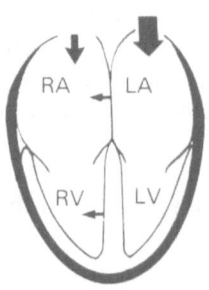 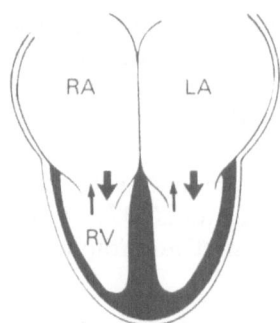

Fig. 4.15. Schematic diagram illustrating differences in cardiac filling dynamics in restrictive cardiomyopathy and constrictive pericarditis. Left panel: In constrictive pericarditis the limitation to cardiac filling is imposed by the rigid pericardium which surrounds all four cardiac chambers as illustrated by the dark solid line. This limitation includes the atria as well as the ventricles, so that an increase in filling on one side of the heart (large black arrow) will shift the interatrial and interventricular septum (small arrows) and impede simultaneous filling on the opposite side (small black arrow). Flow from the atria to the ventricles is less affected. Right panel: In restrictive cardiomyopathy the limitation to filling is primarily into the non-compliant ventricles (dark black shading) and the four chambers do not have a common volume limitation imposed by the pericardium. In this case the ventricles act more independently of each other because the intraventricular septum is affected by the disease process and is non-compliant and therefore does not easily shift back and forth between the ventricles. With an increase in filling in either ventricle (large arrows) pressure rises rapidly and may exceed the pressure rise in the atrium resulting in diastolic flow reversal (regurgitation, small arrows).

Central venous flow velocities. Abnormal venous flow velocity patterns are present in virtually all patients with restrictive cardiomyopathy and constrictive pericarditis. In restrictive cardiomyopathy the most common pattern is diminished or absent atrial filling during systole, with an increase in filling during diastole as shown in Fig. 4.16. This pattern probably occurs in part due to reduced atrial compliance associated with increased pressure in the dilated and poorly contactile atria. Also characteristic are abnormally long or prolonged flow reversals during atrial contraction or systole which increase with inspiration (Fig. 4.17). This increase in reversal is probably the phenomenon associated with Kussmaul's sign in these patients. The inspiratory increase in venous flow reversals appears to be a sensitive indicator of a decrease in right heart distensibility, and is present even in patients with only mild abnormalities in tricuspid deceleration times and hemodynamics (7). In patients with far advanced disease, diastolic flow reversals may preceded atrial contraction indicating that even "passive" right ventricular filling can be associated with reversal of venous flow.

Patients with constrictive pericarditis commonly have venous flow velocity patterns which show both systolic and diastolic filling of the atrium (38, 39). In these patients the increase in flow velocity with inspiration is minimal, and,

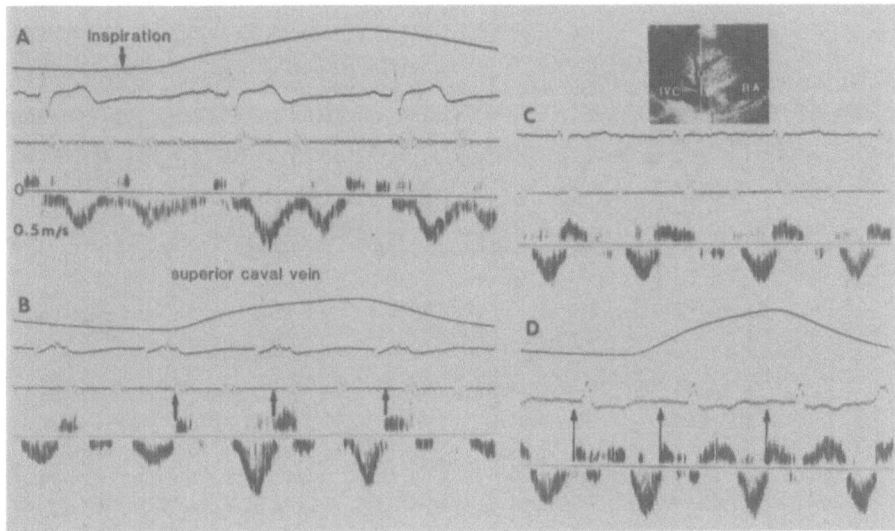

Fig. 4.16. Superior vena cava (SVC, left panels) and hepatic vein (right panels) flow velocity recordings from a normal (nl) subject and three patients with restrictive cardiomyopathy. Panel A: The normal subject demonstrates typical bimodal flow, with systolic flow velocity larger than diastolic velocity, and minimal reversal of flow which does not increase with inspiration. Panel B: An SVC recording from a patient with restrictive cardiomyopathy who has an atrial paced rhythm shows a predominance of diastolic forward flow followed by presystolic flow reversals that occur earlier with inspiration. Panel C: Hepatic vein recording in a restrictive cardiomyopathy patient in atrial fibrillation. Only diastolic forward flow is present which is then followed by pre-systolic flow reversals which extend into systole. Panel D: Hepatic vein recording from a restrictive cardiomyopathy patient in sinus rhythm with moderately severe tricuspid regurgitation. There is forward flow only during diastole, followed by pre-systolic flow reversals that increase and occur earlier in diastole with inspiration (arrows). (Reproduced, with permission, from: Appleton CP, Hatle LK, Popp RL. Demonstration of restrictive ventricular physiology by Doppler echocardiography. J Am Coll Cardiol 1988; 757–768).

in contrast to patients with restrictive cardiomyopathy, there is no increase in reversal during inspiration. Instead, there is a loss of diastolic filling, or a reversal of flow, on the first beat of expiration as shown in Fig. 4.18. The loss of diastolic filling in early expiration is a passive event, which is the result of the marked decrease in tricuspid flow observed at the same time described previously. As shown in Fig. 4.19, this finding disappears after pericardiectomy when tricuspid flow is no longer impeded in early expiration. The reversal of flow in some patients at the onset of expiration has probably also been interpreted as Kussmaul's sign, albeit by a different mechanism than that seen in restrictive cardiomyopathy. Variation in the amount of systolic and diastolic atrial filling is common among patients with constrictive pericarditis and appears to be due in part to differences in atrial function.

Other disease with transvalvular flow velocity variation. Increased respiratory variation in both mitral flow velocity and left ventricular dimension is

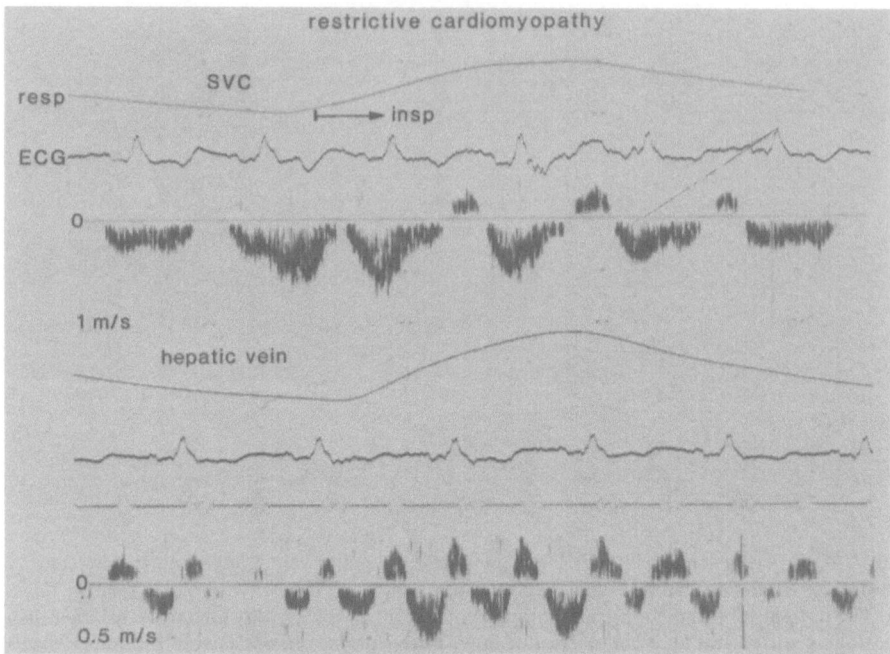

Fig. 4.17. Superior vena cava (SVC) and hepatic vein flow velocity from a patient with restrictive cardiomyopathy. Flow below the zero reference line is toward the heart and flow above is reversal of flow. Upward deflection on respiratory tracing indicates inspiration (insp) and downward deflection expiration. Upper panel: Before inspiration flow is seen to be bi-phasic with systolic and diastolic flow velocities that are approximately equal and there is no reverse flow present. With inspiration forward flow increases but flow reversals are seen at end inspiration and the beginning of expiration. Bottom panel: Hepatic vein recording shows similar findings with an inspiratory increase in flow reversals. These findings indicate that right heart filling increases normally with inspiration but the additional volume cannot be completely accomodated by the non-compliant right ventricle. The increase in reversal of flow in the SVC represents Kussmaul's phenomenon. An increase in reversal of flow in the hepatic vein compared to the SVC is typical of central venous recordings (19).

commonly present in patients with chronic obstructive pulmonary disease (2, 40). However, as shown in Fig. 4.20, the timing of the flow velocity variation in relation to the respiratory cycle is distinctly different in these patients, with the lowest mitral flow velocity often being seen on the second or third beats of inspiration and the highest mitral flow velocity often seen late in expiration. Early tricuspid flow velocity usually continues to increase throughout inspiration and does not decrease on the first beat of expiration to values below those seen at apnea. This marked inspiratory increase in venous return, which indicates that there is no limitation to cardiac filling, is especially apparent in central venous recordings as shown in Fig. 4.21, and appears to be the result of the exaggerated decrease in intrathoracic pressure seen in these patients. Increased respiratory changes in transvalvular flow velocities can also be seen

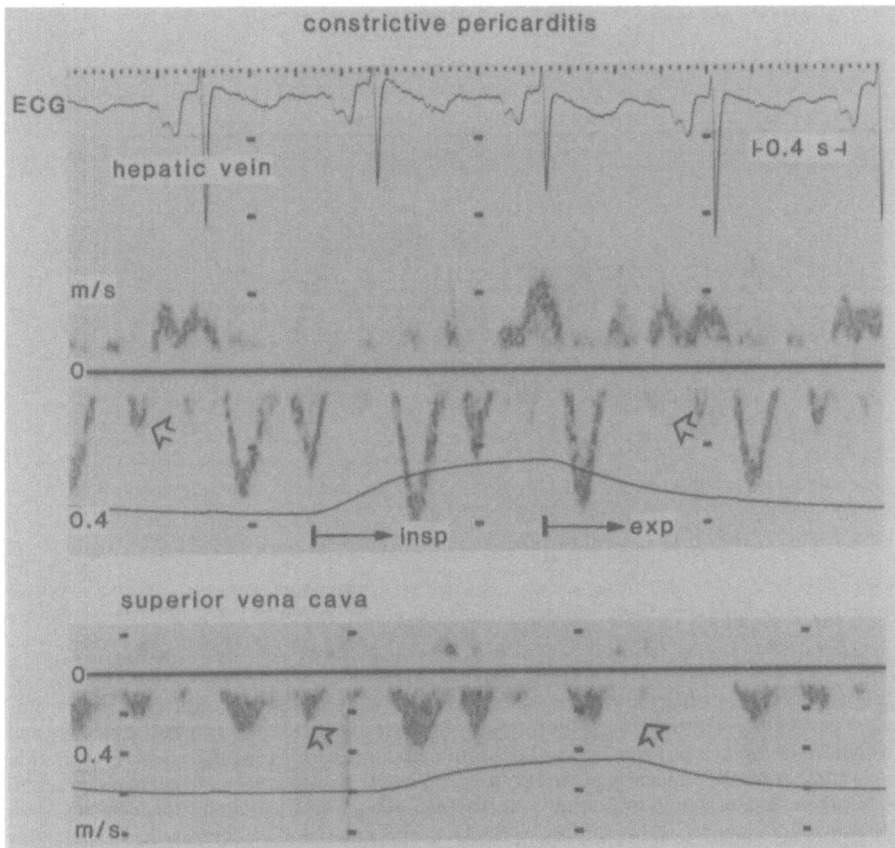

Fig. 4.18. Tracings of superior vena cava (SVC) and hepatic vein flow velocity in a patient with constrictive pericarditis who had well maintained atrial systolic function. Flow below the zero reference line is toward the heart and flow above is reversal of flow. Upward deflection on respiratory tracing indicates inspiration (insp) and downward deflection expiration (exp). In the upper panel the hepatic vein recording shows that systolic velocity is larger than the diastolic velocity. Open arrows show that at the onset of expiration diastolic filling does not occur and in fact there is a reversal of flow. SVC recording shows same findings for forward flow but reversals of flow are typically less prominent. These findings would correlate with a large X descent and less prominent Y descent in the jugular venous pulse. Reversal of flow at the onset of expiration probably represents Kussmaul's sign.

in patients with marked obesity, acute pulmonary emboli or after surgery if the depth of respiration is increased. In these cases the increased depth of respiration may be associated with small changes in the pressure gradient from the pulmonary veins to the right heart and the Doppler findings are similar to those seen in chronic obstructive pulmonary disease.

Limitations. The precise timing of respiratory changes in Doppler flow velocity requires the use of a respiratory thermistor or similar device that has a known relationship to changes in intrathoracic pressure. If not available with

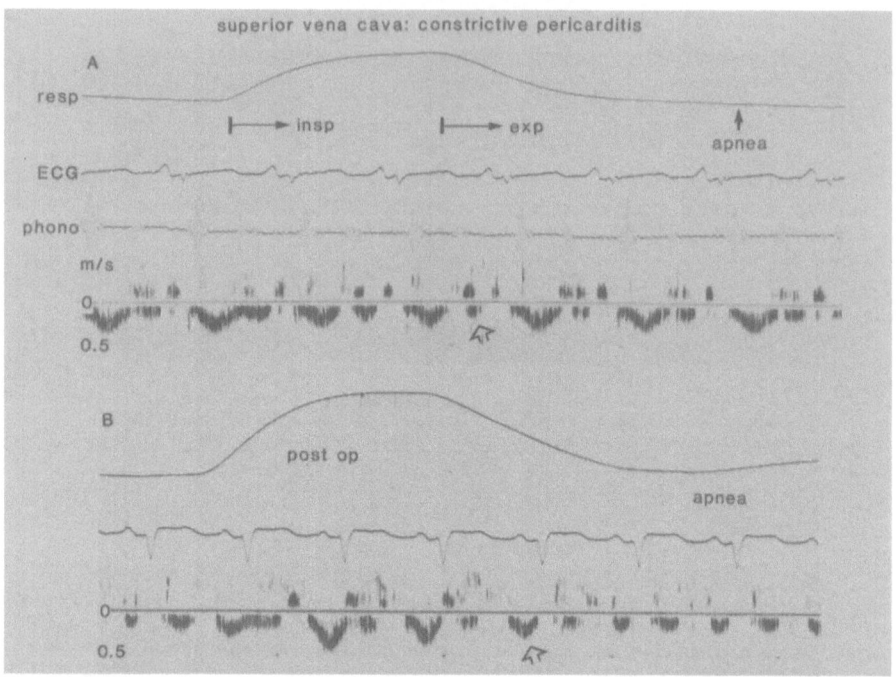

Fig. 4.19. Tracing of superior vena cava flow velocity in a patient with constrictive pericarditis before and after pericardiectomy. Flow below the zero reference line is toward the heart and flow above is reversal of flow. Upward deflection on respiratory tracing indicates inspiration (insp) and downward deflection expiration (exp). Panel A: Before surgery atrial filling is seen to be bi-phasic, again with systolic flow velocity being larger than diastolic flow velocity. With inspiration little increase in forward flow velocity occurs and there is a decrease in diastolic flow velocity at the onset of expiration (open arrow). These findings correlate with a large X descent in the jugular venous pulse and a phasic right atrial pressure that does not decrease normally during inspiration. Panel B: After pericardiectomy diastolic and systolic filling are approximately equal and an inspiratory increase in flow velocity compared to pre-surgical recording is evident. In addition there is no decrease in diastolic filling at the onset of expiration (open arrow). This loss of systolic velocity is common after cardiac surgery and may relate to subclinical injury of the right atrium during the procedure.

the commercial ultrasound and catheterization equipment being used, these devices can be easily made by biomedical engineers.

The presence of atrial fibrillation or other arrhythmias makes interpretation of respiratory changes in transvalvular flow velocity more difficult because peak early flow velocity may vary in these conditions even during suspended respiration. This is a significant problem in both patients with constrictive pericarditis and restrictive cardiomyopathy because most studies report a 20 to 40% incidence of these arrhythmias (5, 18). However, in these cases the respiratory changes in venous Doppler described previously are unaltered and remain helpful in differentiating the two conditions. In patients with rapid heart rates or first degree atrio-ventricular block, an analysis of the

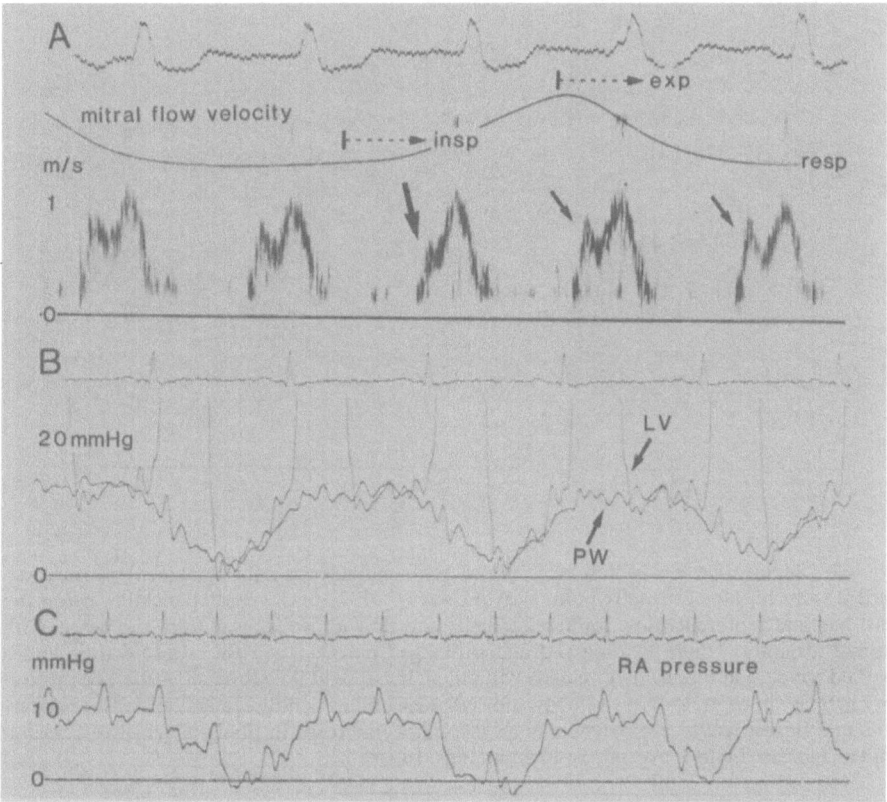

Fig. 4.20. Mitral flow velocity, LV, pulmonary wedge (PW) and right atrial (RA) pressure in a patient with chronic obstructive pulmonary disease. Panel A: Early mitral flow velocity is seen to decrease with inspiration (large arrow) but there is no significant increase in filling on the first beat of expiration as is characteristic of constrictive pericarditis. Panel B: Respiratory variation in intrathoracic and LV pressure is seen to be approximately equal throughout the respiratory cycle with no evidence for "blunting" of LV diastolic pressure changes. Panel C: Large swings in RA pressure with respiration are seen and characteristic of obstructive pulmonary disease.

mitral flow velocity pattern may not be possible if atrial contraction occurs in close proximity to mitral valve opening so that a passive filling phase is not distinctly present. In these cases mild sedation may result in a decrease in heart rate so that the adequate quality recordings can be obtained.

Cardiac catheterization

The recording of intracardiac hemodynamics can help differentiate constrictive pericarditis from restrictive cardiomyopathy provided that the pressure measurements are performed carefully and with high quality recordings.

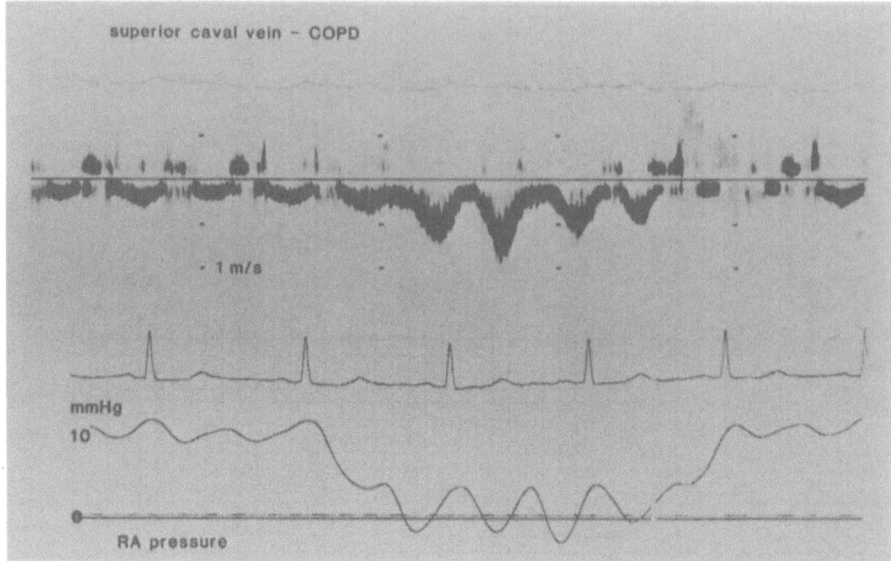

Fig. 4.21. Superior vena cava flow velocity and non-simultaneous right atrial (RA) pressure in a patient with chronic obstructive pulmonary disease (COPD). In the upper panel flow below the zero baseline represents flow toward the heart and flow above is away from the heart. With normal inspiration there is a marked and prolonged decrease in right atrial pressure and a marked increase in venous flow velocity without an increase in flow reversal. A marked inspiratory increase in central venous velocity and right heart filling is not seen in constrictive pericarditis and in restrictive cardiomyopathy an inspiratory increase in filling is usually associated with an increase in flow reversal. Compare to Figs. 16–19.

Ideally, right and left heart pressures should be measured with high fidelity micromanometer tipped catheters to eliminate artifact induced by a fluid filled system (9). However, if these are not available technically adequate pressure recordings can be obtained by using stiff walled, large bore (7–8 Fr) catheters that are attached to manifold micromanometer transducers. In this system the only column of fluid is in the catheter itself. The transducers should be cross-calibrated and carefully leveled and the recorder should have a frequency response that is flat to at least 20 cycles/second. The commonly used flow directed pulmonary artery catheters have soft walls and small lumens and are not adequate for these measurements.

Right atrial, right ventricular, pulmonary artery, pulmonary wedge, left ventricular and aortic pressures should be obtained and labeled during normal breathing, for 10 seconds during apnea and for the first few respiratory cycles immediately after apnea. Simultaneous right atrial-left ventricular, right ventricular-left ventricular and pulmonary capillary wedge-left ventricular pressures should be obtained in a similar fashion. The right ventricular-left ventricular recording should include an expanded scale to examine diastolic pressure relationships and a smaller scale to compare the relationship of peak systolic pressures.

Hemodynamic findings which suggest constrictive pericarditis are: 1) equalization of intracardiac end diastolic pressures; 2) evidence for incomplete transmission of intrathoracic pressure changes to the intracardiac chambers, and 3) evidence for reciprocal ventricular filling. Evidence that intrathoracic pressure changes are abnormally blunted is present when there is little phasic change in right atrial pressure, and respiratory variation of diastolic left ventricular and right ventricular pressure is less than pulmonary capillary wedge pressure. As shown in Fig. 4.3, evidence for reciprocal changes in ventricular filling includes pulsus paradoxus in the aortic recording, peak systolic right ventricular-left ventricular pressures which change in the opposite direction with respiration and respiratory variation in the pulmonary capillary wedge-left ventricular early diastolic pressure gradient which disappears during apnea.

In patients with restrictive cardiomyopathy variation in cardiac diastolic pressures is approximately equal to that seen in pulmonary capillary wedge pressure (Fig. 4.1) so that the pulmonary capilar wedge-left ventricular early diastolic pressure gradient remains approximately the same throughout the respiratory cycle. In addition, right ventricular and left ventricular peak systolic pressures change in the same direction throughout the respiratory cycle. Intracardiac end diastolic pressures may be equalized in some patients but more often they are dissociated by at least 5 mmHg. Marked elevation in pulmonary artery systolic pressure (> 50 mmHg) is sometimes seen in restrictive cardiomyopathy but is not present in constrictive pericarditis unless coexistent pathology is present (5).

Endomyocardial biopsy

Endomyocardial biopsy may be helpful in establishing the diagnosis in patients with infiltrative cardiomyopathies (41). Other findings which may be clinical important include unsuspected myocarditis, severe interstitial fibrosis or smoldering rejection in cardiac transplant recipients. However, in our experience right ventricular endomyocardial biopsies may be negative in patients with restrictive cardiomyopathy, despite obtaining an adequate amount of tissue for analysis (7). This is presumably due to sampling error in a process which does not uniformly affect all parts of the myocardium. Therefore, a positive biopsy appears to be of greater diagnostic value than a negative biopsy in differentiating restrictive cardiomyopathy from constrictive pericarditis.

Radionuclide ventriculography

It has recently been suggested (16, 42) that radionuclide ventriculography may provide useful data for the differentiation between restrictive cardiomyopathy and constrictive pericarditis. The pattern of ventricular filling has been reported as different in both conditions, with higher filling fractions in earlier parts of diastole and shorter times to peak filling rate in constrictive pericarditis than in restrictive cardiomyopathy among other findings. Although these data are in agreement with previous hemodynamic findings based on angiography (14), their definitive clinical value should be validated with larger series.

Computerized tomography and nuclear magnetic resonance

Cardiac and pericardial imaging with computerized tomography and magnetic resonance imaging is a rapidly evolving field. These techniques, which are able to examine the thorax with a slice thickness of 3 mm, have become the method of choice for determining the presence and extent of pericardial thickening. Other advantages of these techniques compared with echocardiography include a global view of thoracic structures and their relationship to each other, the possibility of three dimensional reconstruction of cardiac chambers and the calculation of accurate cardiac volumes. Magnetic resonance imaging, which does not require ionizing radiation or the infusion of contrast media, is particularly appealing for the study of cardiac and pericardial physiology, although image artifacts are more common than with computerized tomography. It can be expected that these imaging techniques will pay an increasingly important role in the evaluation of suspected pericardial disease in the future. A more complete discussion of these techniques, including their use in pericardial disease, can be found in reference 43.

Unresolved issues and directions for future clinical research

As discussed in this chapter, we currently believe that evidence for reciprocal ventricular filling during the respiratory cycle is the most specific finding which differentiates constrictive pericarditis from restrictive cardiomyopathy. However, it should be emphasized that this assumption is based on findings in a relatively small number of patients with constrictive pericarditis. Therefore, larger studies are now needed to confirm if these altered pressure relationships are present in all cases of constrictive pericarditis and to determine the sensitivity and specificity of the hemodynamic and echocardiographic criteria described in this chapter. The importance of depth of respiration for bringing out these findings also needs further investigation. During these studies special attention should be paid to the relationship of reciprocal ventricular filling with the presence of pulsus paradoxus. This will show whether Doppler techniques are more sensitive in detecting abnormal respiratory variation in cardiac filling volumes than an inspiratory drop in systemic blood pressure.

Further study is also needed to determine whether the echocardiography techniques described are also helpful in identifying constriction limited to a specific chamber of the heart or other forms of less common pericardial disease such as effusive-constrictive pericarditis. Finally, future investigation will still be necessary to establish the exact mechanisms involved in the generation of pulsus paradoxus.

References

1. Seifert FC, Miller DC, Oesterle SN, Oyer PE, Stinson EB, Shumway NE. Surgical treatment of constrictive pericarditis: analysis of outcome and diagnostic error. Circulation 1985; 72 (suppl II): 264–273.
2. Hatle LK, Appleton CP, Popp RL. Differentiation of constrictive pericarditis and restrictive cardiomyopathy by Doppler echocardiography. Circulation 1989; 79: 357–370.
3. Abelmann WH, Lorell BH. The challenge of cardiomyopathy. J Am Coll Cardiol 1989; 13: 1219–1239.
4. Roberts WC, Ferrans VJ. A survey of causes and consequences of pericardial disease. In: Reddy PS, Leon DF, Shavers JA, eds. Pericardial Disease. New York, Raven Press Books Ltd., 1982; 49–76.
5. Fowler NO. Constrictive pericarditis. In The Pericardium in Health and Disease. Mt. Kisco, New York, Futura Publishing Co., 1985; 301–329.
6. Copeland JG, Riley JE, Fuller JK. Pericardiectomy for effusive-constrictive pericarditis after heart transplantation. J Heart Transplant 1986; 5: 171–172.
7. Appleton CP, Hatle LK, Popp RL: Demonstration of restrictive ventricular physiology by Doppler echocardiography. J Am Coll Cardiol 1988; 11: 757–768.
8. Valentine HA, Appleton CP, Hatle LK, Hunt SA, Billingham ME, Shumway NE, Stinson EB, Popp RL. A hemodynamic and Doppler echocardiographic study of ventricular function in long-term cardiac allograft recipients: etiology and prognosis of restrictive/constrictive physiology. Circulation 1989; 79: 66–75.
9. Hirota Y, Kohriyama T, Hayashi T, Kaku K, Nishimura H, Saito T, Nakayama Y, Suwa M, Kino M, Kawamura K. Idiopathic restrictive cardiomyopathy: differences of left ventricular relaxation and diastolic wave forms from constrictive pericarditis. Am J Cardiol 1983; 52: 421–423.
10. Ishida Y, Meisner JS, Tsujioka K, Gallo JI, Yoran C, Frater RWM, Yellin EL. Left ventricular filling dynamics: influence of left ventricular relaxation and left atrial pressure. Circulation 1986; 74: 187–196.
11. Appleton CP, Hatle LK, Popp RL: The relationship of transmitral flow velocity patterns to left ventricular diastolic function: new insights from a combined hemodynamic and Doppler echocardiographic study. J Am Coll Cardiol 1988; 12: 426–440.
12. Klein AL, Oh JK, Miller FA, Seward JB, Tajik J. Two-dimensional and Doppler echocardiographic assessment of infiltrative cardiomyopathy. J Am Soc Echo 1988; 1: 48–59.
13. Klein AL, Hatle LK, Burstow DJ, Seward JB, Kyle RA, Bailey KR, Luscher TF, Gertz MA, Tajik AJ. Doppler characterization of LV function in cardiac amyloidosis. J Am Coll Cardiol 1989; 13: 1017–1026.
14. Tyberg TI, Goodyer AVN, Hurst VW, Alexander J, Langou RA. Left ventricular filling in differentiating restrictive amyloid cardiomyopathy and constrictive pericarditis. Am J Cardiol 1981; 47: 791–796.
15. Janos GG, Arjunan K, Meyer RA, Engel P, Kaplan S. Differentiation of constrictive pericarditis and restrictive cardiomyopathy using digitized echocardiography. J Am Coll Cardiol 1983; 1: 541–549.
16. Aroney CN, Ruddy TD, Dighero H, Fifer MA, Boucher CA, Palacios IF. Differentiation of restrictive cardiomyopathy from pericardial constriction: assessment of diastolic function by radionuclide angiography. J Am Coll Cardiol 1989; 13: 1007–1014.
17. Hansen AT, Eskildsen P, Gotzsche H: Pressure curves from the right auricle and the right ventricle in chronic constrictive pericarditis. Circulation 1951; 3: 881–888.

18. Wood, P. Chronic constrictive pericarditis. Am J Cardiol 1961; 7: 48–61.
19. Shabetai R, Fowler NO, Guntheroth WG: The hemodynamics of cardiac tamponade and constrictive pericarditis. Am J Cardiol 1970; 26: 480–489.
20. Shabetai R: The pathophysiology of constrictive pericarditis. In: Reddy PS, Leon DF, Shavers JA, eds. Pericardial Disease. New York, Raven Press Books Ltd., 1982; 267–274.
21. Appleton CP, Hatle LK, Popp RL. Superior vena cava and hepatic vein Doppler in healthy adults. J Am Coll Cardiol 1987; 10: 1032–1039.
22. Patton JN, Tajik AJ, Reeder GS, Edwards WD, Seward JB. Echocardiographic nondilated, nonhypertrophic (restrictive) cardiomyopathy: clinical profile and natural history. J Am Coll Cardiol 1983; 1: 738 (abstr).
23. Santamore WP, Bartlet R, Van Buren SJ, Dowd MK, Kutcher MA. Ventricular coupling in constrictive pericarditis. Circulation 1986; 74: 597–602.
24. Tyberg TI, Goodyer AVN, Langou RA. Genesis of pericardial knock in constrictive pericarditis. Am J Cardiol 1980; 46: 570–575.
25. Lewis BS, Gotsman MS: Left ventricular function in systole and diastole in constrictive pericarditis. Am Heart J 1973; 86: 23–41.
26. Fowler NO: Constrictive pericarditis: new aspects. Am J Cardiol 1982; 50: 1014–1017.
27. Schnittger I, Bowden RE, Abrams J, Popp RL: Echocardiography: Pericardial thickening and constrictive pericarditis. Am J Cardiol 1978; 42: 388–395.
28. Isner JM, Carter BL, Bankoff MS, Pastore JO, Ramaswamy K, McAdam KPWJ, Salem ND. Differentiation of constrictive pericarditis from restrictive cardiomyopathy by computed tomographic imaging. Am Heart J 1983; 105: 1019–1025.
29. Gibson TC, Grossman W, McLaurin LP, Moos S, Craige E. An echocardiographic study of the interventricular septum in constrictive pericarditis. Br Heart J 1978; 38: 738–743.
30. Candell-Riera J, del Castillo HG, Permanyer-Miralda G, Soler-Soler J: Echocardiographic features of the interventricular septum in chronic constrictive pericarditis. Circulation 1978; 57: 1154–1158.
31. Tei C, Child JS, Tanaka H, Shah PM: Atrial systolic notch on the interventricular septal echocardiogram: an echocardiographic sign of constrictive pericarditis. J Am Coll Cardiol 1983; 1: 907–912.
32. Voelkel AG, Pietro DA, Folland ED, Fisher ML, Parisi AF. Echocardiographic features of constrictive pericarditis. Circulation 1978; 58: 871–875.
33. Engel PJ, Fowler NO, Tei C, Shah PM, Driedger HJ, Shabetai R, Harbin AD, Franck RH. M-mode echocardiography in constrictive pericarditis. J Am Coll Cardiol 1985; 6: 471–474.
34. Lewis BS. Real time two-dimensional echocardiography in constrictive pericarditis. Am J Cardiol 1982; 49: 1789–1793.
35. Thompson CR, Kingma I, MacDonald RPR, Balenkie I, Tyberg JV, Smith ER. Transeptal pressure gradient and diastolic ventricular septal motion in patients with mitral stenosis. Circulation 1987; 76: 974–980.
36. Simonson JS, Schiller NB. Sonospirometry: a new method for non-invasive estimation of mean right atrial pressure based on two-dimensional echocardiographic measurements of the inferior vena cava during measured inspiration. J Am Coll Cardiol 1988; 11: 557–564.
37. Tanaka C, Nishimoto M, Takeuchi K, Fukukawa K, Kawai S, Oku H, Ikuno Y. Presystolic pulmonary valve opening in constrictive pericarditis. Jpn Heart J 1979; 20: 419–425.
38. Appleton CP, Hatle L, Popp RL: Central venous flow velocity patterns can differentiate constrictive pericarditis from restrictive cardiomyopathy. J Am Coll Cardiol 1987; 9 (suppl A): 119A (abstr).
39. von Bibra H, Schober K, Jenni R, Busch A, Sebening H, Blömer H. Diagnosis of constrictive pericarditis by pulsed Doppler echocardiography of the hepatic vein. Am J Cardiol 1989; 63: 483–488.
40. Hoit B, Sahn DJ, Shabetai R. Doppler-detected paradoxus of mitral and tricuspid valve flows in chronic lung disease. J Am Coll Cardiol 1986; 8: 706–709.

41. Schoenfeld MH, Supple EW, Dec GW, Fallon JT, Palacios IF. Restrictive cardiomyopathy versus constrictive pericarditis: role of endomyocardial biopsy in avoiding unnecessary thoracotomy. Circulation 1987; 75: 1012–1017.
42. Gerson MC, Colthar MS, Fowler NO. Differentiation of constrictive pericarditis and restrictive cardiomyopathy by radionuclide ventriculography. Am Heart J 1989; 118: 114–120.
43. Marcus ML, Schulbert HR, Skorton DJ, Wolf G. Cardiac imaging: principles and practice. WB Saunders, Philadelphia (in press).

5. Transient cardiac constriction

J. ANGEL-FERRER, M.D.

Definition

The development of constrictive pericarditis is a common feature in some etiologic types of acute pericarditis, such as purulent and tuberculous pericarditis (1, 2). By contrast, in acute idiopathic pericarditis, evolution to cardiac constriction is quite uncommon; indeed, only isolated cases have been reported (1–5). In our own prospective series, only two of 252 patients with idiopathic pericarditis required pericardiectomy for constrictive pericarditis.

Atypical forms of cardiac constriction, such as elastic (6) and occult (7) constriction, have been reported in recent years. These forms of constriction have their own clinical and hemodynamic features and are less common than the classical type. Accordingly, if the clinician is not aware of their existence, significant constriction may be overlooked. The reported cases (6, 7) are too few to give a clear picture of the natural history of these types of constrictive pericarditis. It is assumed that once constrictive pericarditis of any type is established its course is irreversible and probably progressive.

We have observed 16 patients with acute idiopathic effusive pericarditis in whom features of constriction developed during the resolution of effusion, but later spontaneously subsided. As a rule, constriction was mild and resulted in obvious clinical findings in just a few patients; therefore, it might have initially been overlooked before we became attuned to the syndrome. Accordingly, the prevalence of transient constriction in our series of acute idiopathic pericarditis may have been underestimated. However, we think it is not rare as we documented transient constriction in seven (20%) of 34 consecutive patients with acute idiopathic effusive pericarditis in whom this type of evolution was systematically looked for.

The observation of transient cardiac constriction had not been made before our reports (8, 9). We feel that our findings should be known because they document a hitherto unknown pattern of evolution of acute idiopathic

J. Soler-Soler et al. (Eds.), Pericardial Disease, pp. 95–108.

pericarditis and the awareness of the possible transient character of constriction may prevent unnecessary pericardiectomy.

Description of the syndrome

The 16 patients reported in the present chapter had been included in a series of 292 consecutive patients admitted to our Service for acute pericardial disease (acute pericarditis and/or cardiac tamponade). All patients were investigated following a systematic, previously reported protocol (2). A diagnosis of acute idiopathic pericarditis was made in 252 patients and pericardial effusion was demonstrated in 177 of them. Sixteen of these had transient cardiac constriction and constitute the basis of the present report. There were ten males and six females, with ages ranging between 8 and 59 years (mean

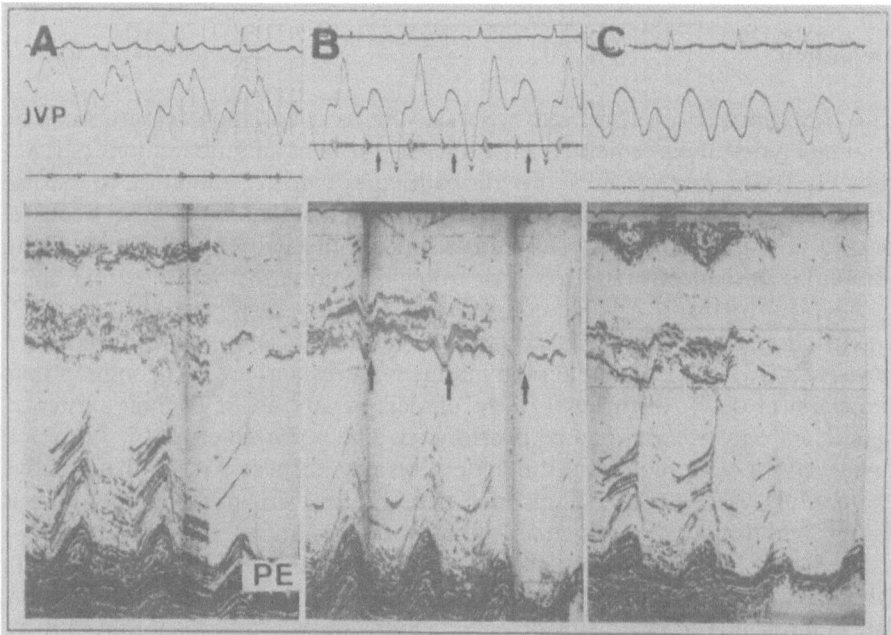

Fig. 5.1. Patient 8. A. Phase I: jugular venous pulse (JVP) recorded simultaneously with phonocardiogram (both are normal). In the lower panel the echocardiogram shows pericardial effusion (PE) in the posterior space. B. Phase II: in the upper panel arrows point to pericardial knock, followed by a marked "y" trough in the jugular venous pulse. The echocardiogram shows an early diastolic notch (arrows) in the interventricular septum. All these findings strongly suggest cardiac constriction. C. Phase III: in the upper panel, the "x" and "y" troughs have become similar and the pericardial knock of the echocardiogram has disappeared. The lower panel shows normalization of septal motion, with disappearance of early diastolic notch. (Reproduced with permission from Permanyer-Miralda G, Candell-Riera J, Sagristà-Sauleda J, Soler-Soler J. Constricción cardiaca transitoria: una forma peculiar de evolución de la pericarditis aguda exudativa. Rev Latina Cardiol 1983; 4: 187–192).

38 years). The first nine patients were diagnosed retrospectively. After these initial observations made us aware that constriction is sometimes transient, all patients with acute idiopathic effusive pericarditis were prospectively followed with clinical findings, jugular venous pulse recordings, phonocardiogram and echocardiogram. Whenever pericardial effusion was identified, external recordings were repeated weekly; if constrictive features were found, the recordings were periodically performed until a steady state was considered to have been achieved. In 34 patients seven new instances of transient constriction were identified.

The 16 patients presented because of acute pericarditis lasting for 1–20 days; three of them had had a probable previous episode of acute pericarditis in the preceding 20–30 days. On admission, the diagnosis of acute pericarditis was made on the basis of symptoms, pericardial friction rub and characteristic ECG changes. In all, the following evolution phases were identified.

Phase I: pericardial effusion

All patients had echocardiographic features of moderate to severe pericardial effusion (Table 5.1, Fig. 5.1) in both anterior and posterior spaces. In addition, nine patients had pleural effusion. Three patients had cardiac tamponade. No findings of cardiac constriction were apparent in this phase in any

Table 5.1. Phase I. Pericardial effusion.

		Echo		
Pt	Tamp	PE	VS	JVP
1	0	+	N	–
2	0	+	N	Xy
3	+	+	N	–
4	0	+	N	Xy
5	0	+	N	Xy
6	0	+	N	–
7	+	+	N	–
8	0	+	N	–
9	0	+	N	–
10	+	+	N	Xy
11	0	+	N	Xy
12	0	+	N	–
13	0	+	N	Xy
14	0	+	N	–
15	0	+	N	–
16	0	+	N	–

Tamp: tamponade; Echo: echocardiogram; PE: pericardial effusion; VS: ventricular septum; JVP: jugular venous pulse; Xy: "x" trough deeper than "y" trough'; 0: absent; N: normal; –: not done.

patient. In six patients an external recording of the jugular venous pulse was obtained, showing an "Xy" pattern in all. The three patients with tamponade required pericardiocentesis, which yielded 130, 150 and 400 ml of pericardial exudate. All patients were treated with bed rest and acetylsalicylic acid (2–3 g/day); all of them experienced a rapid clinical improvement, with a progressive reduction of pericardial effusion.

Phase II: cardiac constriction

In six patients the development of constriction (Table 5.2, Fig. 5.1) was clinically suspected because a prominent "y" trough and an early diastolic sound developed. In the remaining ten patients the features of constriction were discovered on routine phonocardiograms and echocardiograms. All patients showed a deep and brisk "y" wave in the jugular pulse recording; a pericardial knock was recorded in the phonocardiogram in eight patients, and an abnormal early diastolic notch was apparent in the M mode echocardiogram in 15 patients. All patients but one had either two or all three of these findings. In one instance (patient 12) a deep "y" wave in the jugular pulse recording was the only manifestation. By this time, the clinical signs of inflammation

Table 5.2. Phase II. Cardiac constriction.

Pt	T1	Echo		Phono	JVP	1st cath
		PE	VS			
1	8 d	0	notch	p. knock	xY	–
2	15 d	0	notch	p. knock	xY	–
3	10 d	0	notch	p. knock	xY	–
4	5 d	0	notch	N	xY	–
5	18 d	0	notch	p. knock	xY	–
6	10 d	+*	notch	N	xY	–
7	9 d	+*	notch	N	xY	–
8	30 d	+	notch	p. knock	xY	–
9	10 d	+*	notch	N	xY	–
10	17 d	+*	notch	N	xY	constr.
11	11 d	+	notch	p. knock	xY	constr.
12	14 d	0	N	N	xY	constr.
13	7 d	+*	notch	N	xY	constr.
14	20 d	+	notch	p. knock	xY	–
15	18 d	+*	notch	p. knock	xY	constr.
16	3 d	+	notch	N	xY	–

PE: pericardial effusion; VS: ventricular septum; Phono: phonocardiogram; JVP: jugular venous pulse; 1st cath.: first catheterization; T1: time between the first echocardiogram showing effusion and the first recordings showing constriction (d: days); 0: absent; P. knock: pericardial knock; xY: "y" trough deeper than "x" trough; N: normal; constr.: constriction; –: not done; *: pericardial effusion disappeared while constriction was still present.

had subsided and the condition of the patients was good. However, in this phase two patients developed features of venous congestion (distended neck veins, hepatomegaly and peripheral edema). The interval between the first echocardiogram showing pericardial effusion and the first recordings suggesting constriction ranged between 5 and 30 days (mean 11 days). When the signs of constriction developed, pericardial effusion had disappeared in six patients, but a small effusion persisted in nine patients and moderate effusion in the remaining one. Subsequently, in six of these ten patients effusion disappeared, whereas the constrictive features persisted. No patient was treated with diuretics or corticosteroids.

The last seven patients of the series were asked to undergo cardiac catheterization, and five of them consented. At the time of catheterization, pericardial effusion was absent in three patients and mild in two. All five patients underwent standard right and left heart catheterization. Cardiac output was measured by thermodilution. Left and right ventricular pressures were always recorded simultaneously. In four of the five patients measurements were repeated after the rapid infusion (8 min) of 1000 ml of isotonic saline. The following findings were considered for the diagnosis of cardiac constriction:

1. Right ventricular end-diastolic pressure higher than 10 mmHg (in our laboratory, the maximal normal values of right ventricular end-diastolic pressure are 8 mmHg at baseline and 10 mmHg after fluid overload (10–12).

2. In the presence of criterion 1, equalization of diastolic pressures of right and left ventricles (difference not greater than 5 mmHg).

Table 5.3. Catheterization data.

Patient no.	Cath	$T_{(w)}$	HR (bpm)		CI (l/min/m²)		RVEDP (mmHg)		LVEDP (mmHg)		RA (mmHg)	
			Ba	PS	Ba	PS	Ba	PS	Ba	PS	Ba	PS
10	First		117	102	3.30	3.69	5	17*	8	18*	7	18**
	Second	2	85	87	3.50	3.75	4	7	7	10	4	6
11	First		62	64	2.87	3.16	12	16	15*	20*	9	14
	Second	2	55	57	3.30	3.88	4	9	8	13	3	5
12	First		98	98	3.73	4.43	9	13	16	21	7	10**
	Second	4	115	113	3.94	4.43	3	8	5	13	2	4
13	First		100	–	2.79	–	16	–	16*	–	15**	–
	Second	48	75	70	3.15	3.50	8	10	13	15	7	9
15	First		110	120	2.90	3.80	16*	19*	22*	25*	10**	20**
	Second	8	120	120	3.50	4.60	3	8	5	14	1	6

Cath.: catheterization; T: time (weeks) between the first and the second catheterization studies; Ba: baseline state; PS: post saline perfusion; HR: heart rate; CI: cardiac index; RVEDP: right ventricular end diastolic pressure; LVEDP: left ventricular end diastolic pressure; RA: mean right atrial pressure; *: dip-plateau morphology; **: "W" morphology or very prominent "y" trough; –: not done.

3. Dip-plateau configuration of one or both ventricular pressure curves, with right ventricular end-diastolic pressures higher than 10 mmHg or left ventricular end-diastolic pressures higher than 15 mmHg (10–12).

4. Definite "W" morphology or very prominent "y" trough in the right atrial pressure curve.

The results are shown in Table 5.3. Three patients met constriction criteria in the baseline state: typical in two patients (Figs. 5.2 and 5.3) and atypical in one (Fig. 5.4), who did not show equalization of right and left diastolic pressures. After the saline infusion right and left diastolic pressures showed hemodynamic criteria of constriction, ostensible in one (Fig. 5.5) but more subtle in the other (Fig. 5.6). These last two patients, therefore, had an occult constriction. Overall four patients had a dip-plateau appearance of the ventricular pressure curve, and in four patients the right atrial pressure curve was "W" shaped. In Table 5.4 the criteria for constriction of the five patients in baseline conditions are shown; they are also shown for four of them after the saline infusion.

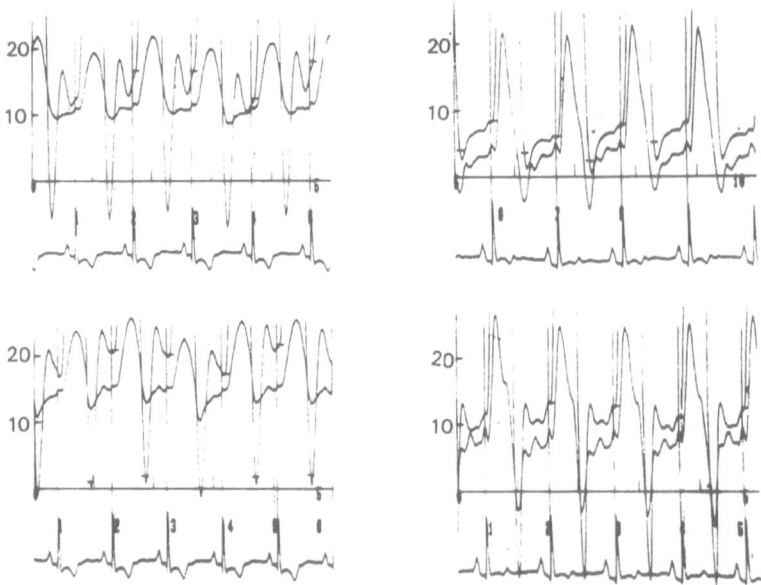

Fig. 5.2. Patient 11. *Left panel.* Right and left ventricular pressures simultaneously recorded during the constriction phase. Above, at baseline the diastolic right ventricular pressure exceeds 10 mmHg, and equals that of the left ventricle. Below, the abnormalities become more marked after fluid overload. The left ventricular pressure curve shows a dip-plateau morphology, but the right ventricular pressure curve does not. *Right panel.* In a study performed two weeks later the filling pressures of both ventricles have become normal, both in the baseline state (above) and after fluid overload (below).

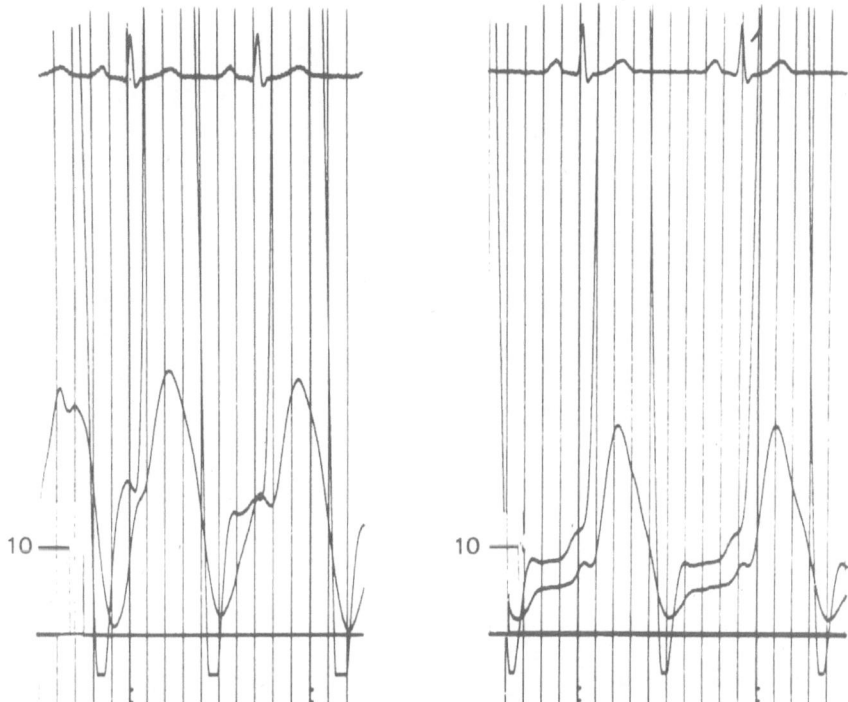

Fig. 5.3. Patient 13. *Left panel*: Right and left ventricular pressure curves. There is a dip-plateau morphology of the left ventricular pressure curve, both end diastolic pressures are 16 mmHg. *Right panel*: in the second study (48 weeks later) all signs of constriction have disappeared. (Reproduced with permission from Sagristà-Sauleda J, Permanyer-Miralda G, Candell-Riera J, Angel J, Soler-Soler J. Transient cardiac constriction: an unrecognized pattern of evolution in effusive acute idiopathic pericarditis. Am J Cardiol 1987; 59: 961–966).

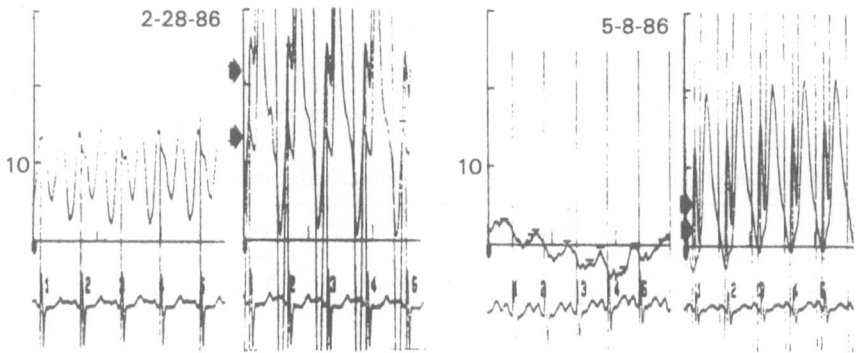

Fig. 5.4. Patient 15. *Left panel*: There is a characteristic "W" morphology of right atrial pressure curve, with high but unequal (arrows) end diastolic left (22 mmHg) and right (12 mmHg) ventricular pressures. *Right panel*: Eight weeks later, the pressures and the morphology of the curves have become normal. (Reproduced with permission from Sagristà-Sauleda J, Permanyer-Miralda G, Candell-Riera J, Angel J, Soler-Soler J. Transient cardiac constriction: an unrecognized pattern of evolution in effusive acute idiopathic pericarditis. Am J Cardiol 1987; 59: 961–966).

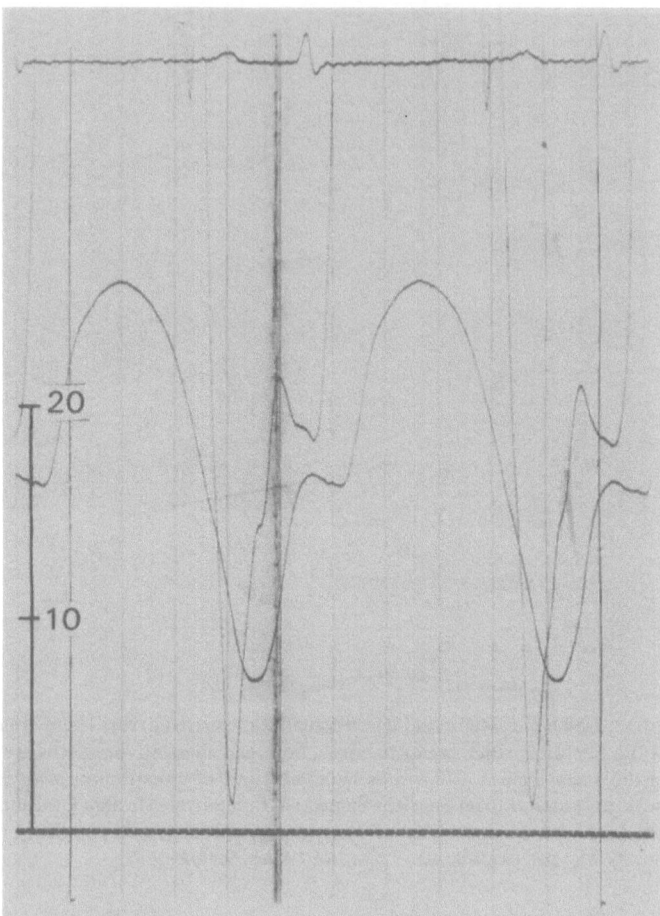

Fig. 5.5. Patient 10. Simultaneous pressures from both ventricles after volume loading. End diastolic pressures are elevated (15–20 mmHg) with a dip-plateau morphology. At baseline the pressures were strictly normal. This case suggests occult constriction.

Table 5.4. Catheterization findings of constriction in individual patients.

No.	Ba	PS
10	0	1, 2, 3, 4
11	1, 2, 3	1, 2, 3
12	0	1, 4
13	1, 2, 3, 4	–
15	1, 3, 4	1, 3, 4

Criterion 1: end diastolic RV pressure > 10 mmHg; criterion 2: criterion 1 + equalization of end diastolic ventricular pressures; criterion 3: criterion 1 + dip-plateau morphology of ventricular pressure curve; criterion 4: right atrial pressure curve with "W" morphology or marked "y" trough; 0: no criteria; Ba: baseline state; PS: post saline perfusion; –: unnecessary because all criteria were fulfilled in baseline.

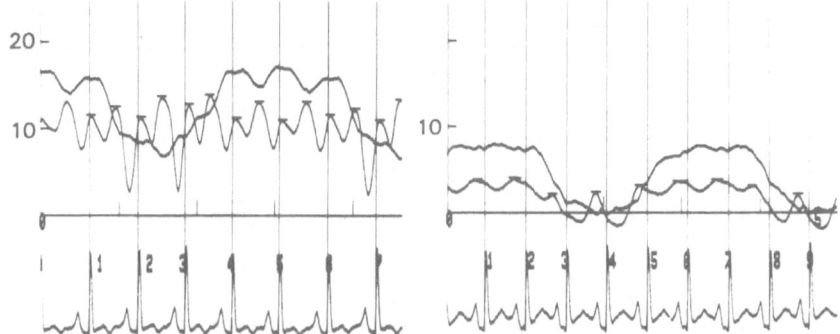

Fig. 5.6. Patient 12. Pulmonary wedge and right atrial pressures after fluid overload. *Left panel*: first study, showing right atrial pressure of 10 mmHg with "W" morphology. Note accentuation of the "y" trough during inspiration (identified by the descent of mean pulmonary wedge pressure). Four weeks later (*right panel*), the right atrial pressure and the curve morphology have become normal.

Phase III: normalization

In three patients the external recordings returned to normal during the hospital admission (7, 12 and 21 days, respectively, after the signs of constriction had appeared). The remaining 13 patients were discharged from the hospital with persistent constrictive features in the external recordings but with full clinical recovery. In these patients, the external recordings became normal during the follow up. This normalization (Table 5.5, Fig. 5.1) was documented between 19 days and 58 months after the constriction features had been recognized. However, if only the seven patients in whom transient constriction was prospectively followed are considered, the interval between the first recordings showing constrictive features and the first normal recordings ranged between 12 days and 10 months (mean 2.7 months). The five patients in whom catheterization had been performed during the constriction phase underwent a second catheterization after the external recordings had become normal. This second catheterization was undertaken between 2 and 48 weeks after the first study. A baseline study and measurements after fluid challenge were performed. The results are shown in Table 5.3. The level and morphology of filling pressure curves of each ventricle had returned to normal. This normalization persisted after saline infusion, despite the fact that the cardiac index was higher than in the first catheterization study. Sinus rhythm was maintained throughout the clinical course.

After hospital discharge, the follow up ranged between 10 and 77 months (mean 31 months). Once the constriction features had disappeared, the physical examination remained normal in all 16 patients. Three patients had recurrent episodes of acute pericarditis that were controlled with acetylsalicylic acid; no patient developed constrictive features in the external recordings performed during recurrences.

Table 5.5. Phase III. Normalization.

		Echo				
Pt	T2	PE	VS	Phono	JVP	2nd cath
1	3 m	0	N	N	xY	–
2	5 m	0	N	N	xY	–
3	7 d	0	N	N	xY	–
4	5 m	0	N	N	xY	–
1	1 m	0	N	N	xY	–
6	58 m	0	N	N	xY	–
7	24 m	0	N	N	xY	–
8	32 m	0	N	N	xY	–
9	5 m	0	N	N	xY	–
10	21 d	0	N	N	xY	normalization
11	12 d	0	N	N	xY	normalization
12	19 d	0	N	N	xY	normalization
13	10 m	0	N	N	xY	normalization
14	3 m	0	N	N	xY	–
15	2 m	0	N	N	xY	normalization
16	1 m	0	N	N	xY	–

JVP: jugular venous pulse; N: normal; PE: pericardial effusion; 2nd Cath: second catheterization; T2: interval between the first recordings showing constriction and the first normal recordings (m: months, d: days); VS: ventricular septum; xy: both "x" and "y" troughs of similar magnitude; xY: "y" trough deeper than "x" trough; 0: absent; –: not done.

Pathophysiology

It is apparent that all 16 patients with acute idiopathic effusive pericarditis reported in this chapter developed, during the resolution phase of pericardial effusion, a clinical and hemodynamic disorder consistent with cardiac constriction, and that this disorder was self-limited and transient. This statement is based on the documentation of the following findings: a deep "y" trough in the jugular venous pulse, a pericardial knock in the phonocardiogram and an abnormal early diastolic motion of the interventricular septum in the echocardiogram. These findings are characteristic of cardiac constriction (13–16), and, although each of them may have limitations by itself in a given case, the otherwise unexplained coexistence of several of them in our patients is highly suggestive of constriction. In addition, in all patients who underwent catheterization impaired cardiac filling was suggested, either at baseline (three patients) or after fluid load (two patients), by abnormalities in the level and morphology of ventricular diastolic and right atrial pressures. It should be emphasized that, at the end of follow-up, in all 16 patients the external recordings returned to normal; in particular, in the five patients undergoing catheterization the diastolic pressures and the pressure curves returned to absolutely normal values both in the basal state and after fluid overload, despite similar heart rate and cardiac index. One may wonder whether the diastolic abnormalities documented in phase II did not correspond with tamponade rather than constriction as all patients had pericardial effusion at admission, the effusion persisted at the beginning of phase II in 10 patients, and at the time of the first catheterization there was still mild effusion in two patients. However, in this phase pericardial effusion was clearly subsiding in all patients and, in six, had completely disappeared while constriction signs remained unchanged. In addition, three of the five patients who underwent catheterization were studied at a time when effusion had altogether disappeared. Moreover, all the abnormalities in the external recordings and in the catheterization studies suggested constriction rather than tamponade. We think, accordingly, that our patients really had cardiac constriction in phase II. However, the hemodynamic pattern of some of our patients was atypical (1, 17), particularly showing the lack of equal diastolic pressures and of dip-plateau morphology in the pressure curves of both ventricles. Although these atypical hemodynamic patterns may be found in patients with definite constrictive pericarditis (even with calcification) (11, 18), they suggest that our patients could have a type of cardiac constriction different from the classical one. The hemodynamic pattern of some of our patients corresponded to that reported by Hancock in patients with subacute constriction (6). This author emphasized the absence of a definite dip-plateau pattern in those patients, even in the absence of concomitant pericardial effusion. He attributed this finding, which he called "elastic" constriction, to the restriction to diastolic filling brought about by a fibroelastic pericardium that would compress the heart throughout the diastole, as opposed to the more classical constriction exerted by a rigid and wholly inextensible pericardium that limits the filling only in middle and end diastole. We think, therefore, that some of our patients had elastic constriction.

Our findings provide new insights into the spectrum of evolution of acute idiopathic pericarditis. It is well known that the great majority of patients recover from this condition without any sequel, and that the development of constrictive pericarditis requiring pericardiectomy is uncommon, only isolated cases having been reported (1–5). As mentioned before, Hancock (6) described another type of constrictive pericarditis ("elastic" constriction) with or without concomitant effusion. On the other hand, Bush et al. (7) introduced the notion of occult constriction, where the hemodynamic abnormalities are only brought to light after the rapid infusion of saline. In some cases of both elastic and occult constrictive pericarditis, there is an implicit relationship between constriction and acute pericarditis. Our study has documented, for the first time, the possible transient character of these abnormalities and it has widened the range of possible evolution from acute idiopathic effusive pericarditis.

Another interesting feature is the persistence of a small pericardial effusion during the phase of constriction in ten of our patients. In six of them the course followed four stages: acute pericarditis with effusion, constrictive pericarditis with persisting effusion, pure constrictive pericarditis, and resolution. Some of these stages may go unnoticed, as they can be short lived and a high suspicion index is required for their identification. However, the whole sequence raises the possibility of a *continuum* from the stage of uncomplicated effusive pericarditis. Most patients with effusive pericarditis proceed directly to complete resolution, but in some recovery may be preceded by transient constriction, with or without an intermediate phase of concomitant constriction and effusion. Rare patients may directly develop constrictive pericarditis, with or without concomitant effusion. This spectrum widens the range of hemodynamic possibilities considered by Hancock (6, 19), who placed tamponade and rigid constriction at each end and elastic constriction in the middle. In some of the patients reported by this author acute effusive pericarditis developed into effusive-constrictive pericarditis, and, subsequently, into constrictive pericarditis requiring pericardiectomy. Our patients (Fig. 5.7) seem to follow a parallel evolution, with a lesser severity degree in each stage, but proceeding to spontaneous resolution.

In our series constriction was, as a rule, mild and sometimes of short duration; therefore, it may be overlooked if the index of suspicion is not high and serial external recordings are not carried out. However, overt features of venous congestion developed in two of our patients, leading to a consideration of pericardiectomy; in another four patients the findings of constriction were sufficiently apparent to be revealed at physical examination. In some patients, signs of constriction may persist for several months, which is clinically relevant for their management.

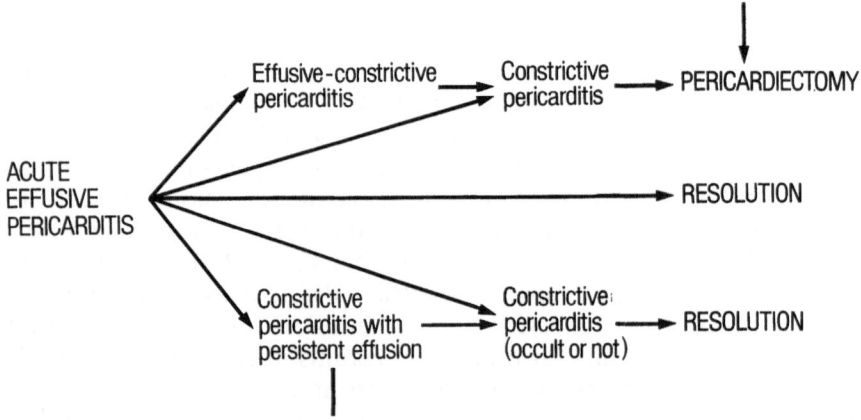

Fig. 5.7. Possible patterns of evolution of acute effusive pericarditis. In the upper part the possibilities described by Hancock (6) are depicted. The lower part of the figure represents the possible patterns of evolution of transient cardiac constriction. Note the parallelism between both types, although with a lesser degree of severity in the latter, which, on the other hand, eventually returns to normal. In the middle, the most common pattern of evolution (direct resolution) is depicted.

The underlying pathological basis of transient constriction is unknown. We speculate, however, that the pericardium may undergo anatomical and functional changes related with reversible fibrin deposition. In fact, two of our patients were studied with computed tomography scan during the phase of constriction, and a mild thickening of parietal pericardium was found; this thickening subsequently disappeared.

Clinical implications

The importance of our findings is not only academic but has implications for the clinical practice. They document a hitherto unreported type of evolution of acute idiopathic pericarditis, bringing to light the previously unknown occurrence of transient cardiac constriction. Knowledge of this type of evolution may prevent the performance of an unnecessary pericardiectomy. When signs of cardiac constriction develop during the resolution of acute idiopathic pericarditis, it is wise to adopt a conservative approach and not to advise pericardiectomy unless severe and progressive signs of venous hypertension develop.

References

1. Shabetai R. The pericardium. New York, Grune & Stratton, 1981; 154–223.
2. Permanyer-Miralda G, Sagristà-Sauleda J, Soler-Soler J. Primary acute pericardial disease: A prospective series of 231 consecutive patients. Am J Cardiol 1985; 56: 623–630.
3. Azar GJ. Acute nonspecific pericarditis complicated by the development of constrictive pericarditis. Am Heart J 1963; 65: 474–481.
4. Robertson R, Arnold CR. Acute constrictive pericarditis. J Thorac Cardiovasc Surg 1965; 49: 91–102.
5. Howard EJ, Maier HC. Constrictive pericarditis following acute Coxsackie viral pericarditis. Am Heart J 1968; 75: 247–250.
6. Hancock EW. On the elastic and rigid forms of constrictive pericarditis. Am Heart J 1980: 100: 917–923.
7. Bush CA, Stang JM, Wooley CF, Kilman JW. Occult constrictive pericardial disease. Diagnosis by rapid volume expansion and correction by pericardiectomy. Circulation 1977; 56: 924–930.
8. Permanyer-Miralda G, Candell-Riera J, Sagristà-Sauleda J, Soler-Soler J. Constricción cardíaca transitoria: una forma peculiar de evolución de la pericarditis aguda exudativa. Rev Latina Cardiol 1983; 4: 187–192.
9. Sagristà Sauleda J, Permanyer Miralda G, Candell Riera J, Angel J, Soler-Soler J. Transient cardiac constriction: Un unrecognized pattern of evolution in effusive acute idiophatic pericarditis. Am J Cardiol 1987; 59: 961–966.
10. Angel J, Anivarro I. Cateterismo cardíaco. In: Soler Soler J, Bayés de Luna, A, eds. Cardiología. Barcelona, Ed. Doyma, 1986; 202.
11. Serrat R, Angel J, Domingo E, Anivarro I, Soler Soler J. Detection and diagnosis between occult pericardial constriction and restrictive cardiomyopathy. X World Congress of Cardiology, Abstract book, 1986; 5.
12. Angel Ferrer J, Anivarro Blanco I. Manometrías, flujos y áreas valvulares. In: López

Bescós L, ed. Avances en hemodinámica y angiocardiografía. Sociedad Española de Cardiología. Barcelona; Ed. Doyma, 1988; 36–57.

13. Wide D, Conti CR. Constrictive pericarditis. In: Spodick DH, ed. Pericardial diseases. Philadelphia, FA Davis Co. 1976; 197–209.

14. Spodick DH. Acoustic phenomena in pericardial disease. Am Heart J 1971; 81: 114–124.

15. Candell-Riera J, García del Castillo H, Permanyer-Miralda G, Soler-Soler J. Echocardiographic features of the interventricular septum in chronic constrictive pericarditis. Circulation 1978; 57: 1.154–1.158.

16. Engel PJ, Fowler NO, Tei C, Shah PM, Driedger HJ, Shabetai R, Harbin AD. M mode echocardiography in constrictive pericarditis. J Am Coll Cardiol 1985; 6: 471–474.

17. Shabetai R, Fowler NO, Guntheroth WG. The hemodynamics of cardiac tamponade and constrictive pericarditis. Am J Cardiol 1970; 26: 480–489.

18. Anderson PAW. Diagnostic problem: Constrictive pericarditis or restrictive cardiomyopathy? Cath Cardiovasc Diag 1983; 9: 1–7.

19. Hancock EW. Subacute effusive constrictive pericarditis. Circulation 1971; 43: 183–192.

6. Tuberculous pericarditis

J. SAGRISTÀ-SAULEDA, M.D.

Incidence

The true incidence of tuberculous pericarditis is not accurately known. Most available studies were performed before the introduction of modern chemotherapy, and some series include cases classified as tuberculous without proof but on the basis of indirect evidence. In Wood's series (1), the incidence of pericardial involvement in patients who died of tuberculosis was 7.8%. In his comprehensive review of the disease, Schepers (2) remarked that 7–10% of pericarditis were tuberculous. In addition, there are wide geographic and racial variations (3, 4), and an increasing incidence has been recently reported in some populations (5, 6). The incidence of tuberculous pericarditis in Spain is not known, as recent reports are based on isolated observations of small numbers of patients (7, 8). However, it is likely that the prevalence has remained constant for many years, particularly if pericarditis behaves like other extrapulmonary manifestations of tuberculosis, the incidence of which has not changed over the last several years. Tuberculous pericarditis complicating acquired immunodeficiency syndrome has been recently reported (9–11) raising the possibility that some other cases have gone undiagnosed. Between January 1977 and June 1986 we had seen 13 patients with tuber-

J. Soler-Soler et al. (Eds.), Pericardial Disease, pp. 109–121.

culous pericarditis (12), among 294 consecutive patients with primary acute pericardial disease, that is, acute pericardial disease without evidence of its etiology at the time of admission. This represents a prevalence of 4.4%. From June 1986 to September 1988 we have seen three additional patients. Therefore, in our part of the world tuberculous pericarditis is a relatively uncommon cause of acute pericardial disease.

Pathogenesis

Although tuberculous pericarditis may be acquired through direct contact with foci of pulmonary tuberculosis or as a feature of miliary dissemination, it is commonly caused by a reactivation of latent tuberculous infection in mediastinal lymph nodes, with direct extension into the pericardium. The most common source is the lympth nodes in the carina. Although clinical and pathological findings may be confined to the pericardium, it is believed that tuberculous pericarditis is always secondary to an extrapericardial focus and that primary tuberculous pericarditis does not exist.

Prognosis

Before the specific chemotherapy was introduced, the prognosis of tuberculous pericarditis was very poor: 80–90% of patients died in the acute phase and many of those remaining subsequently died from constrictive pericarditis or dissemination. The introduction of streptomycin resulted in a reduction of mortality from 90% to 43% (13). In later years, newer chemotherapeutic agents have induced a dramatic improvement in the prognosis. Nevertheless, in some recent series (3, 4, 14) the mortality is significant, and it still is not rare to discover the existence of tuberculosis at autopsy (15). Tuberculous pericarditis, although uncommon, can still cause severe tamponade during the effusive phase and constriction in the resolution phase. Constrictive pericarditis commonly follows tuberculous infection of the pericardium despite specific chemotherapy, and therefore many of those infected eventually require pericardiectomy. It is possible that this course might be favorably modified by early diagnosis and therapy. Thus, the major challenge now posed by tuberculous pericarditis is diagnosis, and, particularly, early diagnosis.

Diagnosis

Diagnostic criteria

The only absolute evidence of tuberculous pericarditis is the identification of tubercle bacilli in the pericardial fluid or tissue. Clinical practice often falls short of this ideal. Frequently it is not possible to demonstrate tubercle bacilli in the samples, and only in exceptional circumstances is direct staining of pericardial fluid by the Ziehl-Neelsen method diagnostic. Also, isolation of the tubercle bacilli depends on culture in specific media, with the corresponding delay in diagnosis. Liberalising the indications for pericardiocentesis and pericardial biopsy in acute pericarditis in an attempt to establish an early diagnosis of tuberculous pericarditis would result in an excessive number of invasive procedures in patients with idiopathic disease; this would be unacceptable in view of the comparatively small prevalence of tuberculous pericarditis. Therefore, quite often the diagnosis has to be made on the basis of other criteria which cannot be absolute but are highly suggestive. Among these are identification of tubercle bacilli or histological evidence of caseating granulomas elsewhere in the body. It is quite common to find in the literature series where the diagnosis of some patients was made only on the basis of indirect criteria (1, 3–6, 16), such as basically the clinical features, a chest radiogram suggesting tuberculosis, a strongly positive tuberculin skin test, or a favorable response to antituberculous chemotherapy. It should be emphasized, however, that these criteria are not conclusive evidence of tuberculosis. Regarding the clinical features, the insidious development of symptoms with subsequent relapsing effusion after pericardiocentesis has been reported as characteristic of tuberculous pericarditis. However, the clinical presentation of tuberculous pericarditis is highly variable. The initial manifestation may be acute pericarditis simulating viral pericarditis and even, in exceptional cases, recurrent pericarditis (17). To add to the difficulties, viral or idiopathic pericarditis may persist for several weeks and be associated with tamponade. In our series of primary acute pericardial disease (18), 23 patients out 192 with acute idiopathic pericarditis had been ill for more than three weeks before admission and 32 had cardiac tamponade. In the individual patient, therefore, clinical features may not be particularly helpful, although it is obvious that in patients with acute rapidly self limited pericarditis the possibility of tuberculosis is remote. We have a strong tendency not to pay much attention to a positive tuberculin skin test because in Catalonia about 40% of adult individuals have positive reactions to tuberculin (19). Furthermore, five of our patients with tuberculous pericarditis had a negative reaction, whereas in 41% of our patients with idiopathic pericarditis the reaction was positive (20). Finally, the response to antituberculous therapy is unsatisfactory evidence. Indeed, we considered including blind antituberculous chemotherapy in the initial version of our study protocol (20); in the event we have never found it necessary.

For the unequivocal diagnosis of tuberculous pericarditis we required one of three criteria: isolation of tubercle bacilli in the pericardial fluid or tissue, isolation of tubercle bacilli elsewhere in the body, or caseating pericardial lesions or caseation elsewhere. Seven patients fulfilled the first criterion. Isolation of tubercle bacilli elsewhere in the body was achieved in six patients; in four, tubercle bacilli grew from the sputum and in two from axillary and mediastinal node biopsy. Caseating granulomas of the pericardium were detected in two patients and caseation was present in the pleural biopsy of another.

Study protocol

A brief review of the algorithm for the diagnosis of tuberculous pericarditis in our initial protocol for primary acute pericardial disease (20) is now pertinent. The first 13 patients of our present series were evaluated following this approach (12). Subsequently, however, due to analysis of our initial results, the study protocol was modified. In *stage I*, a tuberculin skin test with 10 units of PPD was applied and three samples of sputum or gastric aspirate were obtained. Any other investigation such as thoracentesis and pleural or node biopsy suggested by the clinical picture was carried out at this stage. In *stage II*, pericardiocentesis was performed in all patients with cardiac tamponade and in those in whom pericardial effusion had persisted, unchanged or larger, longer than one week. In *stage III*, surgical pericardial drainage was carried out in all patients in whom tamponade relapsed after pericardiocentesis, and also in those with persistent clinical activity three weeks after hospital admission. Finally, in *stage IV* blind antituberculous chemotherapy was contemplated when a diagnosis had not been established and clinical activity persisted five to six weeks after admission. Subsequently we modified the study protocol and limited pericardiocentesis to patients with tamponade. The last three patients of the series reported in this chapter were studied following this new protocol.

Overall yield of the study protocol

Table 6.1 shows the methods whereby the diagnosis of tuberculous pericarditis was made in the 16 patients. The positive results are rather evenly distributed throughout all the studies. Sputum culture was the most commonly positive investigation, being positive in six of 14 patients in whom it was available, including four in whom the chest radiogram was normal. In four patients the sputum culture was the first investigation to disclose the diagnosis. Pericardiocentesis was carried out in nine patients. Tubercle bacilli were demonstrated in six of them (all by culture) but it was the first procedure to demonstrate the diagnosis in only four, as, before the culture results were available,

Table 6.1. Diagnostic yield of the different studies.

No	TBS	P-cent	ADA	P. biop	P-tomy	Pl. biop	LN biop
1	⊕	−	−	−	−	−	−
2	−	neg	−	⊕	−	−	−
3	−	+	−	⊕	?	−	−
4	neg	⊕	−	−	+	−	−
5	neg	−	−	−	−	⊕	−
6	+	neg	−	−	+	−	⊕
7	⊕	−	−	−	+	−	−
8	⊕	−	−	−	−	−	−
9	neg	⊕	−	−	−	neg	−
10	neg	neg	96	−	+	−	⊕
11	⊕	−	−	−	−	−	−
12	−	⊕	95	−	+	−	−
13	+	−	162	⊕	+	−	−
14	neg	+	140	−	⊕	−	−
15	neg	⊕	36	−	−	−	−
16	neg	−	−	−	⊕	−	−

+: positive diagnostic study; O: first study which identified the diagnosis; −: not done; neg: negative diagnostic study; ?: not available; TBS: culture of tubercle bacilli in sputum or gastric aspirate; P-cent: pericardiocentesis; ADA: adenosine deaminase measurement in pericardial fluid; P. biop: pericardial biopsy; P-tomy: pericardiectomy; Pl. biop: pleural biopsy; LN biop: lymph node biopsy.

one required pericardial biopsy and another pericardiectomy and the diagnosis was first achieved as a result of these procedures. Pericardiocentesis was not performed in seven of the 16 patients with tuberculous pericarditis because in six of them effusion was small or absent, and in another the diagnosis had already been made. Therefore, in more than one third of patients with tuberculous pericarditis effussion was too little for pericardiocentesis. Pericardial biopsy was performed in only three patients; in one because tamponade relapsed after pericardiocentesis and in the other two because clinical features persisted, although without hemodynamic compromise, three weeks after admission. In all three patients biopsy was positive, being the first study to give the diagnosis. Therefore, in contrast to our initial idea that many patients with tuberculous pericarditis would present with prolonged illness, often requiring pericardial biopsy for diagnosis, we found that only two of our 16 patients had this kind of clinical evolution. Pericardiectomy also confirmed the diagnosis in nine cases (in one patient the surgical specimen was not examined), being the first study to disclose the diagnosis in two cases. The first of these (patient 14) had previously required pericardiocentesis for cardiac tamponade and the culture of the pericardial fluid was subsequently positive. However, in the meantime, the patient developed subacute constrictive pericarditis and tuberculous pericarditis was first disclosed by the surgical specimen. In the second patient (patient 16), pericardiectomy, carried

out for constrictive pericarditis, was the only procedure that yielded the etiologic diagnosis. This patient had, on admission, a moderate pericardial effusion, but no tamponade. Accordingly, following the recommendations of our
current protocol, pericardiocentesis was not carried out. The initial course
was satisfactory, with spontaneous disappearance of fever and a significant
reduction in pericardial effusion after two weeks. The patient was discharged
with a diagnosis of acute idiopathic pericarditis, but readmitted when he
developed constriction. This was our only patient in whom the diagnosis of
tuberculosis was achieved only through pericardiectomy, thus representing a
failure of our present diagnostic approach. Finally, pleural biopsy in one case
and lymph node biopsy in another two (axillary and mediastinal, respectively)
were the studies which provided the correct diagnosis. Table 6.1 illustrates
that the diagnosis of tuberculous pericarditis can be disclosed by different
studies in individual patients. Therefore, a multiple approach should be
undertaken to achieve early diagnosis.

Measurement of adenosine deaminase activity in pericardial and pleural
fluids

This technique deserves separate comment. Although our experience with
this measurement in pericardial fluid is still limited, it should be remarked
that in the five patients with tuberculous pericarditis in which it was carried
out, the values were 36, 95, 96, 140 and 162 U/l, whereas they were lower
than 30 U/l in 53 specimens of pericardial fluid from patients with pericarditis of other etiology (21). This measurement may, therefore, permit a simpler
approach to the diagnosis of tuberculous pericarditis when its diagnostic
accuracy is adequately validated. To this end, our current policy (22) is to
indicate pericardial biopsy when a high adenosine deaminase content is
found in pericardial fluid. The diagnostic value of adenosine deaminase
measurement in pleural fluid has been clearly shown. Experience from our
institution (23) suggests that an adenosine deaminase value higher than 45
U/l in pleural fluid has a sensitivity and specificity over 90% for the diagnosis
of pleural tuberculosis. This observation is of great interest considering that
the measurment of adenosine deaminase is easy, nonexpensive and quick.
Pleural fluid is common in pericarditis, particularly tuberculous pericarditis
(10 of the 16 patients in our series), and is easily obtained. Therefore, the
measurement of adenosine deaminase in pleural exudate seems to be very
promising as a screening tool for tuberculous pericarditis. However, the following shortcomings call for caution when interpreting adenosine deaminase
activity measurements in pleural fluid. First, some authors (24) have reported
lower sensitivity values. Second, high adenosine deaminase activity has been
found in empyema (25), rheumatoid arthritis (25, 26) and lymphoma (27).
Finally, low adenosine deaminase values may be found when the pleural fluid
is a transudate, which is a common finding in tuberculous pericarditis when
tamponade or constriction have developed.

It should be emphasized that these studies were made in immunologically competent patients. The values of adenosine deaminase, which are related to the activity of T-lymphocytes, may not have the same meaning in immunologically compromised patients. In fact, in two patients with AIDS and tuberculous pericarditis seen after the present series was collected, the adenosine deaminase activity in pericadial fluid was lower (31 and 28 U/l, unpublished observations).

Diagnostic yield of pericardiocentesis and pericardial biopsy

Pericardiocentesis

Pericardiocentesis made the diagnosis in six of the nine patients in whom it was carried out. The shortcomings of pericardiocentesis for the diagnosis of tuberculous pericarditis have been recognized by other authors. Thus, Wood (1) identified tubercle bacilli in four of eight patients. Spodick (16), in a review of the literature in 1956, reported a rate ranging between 44 and 71%. Schepers (2), in his review of the literature in 1962, considered pericardiocentesis clearly insufficient for the diagnosis of tuberculous pericarditis. He attributed the high frequency of false negative results to the supposedly allergic character of the tuberculous exudate, in which the number of tubercle bacilli is small. Rooney et al. (14) made nine diagnoses by culture of pericardial fluid in 18 patients with tuberculous pericarditis undergoing pericardiocentesis, and Fowler and Manitsas (28) made 10 diagnoses in 13 patients. Gooi et al. (5) isolated tubercle bacilli from pericardial fluid in only 4 of 13 patients. Finally, in the series by Strang et al. (4), from South Africa, culture of pericardial fluid was positive in 56% of 189 patients. In all studies except that of Fowler and Manitsas (28) the identification of tubercle bacilli in the pericardial fluid depended on culture, thereby delaying diagnosis for several weeks. Our experience is the same, as in none of our patients was tubercle bacillus identified by stained smears.

The diagnostic value of adenosine deaminase activity measurement in pericardial fluid has already been discussed.

Pericardial biopsy

In our series, pericardial biopsy was diagnostic in all three cases in which it was carried out. In addition, tuberculosis was demonstrated in all eight pericardiectomy specimens that were investigated. The diagnostic yield of the histological study of the pericardium was, therefore, very high. Information in the literature regarding the diagnostic yield of pericardial biopsy for tuberculous pericarditis in developed countries is scanty. The report by Cheitlin et al. (29), often quoted as an example of the shortcomings of biopsy for the diagnosis of tuberculous pericarditis, described only two patients, in one of

whom the result of histologic study was a false negative. In the series by
Fowler and Manitsas (28), biopsy was carried out in only three of the 19
patients. Hageman et al (30) made the histologic diagnosis of tuberculous
pericarditis in 10 out of 44 patients, but it is unclear whether by biopsy or
pericardiectomy. Rooney et al (14) reported only three biopsies in 35
patients. In the study with the highest number of pericardial biopsies (4), carried out in an African population, biopsy was positive in 27 of 32 patients
(84%) with positive culture of tubercle bacillus in pericardial fluid. Therefore,
it seems that histologic examination of the pericardium has a high diagnostic
yield for the diagnosis of tuberculous pericarditis.

With our study protocol, the interval between admission and diagnosis
ranged between one and 14 weeks (mean 6.1). This long delay was due in the
main to the time required for the organism to grow on culture medium. The
cases diagnosed earliest (1–2 weeks) were those in whom the diagnosis was
made by pleural or lymph node biopsy. The delay in diagnosis was unaccept-
ably long in most other cases, even though we followed a systematic prospective protocol. This delay may have played a part in the frequent progression to
constrictive pericarditis, which developed in nine of our patients. Reduction
of this delay is a major challenge in tuberculous pericarditis. We hope that the
measurements of adenosine deaminase activity in pleural or pericardial fluid
or both may prove of substantial help in this regard.

Clinical features

The 16 patients in our series were whites. Fourteen were males and two females. They were not immunologically compromised, and their ages ranged
between 13 and 70 years (mean 44 years). Male predominance had also been
pointed out by Schepers (2). Three patients had had symptoms for less than
two weeks before admission, one between two weeks and one month, seven
between one and three months, and five more than three months. The interval
between the onset of symptoms and admission ranged between one day and
four months (mean 8 weeks).

Eleven patients had chest pain suggestive of pericarditis, 8 had dyspnea, 7
had cough, 8 had lost weight and 4 had increased perspiration. The major
clinical findings are listed in Table 6.2. The tuberculin skin test was negative
in 5 of the 15 patients in which it was performed. The chest radiogram
showed pulmonary infiltrate or lymph node enlargement in four patients; in
the other 12 the only abnormality was pleural effusion in 10. The frequency
of these signs and symptoms was somewhat variable in three large series (14,
28, 30). Thus, in the series by Fowler and Manitsas (28), 94% of the patients
had cough and 76% chest pain, whereas these symptoms were present in only
48% and 39% of the patients in the series by Hageman et al (30). In addition,
Fowler and Manitsas (28) reported cardiomegaly in 95% of their patients
(assumed to be caused by pericardial effusion), while it was reported in 85%

Table 6.2. Clinical findings (n: 16).

Fever	15 (94%)
Pericardial effusion	15 (94%)
Pericardial rub	12 (75%)
Pleural effusion	10 (62%)
Cardiac tamponade	7 (44%)

of the patients by Rooney et al. (14) and in only 48% of those in the series by Hageman et al. (30). In these series, pericardial rub was present in 37%–84% and hemodynamic compromise in 46%–71%. In the series by Fowler and Manitsas (28), 32% had pulmonary infiltrates. The rate of positive tuberculin skin tests in our series was similar to that reported by Fowler and Manitsas (28), but much lower than that reported by Rooney et al. (14) (100%). The high prevalence (58–71%) of pleural effusion in these series is in agreement with our findings, and we emphasize its importance as it may point the way to earlier diagnosis of tuberculosis.

Clinical course

The presentation and clinical course of our 16 patients with tuberculous peri-carditis was remarkably variable. Virtually all acute pericardial syndromes were observed. Thus, one patient had acute dry pericarditis, 4 had apparently self limited effusive pericarditis, one patient had recurrent tamponade, 5 had tamponade effectively managed by pericardiocentesis, and one had tam-ponade but developed subacute constriction after pericardiocentesis. Finally, 4 had toxic symptoms with persistent fever. In six patients the course looked as though it would be self limited. In these instances, the initial diagnosis was idiopathic pericarditis. The correct diagnosis was made after the result of cul-ture of sputum or pericardial fluid, or examination of the pericardiectomy specimen (one patient) became available. The possibility of tuberculous peri-carditis of acute onset and apparently self limited features has already been pointed out (1, 2), even with recurrent evolution (17). Our experience is in agreement with others (16, 31) who point out that one of the features of tuberculous pericarditis is its variability and that there is no characteristic pat-tern or combination of symptoms and signs. Accordingly, tuberculous peri-carditis should always be considered in the differential diagnosis of pericar-ditis of unknown origin.

Pericardial effusion may be a prominent feature at presentation, but even without specific treatment, may diminish or disappear in the weeks preceding the availability of the results of culture. We observed this phenomenon in four cases, three of which went on to constrictive pericarditis. We established the correct diagnosis early in two other cases and therefore we were not in a posi-tion to observe the spontaneous course of their pericardial effusion. We never observed evolution to a large chronic pericardial effusion, probably as a result of treatment, but conceivably because of the natural course of the disease.

Treatment

All patients received triple antituberculous chemotherapy with isoniazid (5 mg/kg/day for nine months), rifampin (10 mg/kg/day for nine months), and ethambutol (25 mg/kg/day for three months). Six patients received prednisone as advised by the attending physician. On this point the protocol was not strict, and no firm conclusion can be drawn about the possible usefulness of treatment with prednisone. It should be pointed out, however, that three of the six developed constriction as compared with six of the ten who were not treated with that drug. Rooney et al. (14) compared 28 patients from their series who received only antituberculous chemotherapy with 18 who also received prednisone, and insisted on the beneficial effect of steroid treatment on the suppression of inflammatory features and the reabsorption of pericardial fluid. They went so far as to suggest that the overall outcome was better and the mortality rate less in the patients treated with prednisone. Likewise, Strang et al (4), reporting a controlled study, suggested that corticosteroids improved the outcome of the patients with tuberculous pericardial effusion. Although these authors (4, 14) recommend the use of corticosteroids in all patients with tuberculous pericarditis, there is no evidence that constriction was prevented in their patients.

Late course

Eight of our 16 patients developed classical constrictive pericarditis and one developed effusive constrictive pericarditis within six months after admission. This high incidence of constriction is striking, but it is in agreement with the experience of most authors. This complication appeared in six of Wood's 21 patients (1), in 21 of 44 patients in the series of Hageman at al (30), and in seven of the 19 patients in the series by Fowler and Manitsas (28), and in 22 of 198 in the series by Strang et al. (4). The development of constriction is virtually always subacute, occurring within the first few months; later constriction is much less common. In the 9 patients of our series in whom pericardiectomy was carried out, the operation was indicated for severe constriction. Pericardiectomy was not indicated in any of our cases for persistence of effusion or the lack of response of fever or symptoms to medical treatment. Although some authors (32, 33) have advocated a more aggressive approach, advising pericardiectomy in all patients who do not show a prompt response to pharmacologic treatment, a recent series (33a) points to the contrary.

Analysis of the interval between the onset of symptoms and starting specific therapy (Fig. 6.1) does not separate the patients who required pericar-

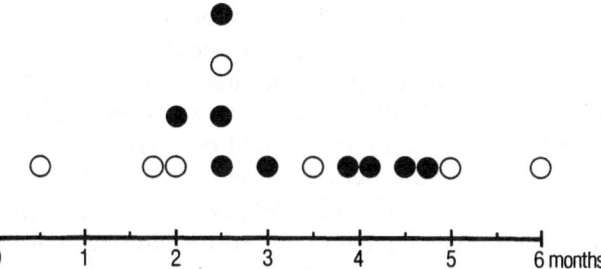

Fig. 6.1. Interval between the onset of the disease and the institution of chemotherapy. The empty circles indicate the patients who did not require pericardiectomy, while the black circles indicate those who did require it.

diectomy from those who did not. It should once more be emphasized, however, that the diagnosis usually required several weeks after the onset of symptoms. It is possible that earlier diagnosis migh favorably influence this outcome. Hageman et al. (30) concluded that early therapy reduced the need for pericardiectomy: only four of the 13 patients in their series in whom the diagnosis was made within the first four weeks required pericardiectomy, while it was required in 11 of the 19 in whom the diagnosis was delayed longer than 12 weeks.

After hospital discharge all patients were followed in the outpatient clinic. Follow up has ranged between one month and six years (mean 28.5 months). No patient developed constrictive pericarditis later than 3.5 months after admission. The patients who had undergone pericardiectomy also had a satisfactory clinical evolution; however, residual features of constriction were seen in the echocardiogram and external recordings in three patients (6, 12 and 12 months, respectively, after pericardiectomy). However, none of these patients had elevated venous pressure. Pericardiectomy was technically difficult in these patients because of the tight adhesion between the pericardial layers. No patient of the series died.

Clinical recommendations

Although tuberculous pericarditis is a comparatively uncommon condition (5.2% of primary acute pericardial disease in our most recent experience), it still represents a serious clinical challenge. The variability of the clinical presentation makes it mandatory to consider tuberculosis in all instances of pericarditis which do not quickly show spontaneous resolution. The major problem is to arrive expeditiously at the correct diagnosis. Diagnosis should be based on a systematic approach.

On the basis of our experience (12, 18, 20, 22, 34) we think that the following workup might be the most effective for the identification of tuberculous pericarditis: In all patients with acute pericarditis persisting for more than one week, or with tamponade or other severe clinical features, three examinations of sputum or gastric aspirate should be carried out. In addition, adenosine deaminase activity should be measured in the pleural fluid when present. Pleural biopsy should be considered when adenosine deaminase activity is high. Lymph node biopsy should be carried out in all patients with prominent lymphadenopathy. Pericardiocentesis should be limited to patients with cardiac tamponade. Pericardial biopsy should be performed for tamponade persisting or relapsing after pericardiocentesis and for failure to remit after three weeks; it might be considered for cases with high adenosine deaminase activity in the pleural or pericardial fluid. Further experience is needed to establish the definitive diagnostic value of the latter finding, which might permit to avoid pericardial biopsy in selected patients. In patients with AIDS, the diagnostic approach should be individualized, considering the possibly higher prevalence of tuberculous infection in this population and their lower adenosine deaminase activity.

Following this approach, tuberculous pericarditis may occasionally be missed and not diagnosed until subsequent pericardiectomy, as in one of our patients. Diagnostic pericardiocentesis or biopsy should nonetheless be limited in any geographic region in which the incidence of tuberculous pericarditis is low, as their diagnostic yield is poor when carried out in patients without hemodynamic compromise and wider indications would result in many unnecessary invasive procedures.

References

1. Wood JA. Tuberculous pericarditis. A study of forty-one cases with special reference to prognosis. Am Heart J 1951; 42: 737–745.
2. Schepers GWH. Tuberculous pericarditis. Am J Cardiol 1962; 9: 248–276.
3. Strang JIG, Gibson DG, Nunn AJ, Kakaza HHS, Girling DJ, Fox W. Controlled trial of prednisolone as adjuvant in treatment of tuberculous constrictive pericarditis in Transkei. Lancet 1987; ii: 1418–1422.
4. Strang JIG, Gibson DG, Mitchison DA, Girling DJ, Kakaza HHS, Allen BW, Evans DJ, Nunn AJ. Controlled clinical trial of complete open surgical drainage and of prednisolone in treatment of tuberculous pericardial effusion in Transkei. Lancet 1988; ii: 759–763.
5. Gooi HL, Smith JN. Tuberculous pericarditis in Birmingham. Thorax 1978; 33: 94–96.
6. Williams IP, Hetzel MR. Tuberculous pericarditis in South-west London: an increasing problem. Thorax 1978; 33: 816–817.
7. De Miguel Prieto J, Rivas JJ, Freire D, Campos V, Pérez Alvarez L, Pedreira JD. Pericarditis tuberculosa. Rev Clin Esp 1985; 176: 39–41.
8. Pastor Torres L, Vázquez García R, Caparrós Valderrama J, Peláez Domínguez S, Gómez Mateos JS. Pericarditis tuberculosa primaria. Rev Esp Cardiol 1986; 39: 159–161.
9. Sunderam G, McDonald RJ, Maniatis T, Oleske J, Kapila R, Reichman LB. Tuberculosis as a manifestation of the acquired immunodeficiency syndrome (AIDS). JAMA 1986; 256: 362–366.
10. Dalli E, Quesada A, Juan G, Navarro R, Payá R, Tormo V. Tuberculous pericarditis as the first manifestation of acquired immunodeficiency syndrome. Am Heart J 1987; 114: 905–906.

11. D'Cruz IV, Seńgupta EE, Abrahams C, Reddy HK, Turlapati RV: Cardiac involvement, including tuberculous pericardial effusion, complicating acquired immune deficiency syndrome. Am Heart J 1986; 112: 1100–1101.
12. Sagristà-Sauleda J, Permanyer-Miralda G, Soler-Soler J. Tuberculous pericarditis: ten year experience with a prospective protocol for diagnosis and treatment. J Am Coll Cardiol 1988; 11: 724–728.
13. Shapiro JB, Weiss W. Tuberculous pericarditis with effusion: impact of antimicrobial therapy. Am J M Sc 1953; 229240.
14. Rooney JJ, Crocco JA, Lyons HA. Tuberculous pericarditis. Ann Intern Med 1970; 72: 73–78.
15. Katz I, Rosenthal T, Michaeli D. Undiagnosed tuberculosis in hospitalized patients. Chest 1985, 87: 770–774.
16. Spodick DH. Tuberculous pericarditis. Arch Intern Med 1956; 98: 737–749.
17. Janovsky RC, Boettner JF, Van-Ordstrand HS. Recurrent tuberculous pericarditis. Ann Intern Med 1952; 37: 1268–1274.
18. Permanyer-Miralda G. Estudi etiològic de les malalties agudes del pericardi. Tesi Doctoral. Universitat Autònoma de Barcelona, 1986.
19. March P, Alcaide J. Salleras L, Gili M. Anàlisi epidemiològica de la infecció i malaltia tuberculosa a Catalunya. In: Informe: La tuberculosi a Catalunya. Generalitat de Catalunya. Departament de Sanitat i Seguretat Social. Barcelona, 1983; 33–85.
20. Permanyer-Miralda G, Sagristà-Sauleda J, Soler-Soler J. Primary acute pericardial disease. A prospective series of 231 consecutive patients. Am J Cardiol 1985; 56: 623–630.
21. Martínez Vázquez JM, Ribera E, Ocaña I, Segura RM, Serrat R, Sagristà J. Adenosine deaminase activity in tuberculous pericarditis. Thorax 1986; 41: 888–889.
22. Sagristà-Sauleda J. Permanyer-Miralda G, Soler-Soler J. Tuberculous pericarditis. Cardiol Board Rev 1989; 6: 114–120.
23. Ocaña I, Martínez Vázquez JM, Segura RM, Fernández de Sevilla T, Capdevila JA. Adenosine deaminase in pleural fluids. A test for the diagnosis of tuberculous pleural effusion. Chest 1983; 84: 51–53.
24. Niwa Y, Kishimoto H, Shimokata K. Carcinomatous and tuberculous pleural effusions. Comparison of tumor markers. Chest 1985; 87: 351–355.
25. Pettersson T, Ojala K, Weber TH. Adenosine deaminase in the diagnosis of pleural effusions. Acta Med Scand 1984; 215: 299–304.
26. Pettersson T, Klockars M, Weber T. Pleural fluid adenosine deaminase in rheumatoid arthritis and systemic lupus erythematosus. Chest 1984; 86: 273.
27. Pérez Vidal R, Arán X, Broquetas J. High adenosine deaminase activity level in pleural effusion. Chest 1986; 90: 625.
28. Fowler NO, Manitsas GT. Infectious pericarditis. Prog Cardiovasc Dis 1973; 16: 323–338.
29. Cheitlin MD, Serfas LJ, Abard SS, Glaasser SP. Tuberculous pericarditis: is limited pericardial biopsy sufficient for diagnosis? Am Rev Resp Dis 1968; 98: 287–291.
30. Hageman GH, D'Esopo ND, Glenn WL. Tuberculosis of the pericardium. A long-term analysis of forty-four proved cases. N Eng J Med 1964; 270: 327–332.
31. Gleckman RA. Nonviral infectious pericarditis. In: Spodick DH, ed. Pericardial diseases. Philadelphia, FA Davis Co, 1976: 159–176.
32. Holman E, Willett F. Treatment of active tuberculous pericarditis by pericardiectomy. JAMA 1951; 146: 1–7.
33. Carson TJ, Murray GF, Wilcox BR. The role of surgery in tuberculous pericarditis. Ann Thorac Surg 1974; 17: 163–167.
33a. Long R, Younes M, Patton N, Hershfield E. Tuberculous pericarditis: long-term outcome in patients who received medical therapy alone. Amer Heart J 1989; 117: 1133–1139.
34. Sagristà-Sauleda J, Permanyer-Miralda G, Soler-Soler J. Utilidad clínica de la pericardiocentesis y de la biopsia pericárdica en las enfermedades agudas del pericardio. Rev Esp Cardiol 1987; 40: 94–99.

7. Pericardial involvement in end stage renal disease

M. MORLANS, M.D.

Definition

Our definition of pericardial involvement in end stage renal disease includes all types of pericardial disease in uremic patients, whether or not they have started any modality of dialysis. We therefore agree that the term uremic pericarditis should be reserved for pericardial involvement in advanced uremia, assuming that pericardial disease in patients on hemodialysis might have a different etiology and pathogenesis (1, 2). Uremic pericarditis is an example of the changes brought about by the advances in medicine in the incidence, clinical presentation and outcome of several diseases. The response of the pericardium to far advanced uremia, in the form of a fibrinous exudate with adhesion between the two layers and invasion and organization of the space between them has long been known as a complication that often heralds death (3–6). Its evolution to cardiac tamponade was considered to be exceptional (7), probably because the patients died without the benefit of dialysis. The introduction of dialysis has modified the history of this condition, reducing the incidence of uremic pericarditis while resulting in the more common development of tamponade. Usually, tamponade develops during the dialysis session or immediately afterwards (8–15). This condition, which is potentially lethal, has given rise to a variety of therapeutic approaches

123

J. Soler-Soler et al. (Eds.), Pericardial Disease, pp. 123–139.

ranging from intensification of dialysis (12, 14, 16) to drainage of pericardial effusion (8, 9, 12, 14, 16–22). The introduction of echocardiography has allowed us to detect silent effusion which disappears with dialysis and ultra-filtration in the uremic patients (23–26) and to follow the clinical course of effusive pericarditis (27–30). The nature of these effusions and the etiology and pathogenesis of pericardial disease in patients receiving hemodialysis are controversial, as reflected in several reviews (1, 2, 31–36).

In the present chapter, we analyze the different diagnostic and therapeutic aspects of this condition on the basis of personal experience, gained by following a prospective protocol (p. 223). We compare our results with those in the literature and we propose a clinical classification to permit the identification of subsets who may benefit from given therapeutic approaches. We include 85 patients with end stage renal disease (creatinine clearance of 5 ml/min or less) in whom pericarditis, pericardial effusion or cardiac tamponade were identified between January 1978 to December 1985. For the diagnosis of pericarditis we required at least two of the following: suggestive chest pain, pericardial friction rub and characteristic electrocardiographic changes. We considered cytologic and biochemical inflammatory features in pericardial fluid as diagnostic of pericarditis, even in the absence of clinical criteria. The presence of pericardial effusion was established by M mode echocardiography. We are including in the study only effusions that were considered as moderate or large (sum of the anterior and posterior echo free space, measured at the level of the mitral valve tip, between 10–20 mm or higher than 20 mm, respectively (37)). When, in the presence of significant pericardial effusion, systolic blood pressure was 80 mmHg or less, venous pressure was elevated or pulsus paradoxus was 10 mmHg or more the diagnosis of cardiac tamponade was made unless the findings could be explained by other conditions such as overhydration or heart failure. The statistical differences were evaluated with the Mann-Whitney's U rank test.

Epidemiology

Figures on the incidence of pericardial disease in end stage renal disease are widely variable. It has been stated that its frequency among uremic patients has been reduced since renal failure is treated with dialysis; on the other hand, pericardial involvement among those already treated by dialysis has increased (31). Its reported frequency varies between 12 and 41% (10, 12, 27, 32). This wide difference may depend on the epoch when the series was collected, the size of the population at risk, the duration of follow up, and whether pericardial diseases diagnosed soon after dialysis is started were included as uremic or associated with hemodialysis. In our Service we consider pericarditis diagnosed during the first three months of dialysis as uremic, because we accept that complications of the uremic syndrome are more common during that period (10, 12). The incidence of pericardial dis-

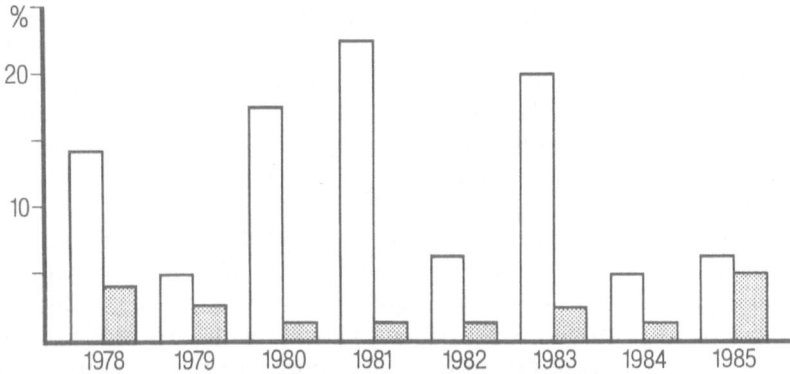

Fig. 7.1. Incidence of pericardial disease in end stage renal disease in untreated patients (open bars) and in patients on hemodialysis (stipled bars) shown as cases/100 patients/year.

ease (Fig. 7.1) varied between 5 and 23 cases/100 patients/year in 444 patients with end stage renal disease identified between January 1978 and December 1985. The frequency of pericardial disease in patients treated with dialysis, as reported in the literature, ranges between 6 and 15% (10, 12, 27, 32). Its incidence in our own patients on hemodialysis varied between 1 and 4 cases/100 patients/year. The number of hemodialysis patients years ranged from 187 to 228 (mean 210). The incidence of pericardial disease was five times greater among uremic patients than in those on hemodialysis. Furthermore, a tendency towards a reduced incidence was not confirmed in either group.

Pericarditis is thought to be commoner among young patients and in females (12, 16). The first aspect, but not the second, was confirmed in our series (Table 7.1). The mean age of the 49 uremic patients with pericardial disease was significantly lower than the mean age of the population at risk.

Table 7.1. Mean age, range and male to female ratio in patients with pericardial involvement in untreated end stage renal disease (UP) and in those on hemodialysis (PHD), as compared with the overall group of untreated uremic patients and the overall group on hemodialysis.

	UP (n: 49)	All untreated (n: 444)	PHD (n: 36)	All hemodialysis (n: 340)
Mean age (range)	$47(17–76) \leftarrow^{*} \rightarrow$	$54(15–80)$	$43(19–65) \leftarrow^{**} \rightarrow$	$49(15–85)$
Male-to-female ratio	23 : 26 (47%)	244 : 200 (55%)	20 : 16 (56%)	204 : 136 (60%)

*: $p < 0.001$,
**: $p < 0.01$.

Forty-seven percent were males and 53% females, while male to female ratio
was 55/45 in our uremic patients. We identified 36 episodes of pericardial
disease in patients who had been treated by hemodialysis from 4 to 116
months (mean 32 months). Their mean age was significantly younger than the
mean age of the population on dialysis. There were no differences in the sex
distribution: 56% males and 44% females in patients with pericarditis, and
60% and 40%, respectively, in patients on dialysis.

Although in previous reports it had been stated that uremic pericarditis
was more common in patients with chronic glomerulonephritis or vascular
nephropathy (32), we did not observe significant differences in the distribution of the type of primary disease among patients with pericardial disease
and the populations at risk, except for the absence of pericardial disease in
patients being dialyzed for vascular nephropathy (Fig. 7.2).

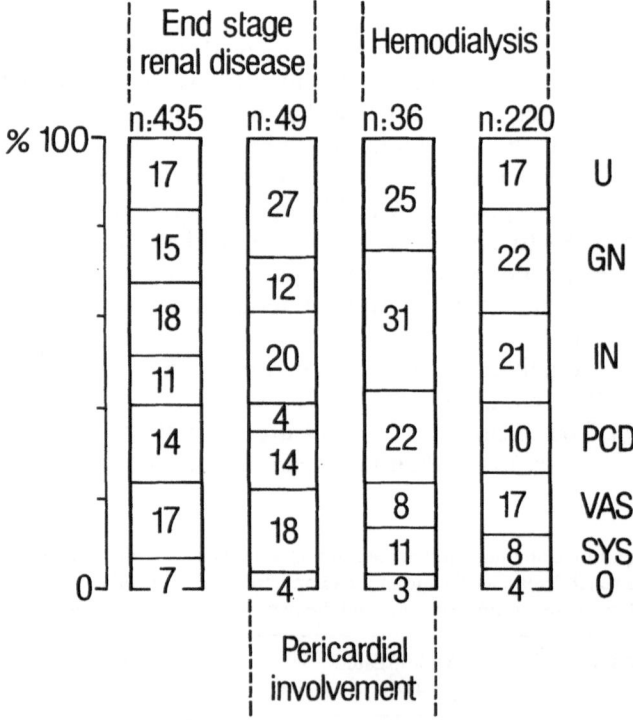

Fig. 7.2. Percent distribution of the underlying renal disease in patients with pericardial involvement in untreated end stage renal disease (second histogram from the left) and in those on
hemodialysis (third histogram), as compared with the same distribution in the overall group of
untreated uremic patients (first histogram) and in the overall group on hemodialysis patients
(fourth histogram). Abbreviations of the underlying renal disease: U: unknown; GN: glomerular
nephropathy; IN: interstitial nephropathy; PCD: polycystic disease; VAS: vascular disease; SYS:
systemic disease; O: other.

Etiology

To date, the mechanisms whereby the pericardium is damaged in uremia are unknown. In studies carried out to correlate the plasma level of retained nitrogen products with the incidence of pericarditis, it has been shown that nitrogen retention is not greater in patients with pericarditis than in the remaining population (12, 27, 30, 32). These studies should be interpreted with caution, as the substances evaluated (urea, creatinine, uric acid and phosphorus), although reflecting the degree of renal failure, are not toxic in themselves. This lack of correlation has given rise to the hypothesis that the culprit might be substances of medium molecular weight (38). These middle molecules could be implicated in the pathogenesis of pericarditis, because their plasma level is higher in the patients with pericarditis (39); pericarditis is also less frequent in patients treated with peritoneal dialysis (16), and it is known that peritoneum is more permeable than artificial membranes to middle molecules (38). The hemorrhagic character of some of the pericardial effusions has raised the hypothesis that the coagulation disorders of uremic patients (impaired platelet aggregation, reduced fibrinolytic activity, etc.) might be implicated in the pathogenesis (35, 40). The institution of hemodialysis, which requires anticoagulation, might result in pericardial hemorrhage and in an increase of the volume of the effusion; this would explain the poor course of these patients despite dialysis. Therefore, techniques to limit the effect of heparin have been devised (12, 14).

There are many factors that have been implicated as possibly precipitating or facilitating pericarditis in hemodialysis patients: poor condition of the vascular access, bacterial infection, trauma, major surgical procedures and secondary hyperparathyroidism (9, 10, 12). All of them result in insufficient dialysis, either because flow via the vascular access is inadequate, or because hypercatabolism precipitated by infection, trauma or surgical procedure requires a greater number of dialysis hours per week to remove the catabolic products. Patients who are stable on chronic hemodialysis and show clinical and biochemical criteria of a good control may develop pericarditis without the occurrence of the above mentioned risk factors. In a few patients of this type infective agents such as cytomegalovirus (41), Coxsackie A or B, influenza or echovirus (42) have been recovered, but most authors agree that, in spite of strong clinical suspicion, it is difficult to identify a specific causative organism (12, 17, 27, 29, 30). This was also our experience, as all cultures from our patients were negative. The only indirect evidence was the demonstration of an epidemic of pericarditis concomitant with the seroconversion of the surface antigen of the hepatitis B virus (43), for which a possible etiologic role has been recently claimed (44). An epidemic of pericarditis was detected in another dialysis unit. A viral etiology was suspected although serologic studies for respiratory syncytial virus were positive in only one patient (45). The problems of identifying the cause of pericarditis associated with hemodialysis are similar to those of primary acute pericardial disease

128 M. MORLANS

(46). Purulent pericarditis is extremely uncommon in the uremic patient (8), and it was not identified in any of our cases.

Recent studies have emphasized that immunological mechanisms mediated by immunocomplexes may have a causative role in serositis in the uremic patient (47), particularly in the case of pericarditis (48).

In the patient with end stage renal disease, minimally symptomatic pericardial effusion associated with congestive heart failure or fluid overload may appear (26, 27, 29, 30, 32). These effusions disappear with dialysis and ultrafiltration (49), suggesting that these effusions are transudates. Similar effusions are more commonly found at the beginning of the dialysis therapy (23–25).

It is very likely that in many instances of pericardial disease in end stage renal disease several of the mentioned factors may coexist; therefore, the etiology and pathogenesis of this condition should be considered as multifactorial until further information is available.

Clinical features

Although in some patients the clinical picture of pericarditis is full blown (chest pain, fever, pericardial friction rub and characteristic electrocardiographic changes), in others most symptoms are absent and the only feature of pericardial disease may be a friction rub. In fact, this is the most commonly reported finding (12, 16), as it was in our series (Table 7.2). Our series confirmed previous observations that fever is more common among patients receiving hemodialysis than in untreated uremic patients (12, 32). In our cases, characteristic chest pain and fever were significantly more common in patients treated by hemodialysis (Table 7.2), supporting our impression that pericardial disease is more silent in uremic patients than in those on a hemodialysis regimen. However, in both groups, we observed additional cases where a diagnosis of acute pericarditis was made from the inflammatory character of the pericardial fluid but our clinical criteria were not fulfilled (Table 7.3). We disagree with those authors who attempt to distinguish between exudates and transudates by purely clinical means (27, 29). In addi-

Table 7.2. Frequency of diagnostic criteria for pericarditis in patients with pericardial involvement in the overall group (ESRD), the uremic subset (UP) and the subset on hemodialysis program (PHD).

	ESRD (n: 85)	UP (n: 49)	PHD (n: 36)
Pericardial rub	64 (75%)	36 (73%)	28 (78%)
Chest pain	49 (58%)	23 (47%) ←*→ 26 (72%)	
Fever	32 (38%)	12 (24%) ←*→ 20 (58%)	
ECG changes	29 (34%)	20 (41%)	9 (25%)

* p<0.01.

Table 7.3. Pericarditis, complications and procedures in uremic patients (UP) and patients on hemodialysis (PHD) with pericardial involvement.

	UP (n: 49)	PHD (n: 36)
Pericarditis (clinical criteria)	28 (57%)	26 (72%)
Pericarditis (effusion characteristics criteria)	6 (12%)	4 (11%)
All pericarditis	34 (69%)	30 (83%)
Pericardial effusion	39 (80%)	32 (90%)
Pleural effusion	40 (82%) ←—*—→ 15 (42%)	
Heart failure	27 (55%) ←—*—→ 7 (19%)	
Cardiac tamponade	7 (14%)	11 (31%)
Pericardiocentesis	11 (22%)	15 (42%)
Pericardiectomy	2 (4%)	6 (17%)

* $p < 0.001$.

tion, we emphasize the potential risk of tamponade in barely symptomatic effusions (50).

The most useful laboratory investigation in the management of nephrogenic pericardial disease is echocardiography. It is useful for detecting small clinically silent effusions (23–26) and in following the evolution of effusive pericarditis (27–30).

Associated pleural effusion is common (65%) (12, 16). Some of these effusions are secondary to heart failure or fluid retentin, present in 40% of cases. Not surprisingly, heart failure and pleural effusion are significantly more common in the uremic patients than in those on dialysis (Table 7.3), reflecting the water and sodium retention. When heart failure is absent, we have found that pleural effusion is usually on the left (51), as is true for pericarditis of other etiologies (52).

Classification

We divided pericardial involvement into five categories: uremic, hemodynamic, infective, due to inadequate dialysis and unknown. In end stage renal disease it is particularly helpful to differentiate inflammatory pericarditis of

Table 7.4. Clinical classification of pericardial disease in end stage renal disease.

	Number of cases
Uremic pericarditis	34 (40%)
Pericardial effusion associated with heart failure, overhydration or both	21 (25%)
Possible viral infection	12 (13%)
Inadequate dialysis	9 (11%)
Absence of predisposing factors	9 (11%)

uncertain origin from pericardial transudate due to congestive heart failure or fluid retention and to analyze the outcome and response to therapy of both types separately. Few authors have really done so, but our retrospective classification (Table 7.4) does, and aims to identify subsets that might benefit from a similar therapeutic approach. In addition to our clinical criteria for acute pericarditis, we accept this diagnosis when the fluid obtained by pericardiocentesis is an exudate, containing inflammatory cells.

Uremic pericarditis

We classify as uremic pericarditis patients with the above characteristics and end stage renal disease who have either not been dialysed or are within the first three months of dialysis. They included 40% of our patients.

Pericardial effusion associated with heart failure or overhydration

We saw 21 cases of pericardial effusion, 14 of which were in uremic patients, that were due to heart failure or fluid overload without clinical criteria of pericarditis. Pericardial effusion resolved with dialysis and ultrafiltration, and cardiac tamponade did not develop in any of them. In 12 of these patients a pericardial friction rub was heard but we did not accept this as evidence of inflammation because the remaining clinical criteria for pericarditis were not met. Transudation is the most likely cause of effusion in these patients, and we prefer to include them in a separate category, in which the only instance of effusion shown by pericardiocentesis to be a transudate was included. Twenty-five percent of our patients fell in this category.

Possible viral infections

Patients with clinical features of pericarditis or with inflammatory characteristics in the pericardial fluid who had previously had fever with constitutional symptoms such as pharyngitis or pneumonitis, or who presented during an epidemic, were considered as infective; this was presumed to be viral in spite of negative cultures. They accounted for 13% and were in the group on a stable hemodialysis regimen.

Inadequate dialysis

The following characteristics were required before we adscribed pericardial disease to inadequate dialysis: poor vascular access, previous use of a filter with too small a surface for the patient's height and weight, and hypercata-

bolic states without a corresponding increase in dialysis hours. Eleven percent of our patients were included in this category.

Absence of predisposing factors

There was an additional 11% of instances of pericarditis in patients on hemodialysis who had no preceding clinical findings which would allow us to include them in any of the preceding groups. Fever was present in some of
them, but was not by itself a sufficient reason to include them in the category
of infective pericarditis.

Complications

Cardiac tamponade

Cardiac tamponade due to uremic pericarditis was an exceptional occurrence
before the introduction of dialysis (7, 8), perhaps because the untreated
patients died earlier or perhaps because dialysis itself can induce cardiac
tamponade. Coincident with the widespread use of dialysis, an increase of the
frequence of tamponade has been observed (25%); it has been reported to
occur in 14–55% of all identified instances of uremic pericarditis (13), with a
remarkable temporal relationship with hemodialysis and a high mortality rate
(between 13% and 43% of all instances of tamponade) (9, 12, 14, 16, 19, 20,
29). We saw 18 instances of tamponade, in nine of which it was the presenting
feature of pericardial involvement. One of the 18 died before pericardiocentesis could be carried out, and in two others it had previously been performed
for persistent large pericardial effusion. The overall prevalence of tamponade
in our series was 21%. Although tamponade was more common in the
patients undergoing hemodialysis on a regular basis than in the group of
uremic patients, this difference was not statistically significant (Table 7.3).
    Persistent hypotension, or hypotension associated with hemodialysis, with
or without elevated central venous pressure, is a common presentation of
pericardial disease in end stage renal disease (28, 53, 54). This was true in
half of the instances of tamponade in the present series. In some of these
patients, pulsus paradoxus is not detected (55, 56). Catheterization studies
have proved the absence of pulsus paradoxus in a group of hemodialysis
patients with cardiac tamponade (56). A feature common to all these patients
was the coexistence of left ventricular dysfunction documented by grossly
elevated left ventricular diastolic pressure. Hypertension, anemia, cardiomyopathy, fluid overload and left ventricular failure are common in these
cases.
    Echocardiographic signs of cardiac tamponade increase the diagnostic
reliability of this technique (57–59). Hemodynamic evaluation including the

measurement of pericardial pressure is the most specific method for diagnosing cardiac tamponade (56, 60), but is often unnecessary. We advised catheterization only to confirm the development of constriction or when diagnosis was unusually difficult; for instance, in a case of cardiac tamponade with effusion predominantly localized to the anterior space (61). Thus, in our protocol the diagnosis of tamponade was established when significant pericardial effusion, demonstrated by echocardiography, was present, associated with any of the three previously mentioned clinical signs.

A cornerstone for successful management of pericardial effusion in end stage renal disease is understanding the close relationship between the performance of dialysis and the appearance of tamponade. A clinical report (8) and a catheterization study carried out during a hemodialysis session (11) helped us to elaborate the following hypothesis. In conventional dialysis, two simultaneous phenomena take place through the semipermeable peritoneal or filter membrane; solute diffusion down the concentration gradient and the plasma ultrafiltration, favored by a difference in hydrostatic pressure. In Fig. 7.3 the main elements of an ultrafiltration circuit are represented. Blood from the arteriovenous fistula is propelled by a pump through a filter consisting of a semipermeable membrane. With equivalent levels of blood flow, greater ultrafiltration is obtained by increasing the outflow resistance of the filter with a clamp that regulates the venous return. A great degree of ultrafiltration results when central venous pressure is elevated, such as occurs in overhydration. It is likely that increase in central venous pressure in patients with hemodynamically stable cardiac tamponade undergoing dialysis may induce excessive ultrafiltration with the resulting depletion of intravascular volume, hypotension and development of life threatening tamponade.

Other complications

Rare cases of pericardial effusion with subacute evolution to constrictive pericarditis have been reported after apparent recovery from an episode of acute pericarditis (9). Chronic constrictive pericarditis as a late complication of acute episodes of pericardial disease is exceptional (16, 62) but, when suspected, should be confirmed by cardiac catheterization (60). Specific causes, particularly tuberculosis, it should always be ruled out. We did not find these complications in our patients, although among our last cases we observed, probably as a consequence of a high suspicion index, transient cardiac constriction confirmed by external recordings and echocardiogram in the resolution phase of two episodes of acute pericarditis in patients on hemodialysis. The findings of cardiac constriction disappeared spontaneously, as has been reported in some cases of acute idiopathic effusive pericarditis (63).

Cardiac arrhythmias, mainly atrial fibrillation or flutter, are more common in these patients (uremic and hemodialysis associated pericarditis) than in idiopathic pericarditis (64), being found in 14–37% of cases (32, 43). Ar-

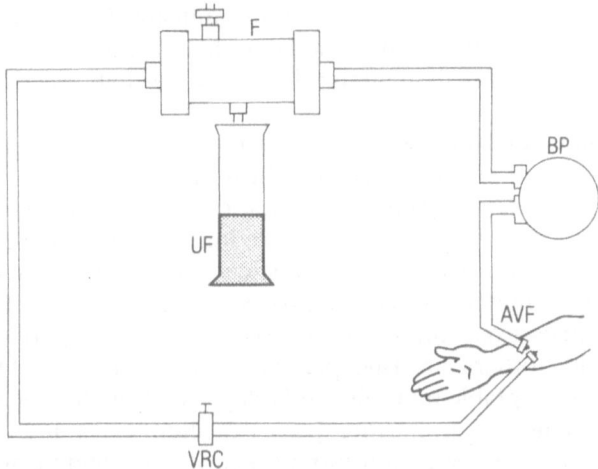

Fig. 7.3. Ultrafiltration circuit. AVF: arteriovenous fistula; BP: blood pump; F: filter; UF: ultra-filtrate; VRC: venous return clamp. See discussion in text.

rhythmia is facilitated by predisposing factors such as cardiomyopathy, hypertension, electrolyte imbalance or sudden changes in circulating blood volume. These factors aggravate the hemodynamic consequences of arrhythmia. Termination of arrhythmia is therefore mandatory. Detection of arrhythmia in uremic patients should suggest the possibility of pericardial involvement.

Treatment

An important controversy in the management of these patients relates to the optimal dialysis regimen to facilitate the resolution of pericardial involvement and to prevent tamponade. Some authors recommend maintaining the usual hemodialysis schedule (19, 20, 27), whereas others favor increasing the frequency of hemodialysis using regional heparinization (12, 14, 17, 29), or even substituting peritoneal dialysis (16). Although this latter procedure reduces the number of instances of cardiac tamponade, tamponade may still occur. the main drawbacks of peritoneal dialysis are two: its longer duration and the consequently decreased patient compliance with the program, and the risk of peritonitis due to the handling of the intraperitoneal catheter. For these reasons we have now limited the indications for peritoneal dialysis, that we initially advocated for all cases of pericardial disease (43, 54), to patients who lack an adequate vascular access.

We believe that corticosteroids and nosteroidal antiinflammatory drugs should be avoided whenever possible because of their side effects, which may be aggravated in these immunologically compromised patients. In our series, the mean time of resolution of pericardial disease in uremic patients was 20 ± 14 days, peritoneal dialysis being started in 33 (67%) and hemodialysis in the remaining 16 (33%). There was no significant difference in the mean time of resolution in patients on stable hemodialysis (26 ± 21 days); of these, one half persisted with hemodialysis while the other half was shifted to peritoneal dialysis.

Another controversial issue is the management of cardiac tamponade and persistent pericardial effusion. Recently, those factors that allow discrimination between patients requiring only initiation or intensification of dialysis from those who will need invasive procedures have been retrospectively analysed (65, 66), and a model of statistical analysis has been developed. Validation of this model will require prospective studies (66). On the other hand, discrepancies exist among authors, some advocating pericardiocentesis (8, 9, 14, 16) and others favoring pericardiectomy (12, 18–21). The latter state that the unacceptable mortality and relapse rates with pericardiocentesis are sound reasons for preferring pericardiectomy. As intermediate approaches, pericardiocentesis with intrapericardial instillation of nonabsorbable steroid (17) or subxiphoid pericardiostomy (22) have been proposed. In practice, this choice depends on local experience, availability and personal preferences rather than on studies that have demonstrated the superiority of one approach over the others. Since the first version of our protocol (43) we have proposed the stepwise use of each procedure in order of increasing complexity. Thus, we advise pericardiocentesis when bacterial or fungal infection are suspected, when tamponade is present or when large pericardial effusion (according to preestablished echocardiographic criteria (37)) shows progressive increase. We reserve pericardiectomy for persisting or relapsing tamponade, or persistent large effusion after pericardiocentesis or the development of cardiac constriction (confirmed by external recordings and catheterization).

In our series, 15 of 26 pericardiocenteses were carried out for tamponade and 11 for large effusion. In 25 cases the fluid was a serosanguinous exudate but did not fulfil criteria for hemopericardium. In the remaining case the effusion was a transudate. Viral cultures and cultures for bacteria or tubercle bacillus were negative. Hepatitis B virus surface antigen was present in the pericardial fluid of three patients. Tamponade developed in two patients after pericardiocentesis, and it could thus be considered a complication of the procedure.

Partial pericardiectomy was carried out in 8 patients. In three of them it was indicated for persistent tamponade after pericardiocentesis. Four patients with persistent effusion also required partial pericardiectomy, in two because tamponade developed after pericardiocentesis and in the other two because large effusion persisted after pericardiocentesis. The remaining pericardiectomy was carried out for relapse of the pericardial disease without effusion. Histological study of the pericardiectomy specimen showed effusive fibrinous pericarditis in six cases; five of them from patients with tamponade, and one from a patient with a large serosanguineous effusion. Granulomas were not found and the cultures were negative. In the two remaining patients, pathological study did not identify any abnormality. One normal surgical specimen came from the only instance of transudative effusion shown at peri-cardiocentesis. The patient died 24 hours after operation with refractory shock. Autopsy showed necrohemorrhagic pancreatitis and disseminated lymphoma. The second normal surgical specimen was found at pericardiec-tomy carried out after a relapsing effusion had resolved. This transgression of the protocol permitted us to identify the case as a transudate due to unrecog-nized heart failure (43).

Out of 11 patients with cardiac tamponade treated with peritoneal dialysis and pericardiocentesis, only one (9%) required subsequent partial pericar-diectomy for persistent tamponade, whereas four of the remaining six treated with hemodialysis and pericardiocentesis (67%) eventually required pericar-diectomy. Although pericardiectomy was required less often for tamponade treated with peritoneal dialysis than with hemodialysis, we believe that the modification of hemodialysis is a superior approach. When patients with effusive pericarditis develop high venous pressure during a hemodialysis ses-sion the anticipated excessive ultrafiltration can be offset by the administra-tion of a plasma volume expander to prevent plasma volume depletion, with consequent hypotension and worsening of cardiac tamponade.

Six patients died during the admission when pericardial involvement was identified, but in three (two from the uremic group and the other one from the hemodialysis group) there was, at the time of death, no clinical or echocardio-graphic evidence of pericardial disease, death being caused by the underlying renal disease. Another patient died during a hemodialysis session, probably from cardiac tamponade. The fifth patient died suddenly without apparent cause. Finally, in the sixth patient, autopsy confirmed the clinical diagnosis of acute pulmonary edema and cardiomyopathy; fibrinous pericarditis with a small amount of pericardial fluid was also found. In no case death was con-sidered to be a consequence of an invasive therapeutic procedure.

Conclusions

Pericardial involvement in end stage renal disease is more common in young patients, either before dialysis therapy or shortly after its institution. In these circumstances, pericarditis is probably a consequence of uremic toxins, per-haps the as yet poorly identified middle molecules. The term uremic pericar-ditis should be reserved for these cases. The cases of pericarditis in patients on a stable hemodialysis regimen can be divided into those where dialysis is inadequate, in which the etiology is probably similar to patients with uremic pericarditis, and the remaining, in which the identification of a causative agent is difficult, although a minority have a specific infection. These in-stances probably represent viral pericarditis in immunologically compro-mised patients.

Renal failure, with resulting fluid and salt retention, and the frequently associated cardiovascular pathology, predispose to cardiac failure, which is common in these patients and might cause some of the pericardial effusions, particularly in the uremic group, where heart failure and pleural effusion are significantly more common than in patients on a stable hemodialysis program. In individual patients several etiologic factors may coexist.

Clinically, pericardial involvement is more commonly silent in the uremic patients than in those treated with hemodialysis for more than three months. There are no differences in the evolution and therapeutic response of both groups, and, although the number of cases of cardiac tamponade and invasive procedures is higher in the patients on stable hemodialysis, the differences are not significant. The higher mortality of uremic patients may be attributed to the greater severity of their underlying disease.

Pericardiocentesis results in effective management of most patients with cardiac tamponade and large persistent effusion; thus, pericardiectomy may be avoided in many cases. We only advise partial pericardiectomy in cases of tamponade or large effusion persisting or relapsing after pericardiocentesis. The use of peritoneal dialysis is associated with significantly fewer pericardiectomies.

We suggest that hypotension induced by an excessive ultrafiltration rate precipitates worsening of cardiac tamponade during hemodialysis. This hypothesis could be tested by performing hemodynamic investigations during hemodialysis sessions.

References

1. Renfrew R, Buselmeier TJ, Kjellstrand CM. Pericarditis and renal failure. Ann Rev Med 1980; 31: 345–360.
2. Shabetai R, Rostand SG. Nephrogenic pericardial disease. In: O'Rourke RA, Brenner BM, Stein JH, ed. The heart and renal disease. New York, Churchill Livingstone 1984; 89–125.
3. Bright R. Tubular view of the morbid appearances in 100 cases connected with albuminous urine: with observations. Guy's Hosp Rep 1836; 1: 388–400.
4. Barach AL, Pericarditis in chronic nephritis. Am J Med Sci 1922; 163: 44–60.
5. Richter A, O'Hara J. The heart in chronic glomerular nephritis. N Engl J Med 1936; 214: 824–830.
6. Wacker W, Merrill J. Uremic pericarditis in acute and chronic renal failure. JAMA 1954; 156: 764–765.
7. Goodner C, Brown H. Report of two cases of cardiac tamponade in uremic pericarditis. JAMA 1956; 162: 1.459–1.461.
8. Hager E. Clinical observations on five patients with uremic pericardial tamponade. N Engl J Med 1965; 273: 304–308.
9. Beaudry C, Nakamoto S, Kolf WJ. Uremic pericarditis and cardiac tamponade in chronic renal failure. Ann Intern Med 1966; 64: 990–995.
10. Bailey G, Hampers C, Hager E, Merrill J. Uremic pericarditis. Circulation 1968; 38: 582–591.
11. Alfrey AC, Goss JE, Ogden DA, Vogel JHK, Holmes JH. Uremic hemopericardium. Am J Med 1968; 45: 391–400.
12. Comty CM, Cohen SL, Shapiro FL. Pericarditis in chronic uremia and its sequels. Ann Intern Med 1971; 75: 173–183.

13. Baldwin JJ, Edwards JE. Uremic pericarditis as a cause of cardiac tamponade. Circulation 1976; 53: 896–901.
14. Sevillano R, González V, Tejuca F, Fernández E, Martínez J. El diagnóstico precoz de la pericarditis aguda en las unidades de diálisis. Med Clin (Barc) 1977; 68: 331–334.
15. Carreras L, Caseiro G, Griño JM, Martínez A, Poveda R. Pericarditis en la insuficiencia renal crónica. Rev Soc Esp Dial Trasp 1979; 1: 27–29.
16. Silverberg S, Oreopoulus DG, Wise DJ, Uden DE, Meindok H, Jones M, Rapoport A, de Veber GA. Pericarditis in patients undergoing long-term hemodialysis and peritoneal dyalisis. Incidence, complications and management. Am J Med 1977; 63: 874–879.
17. Buselmeier TJ, Simmons RL, Najarian JS, Maver SM, Matas AJ, Kjellstrand CM. Uremic pericardial effusion. Nephron 1976; 16: 371–380.
18. Sánchez Lloret J, Capdevila J, Zurita M, Saura E. La pericardiectomía como tratamiento del taponamiento cardíaco en las pericarditis urémicas en curso de diálisis. Med Clín (Barc) 1973; 60: 132–143.
19. Ali-Regiaba S, White RP, Gay WA, Stenzel KH, Sullivan JF, Riggio RR, Tapia L., Cheigh JS, David DS, Rubin AL. Treatment of uremic pericarditis by anterior pericardiectomy. Lancet 1974; 2: 12–14.
20. Wray TM, Humphreys J, Perry JM, Stone WJ, Bender HW. Pericardiectomy for treatment of uremic pericarditis. Circulation 1974; S-II 49–50: 268–271.
21. Valles M, Torras A, Darnell A, Letang E, Sánchez Lloret J, Pascual R, Montoliu J, Revert L. Segmental pericardiectomy in the treatment of uremic pericarditis. Dial & Transplant 1981; 10: 432–436.
22. Leehey DJ, Daugirdas JT, Ing TS. Early drainage of pericardial effusion in patients with dialysis pericarditis. Arch Intern Med 1983; 143: 1.673–1.675.
23. Goldstein DH, Hagar CH, Srivastara N, Schacht RA, Ferris FZ, Flowers NC. Clinically silent pericardial effusions in patients on long-term hemodialysis. Chest 1977; 72: 744–747.
24. Horton JD, Gelfand MC, Sherber HS. Natural history of asymptomatic pericardial effusions in patients on maintenance hemodialysis. Proc Dial Transplant Forum 1977; 76–81.
25. Kleiman JH, Motta J, London E, Pennell JR, Popp RL. Pericardial effusions in patients with end-stage disease. Br Heart J 1978; 40: 190–193.
26. Frommer JP, Young JB, Ayus JC. Asymptomatic pericardial effusion in uremic patients: effect of long term dialysis. Nephron 1985; 39: 296–301.
27. Wray TM, Stone WJ. Uremic pericarditis: a prospective echocardiographic and clinical study. Clin Nephrol 1976; 6: 295–302.
28. Winney RJ, Wright N, Sumerling MD, Lambie AT. Echocardiography in uremic pericarditis with effusion. Nephron 1977; 18: 201–207.
29. Luft FC, Gilman JK, Weyman AE. Pericarditis in the patients with uremia: clinical and echocardiographic evaluation. Nephron 1980; 25: 160–166.
30. Yoshida K, Shiina A, Asano Y, Hosoda S. Uremic pericardial effusion: detection and evaluation of uremic pericardial effusion by echocardiography. Clin Nephrol 1980; 13: 260–268.
31. Comty CM, Wathen RL, Shapiro FL. Uremic pericarditis. In: Spodick DH, ed. Pericardial diseases. Philadelphia, FA Davis, 1976; 219–235.
32. Drüeke T, le Pailleur C, Jungers P. Cardiomyopathie et pericardite urémiques. In: Hamburger J, Crosnier J, Funck-Bretano JL, ed. Actualités nephrologiques de l'Hôpital Necker. Paris, Flamarion, 1979; 37–70.
33. Shabetai R. The pericardium. New York, Grune & Stratton, 1981; 385–389.
34. Kotler MN, Parry WR. Pericardial disease in chronic renal failure. In: Lowenthal DT, Pennock RS, Likoff W, Onesti G, eds. Management of the cardiac patient with renal failure. Philadelphia, FA Davis, 1981; 85–109.
35. Comty CM, Shapio FL. Cardiac complications of regular dialysis therapy. In: Drukker W, Parsons FM, Maher JF, eds. Replacement of renal function by dialysis. Boston, Martinus Nijhoff, 1983; 595–610.

36. Rutsky EA, Rostand SG. Treatment of uremic pericarditis and pericardial effusion. Am J Kid Dis 1987; 10: 2–8.
37. Galve E, García del Castillo H, Evangelista A, Batlle J, Permanyer-Miralda G, Soler-Soler J. Pericardial effusion in the course of myocardial infarction: incidence, natural history, and clinical relevance. Circulation 1986; 73: 294–299.
38. Babb AL, Johansen PJ, Strand MJ, Tenckhoff H, Scribner BH. Bidirectional permeability of the human peritoneum to middle molecules. Proc Eur Dial Transpl Assoc 1973; 10: 247–251.
39. Bergström J, Fürst P. Uremic middle molecules. Clin Nephrol 1976; 5: 143–149.
40. Cochran M, Lawton S, Rowlands LM. Fibrinous pericarditis and fibrinolysis in chronic dialysis patients. Clin Nephrol 1979; 11: 23–25.
41. Pabico RC, Nanshaw JB, Talley TE. Cytomegalovirus infection in chronic hemodialysis patients. Abstr West Dial and Transplant Soc 1971; 1: 117–123.
42. Osanloo E, Salhorb RJ, Cioffi RF, Parker RH. Viral pericarditis in patients receiving hemodialysis. Arch Intern Med 1979; 139: 301–303.
43. Morlans M, Ballester M, Bartolomé J, Permanyer G, Olmos A, Piera L. Diagnóstico y tratamiento de la pericarditis en pacientes urémicos. Med Clin (Barc) 1981; 77: 269–273.
44. Dave MB, Choi YJ, Cohen BD. Hepatitis B virus: A possible cause of serositis in hemo-dialysis patients. Nephron 1983; 33: 186–188.
45. Joffe P, Johannessen AC. Uraemic pericarditis, an epidemic disease? Dan Med Bull 1987; 34: 117–118.
46. Permanyer-Miralda G, Sagristà-Sauleda J, Soler-Soler J. Primary acute pericardial disease: A prospective series of 231 consecutive patients. Am J Cardiol 1985; 56: 623–630.
47. Twardowski ZJ, Alpert MA, Gupta RC, Nolph KD, Madsen BT. Circulating inmune com-plexes: Possible toxins responsible for serositis (pericarditis, pleuritis and peritonitis) in renal failure. Nephron 1983; 35: 190–195.
48. Maisch B, Kochsiek K. Humoral inmune reactions in uremic pericardits. Am J Nephrol 1983; 3: 264–271.
49. Ahmad R, Goldsmith HJ. Response of pericardial effusion to ultrafiltration and intensified hemodialysis. Dial Transplant 1977; 6: 12.
50. Morlans M. Pericarditis urémica. Med Clín (Barc) 1983; 80: 263–264.
51. Morlans M, Vallés M, Larrousse E. Asociación de derrame pleural izquierdo y enfer-medad pericárica en el paciente urémico. Nefrología 1986; 6: 53–56.
52. Weiss JM, Spodick DH. Association of left pleural effusion with pericardial disease. N Engl J Med 1983; 308: 696–697.
53. Hancock EW. Cardiac tamponade. Med Clin N Am 1979; 63: 223–237.
54. Morlans M, Ballester M, Camps J, Sans A, Permanyer G, Olmos A. Diagnóstico y trata-miento del taponamiento cardíaco secundario a pericarditis en pacientes hemodializados. Rec Soc Esp Dial Transplant 1981; 3: 93–98.
55. Ports TA, Botvinick EH, Schiller NB, Miller SW, Silverman NH, Chatterjee K. Diagnóstico no invasivo del taponamiento cardíaco. Cardiovascular Rev Rep (ed. esp.) 1981; 2: 23–29.
56. Reddy PS, Curtiss EI, O'Toole JD, Shaver JA. Cardiac tamponade: hemodynamic observa-tions in man. Circulation 1978; 58: 265–272.
57. D'Cruz IA, Cohen HC, Prabhu R. Diagnosis of cardiac tamponade by echocardiography: changes in mitral valve motion and ventricular dimensions, with special reference to para-doxical pulse. Circulation 1975; 52: 460–465.
58. Schiller NB, Botvinick EH. Right ventricular compression as a sign of cardiac tamponade. An analysis of echocardiographic ventricular dimensions and their clinical implications. Circulation 1977; 56: 774–779.
59. Engel PJ. Echocardiographic findings in pericardial disease. In: Fowler NO, ed. The peri-cardium in health and disease. New York, Futura Publishing Co., 1985; 99–151.
60. Shabetai R, Fowler NO, Guntheroth WG. The hemodynamics of cardiac tamponade and constrictive pericarditis. Am J Cardiol 1970; 26: 480–489.

61. Ballester M, Serra A, Angel J, Carcía del Castillo H, Morlans M. Derrame pericárdico localizado con taponamiento cardíaco en un enfermo con insuficiencia renal crónica en programa de hemodiálisis. Med Clín (Barc) 1982; 78: 99–103.
62. Lindsay J Jr, Crawley IS, Callaway GM. Chronic constrictive pericarditis following uremic hemopericardium. Am Heart J 1970; 79: 390–393.
63. Sagristà-Sauleda J, Permanyer-Miralda G, Candell-Riera J, Angel J, Soler-Soler J. Transient cardiac constriction: An unrecognized pattern of evolution in acute idiophatic effusive pericarditis. Am J Cardiol 1987; 59: 961–966.
64. Spodick DH. Arrhythmias during acute pericarditis. JAMA 1976; 235: 39–46.
65. Peraino RA, Pericardial effusion in patients treated with maintenance dialysis. Am J Nephrol 1983; 3: 319–322.
66. DePeace NL, Nestico PF, Schwartz AB, Mintz GS, Schwartz JS, Kotler MN, Swartz C. Predicting succes of intensive dialysis in the treatment of uremic pericarditis. Am J Med 1984; 76: 38–46.

8. Significance of pericardial effusion in acute myocardial infarction

ENRIQUE GALVE, M.D.

Introduction

Classically, pericardial effusion during myocardial infarction had been considered rare (1–3). Echocardiography provides an excellent method to establish the prevalence of pericardial effusion (4) in the evolution of myocardial infarction.

The mechanisms of development of pericardial effusion during myocardical infarction are poorly understood; even the origin of the normal pericardial fluid is still controversial (5). Myocardial infarction is a complex condition where several different factors play a role. If necrosis is transmural, the pericardium may become involved, with the resulting so called early postinfarction pericarditis (6); it is not known, however, whether this type of pericarditis leads to effusion (7, 8). On the other hand, a more delayed pericarditis develops in some patients as a component of Dressler's syndrome; concomitant features include pleuritis and pericardial effusion (9). It is unknown, however, whether Dressler's syndrome is related to earlier pericarditis or pericardial effusion in the acute phase of myocardial infarction.

The use of anticoagulants during myocardial infarction is another pertinent issue. There is an increasing consensus on the need to administer heparin to most patients with myocardial infarction to prevent cardiac, coronary and venous thromboembolism (10, 11). Accordingly, it is necessary to know whether anticoagulation influences the development or progression of pericardial effusion and whether it increases the risk of tamponade. Finally, the need for early diagnosis in cases of cardiac rupture is increasingly felt; peri-

J. Soler-Soler et al. (Eds.), Pericardial Disease, pp. 141–152.

cardial effusion may be a finding suggesting rupture (12, 13) although its real diagnostic significance in this respect has not been established.

Considering all these uncertainties, the study reported in the present chapter was designed to determine the precise incidence of pericardial effusion during infarction, its natural history in the acute, subacute and medium term phases, to evaluate the factors involved in its development, and, finally, to evaluate whether any particular therapeutic approach is indicated when pericardial effusion develops (14).

Study design

The study was prospectively designed. Overall 282 patients were studied, distributed in four groups (Table 8.1).

Group I consisted of 138 consecutive patients with acute myocardial infarction admitted to our Coronary Care Unit. For the diagnosis of infarction at least two of the three following criteria were required: suggestive prolonged pain, new Q waves in the electrocardiogram, and abnormal increase in the MB fraction of the serum creatine kinase level. Seven of these 138 patients died during the initial hours after admission, before the first echocardiogram could be taken, and they were excluded from the study. The remaining 131 patients, 115 males and 16 females, ages ranging between 35 and 81 years, (mean 58 ± 12) were included and underwent echocardiographic evaluations on the first, third and 10th day after admission, and again three and six months after discharge. Subsequently, 10 patients were excluded because the quality of their echocardiograms was inadequate. Therefore, the overall number of evaluated patients in group I was 121.

Group II was a control group of 54 patients admitted with unstable angina. The age and sex distributions were similar to those in group I. The diagnostic criteria for unstable angina were clearly progressive exertional angina, or rest angina lasting more than 15 minutes or recurrent anginal attacks; in all cases new Q waves or an increased level of serum myocardial enzymes were absent. None of these patients had sustained previous myocardial infarction or undergone cardiac surgery. In this group, a single echocardiogram was done on the third day. Two patients were excluded due to poor quality recordings.

Table 8.1. Study groups.

		Patients
Group I	Acute myocardial infarction	138
Group II	Unstable angina	54
Group III	Individuals without heart disease	57
Group IV	Correlation echo-surgery	33
Total		282

Group III was another control group, comprising 57 subjects without evidence of any type of heart disease or any other condition that might be associated with pericardial effusion, after complete clinical and laboratory evaluation. Their age and sex distributions were also comparable to those in group I. Two subjects were excluded due to poor quality recordings.

Finally, group IV consisted of 33 patients similar in age and sex to those in group I, in whom echocardiographic recording was carried out within a few hours previous to cardiac surgery. A correlation between echocardiographic findings and the volume of pericardial fluid found at operation was made. A detailed description of this study, which resulted in a modification of the classical criteria of Horowitz at al. (15), can be found in chapter 1. On the basis of that correlation, the criterion we adopted for the echocardiographic diagnosis of pericardial effusion was an echo free posterior space throughout the cardiac cycle. This pattern corresponded to an amount of at least 50 ml of pericardial fluid at surgery.

Initially, all the recordings were made in M mode with an Ekoline 20A device. In all group I patients in whom images consistent with persistent effusion were obtained without significant changes in three consecutive studies (5 patients), or when interpretation was questionable (16 patients), a two dimensional study with an ATL Mark 300 device was performed.

All studies were evaluated by three experienced observers, who were unaware of the clinical findings. A consensus was reached in all instances of discrepancy.

As the overall number of patients with surgical correlation (group IV) was insufficient to establish quantitative criteria of pericardial effusion, these were arbitrarily estimated, as in other studies (16), from the sum of the amplitudes of the anterior and posterior echo free spaces. The measurements were carried out in end diastole, at the level of the mitral valve tips. Thus, pericardial effusion was considered as small when the total sum was less than 10 mm, moderate when it was between 10 and 20 mm, and large when it was higher than 20 mm.

The results of the quantitative variables are presented as mean ± standard deviation. The comparisons were carried out, depending on the variables in each case, with chi-square test, Fisher's exact test, or Student's t test.

Incidence of pericardial effusion

Considering the 121 patients in group I, an echocardiographic diagnosis of pericardial effusion was made at some time during the course in 34 patients (28%). This result is in disagreement with the previously stated opinion that pericardial effusion is a rare finding during infarction (1–3). However, more recent studies designed to evaluate the incidence of effusion during myocardial infarction (17–19) have shown that pericardial effusion is frequent, although Wunderink (20) found an incidence of 5.6% in a series of 90 patients; it is difficult to explain this low incidence because, as discussed below, this is the incidence in healthy individuals. Kaplan at al. (17) found a 37% incidence in a series of 43 patients, while it was 63% in the 46 patients studied by Somolinos et al. (18). These higher incidences might be explained because in both studies less strict criteria than ours were used for the diagnosis of pericardial effusion. In both, Horowitz's C2 pattern (where pericardium and epicardium do not completely separate in diastole) was accepted as indicative of effusion, whereas we do not agree on the basis of our echocardiographic-surgical correlation. Finally, Pierard et al. (19), in the only study where all patients were evaluated with two dimensional technique, found an incidence virtually identicial to ours (26%).

In group II, consisting of 52 patients with unstable angina, pericardial effusion was found in 4 cases (8%); this prevalence was significantly different from that found in patients with myocardial infarction studied on the third day after admission (25%, $p < 0.02$) (Fig. 8.1).

In group III effusion was found in 3 cases (5%, $p < 0.01$ when compared with group I and $p = NS$ when compared with group II) (Fig. 8.1). This prevalence of a posterior echo free space in healthy individuals was identical to that in the Framingham study in patients of similar age and sex (21). It is our opinion that, although some fluid can be found in the pericardial space of healthy individuals (22), its volume does not exceed 25–30 ml and it cannot be usually detected with echocardiography. Quite probably, this 5% may correspond to epicardial fat, as has been shown in some cases (23).

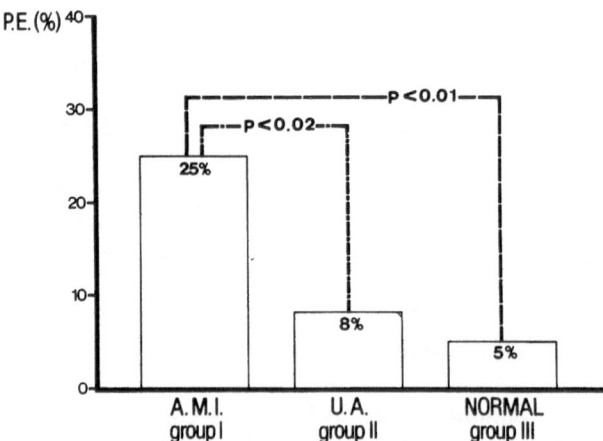

Fig. 8.1. There is a significant difference between the prevalence of pericardial effusion (PE) during the acute phase of myocardial infarction (A.M.I.) and that in patients with unstable angina (U.A.) or free from heart disease. (Reproduced from Galve E, García-del-Castillo H, Evangelista A, Batlle J, Permanyer-Miralda G, Soler-Soler J. Pericardial effusion in the course of myocardial infarction: incidence, natural history, and clinical relevance. Circulation 1986; 73: 294–299. With authorization of the American Heart Association, Inc.).

Evolution of pericardial effusion

Figure 8.2 shows the prevalence of effusion throughout the three evaluations during the acute phase of the disease and in the subsequent periods after discharge. As depicted in the figure, effusion develops early, as it was already present in 17% of patients within the first 24 hours. The highest prevalence was found on the third day (25%). In addition, in those patients in whom effusion was demonstrated on several recordings, there was a tendency for the largest effusion to be found on the third day. Disappearance of the effusion was progressive, its prevalence remaining at 12% at three months and 8% at 6 months. The prevalence at six months was identical to that found in patients with unstable angina, as if this were the prevalence in individuals with coronary artery disease without acute infarction. In any case, if it is accepted that a part of this figure may correspond to individuals with epicardial fat, the prevalence of effusion in these circumstances would be very low.

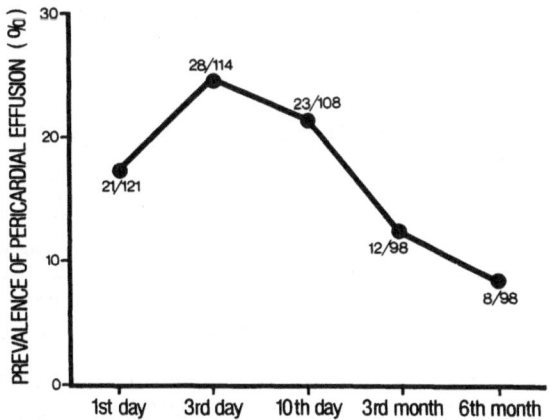

Fig. 8.2. Prevalence of pericardial effusion throughout the successive evaluations in the group of patients with acute myocardial infarction. In each control the numerator indicates the number of patients with effusion and the denominator the number of patients studied. The denominator decreases as a consequence of patient deaths. (Reproduced from Galve E, García-del-Castillo H, Evangelista A, Batlle J, Permanyer-Miralda G, Soler-Soler J. Pericardial effusion in the course of acute myocardial infarction: incidence, natural history, and clinical relevance. Circulation 1986; 73: 294–299. With authorization of the American Heart Association, Inc.).

Quantification and localization of pericardial effusion

On the basis of the previously mentioned quantification criteria, pericardial effusion in patients with infarction was considered to be small in 30 cases (88%) and moderate in 4 (12%); no case of large effusion was found. The patients with effusion could not be identified on the basis of the chest radiogram. The small amount of the effusion in most cases explains why its occurrence has been considered rare. A sensitive and reliable method such as echo-cardiography is therefore required for its identification.

The localization of effusion was not remarkable, being the same as pericardial effusion of other etiology; that is, small effusions were always in the posterior space, while moderate effusions were first in the posterior and then, when the amount in the posterior was sizeable, in the anterior space.

In the 21 patients evaluated with two dimensional echocardiography, localized effusion not accesible to M mode examination was not detected in any case. Intrapericardial masses suggesting blood clots, adhesions or loculations also were not seen.

Factors influencing the development of pericardial effusion

To investigate factors associated with the development of pericardial effusion during myocardial infarction, we examined the correlation between several clinical variables and the occurrence of pericardial effusion. The results are listed in Table 8.2.

Table 8.2. Correlation between clinical findings and the occurrence of pericardial effusion during acute myocardial infarction.

| | Pericardial effusion | | |
	Present	Absent	p
Patients	34 (28%)	87 (72%)	
Age	61.8 ± 9.8	56.7 ± 12.3	NS
Sex			
males	30 (29%)	75 (71%)	
females	4 (25%)	12 (75%)	NS
Peak CK-MB (IU)	83.6 ± 66.2	88.5 ± 51.1	NS
First infarction	31 (28%)	80 (72%)	NS
Reinfarction	3 (30%)	7 (70%)	NS
Temporary pacemaker	1 (10%)	9 (90%)	NS
Ressuscitation maneuvers and/or cardioversion	2 (50%)	2 (50%)	NS
Arrhythmias			
supraventricular	4 (50%)	4 (50%)	NS
ventricular	8 (31%)	18 (69%)	NS
Heart block	1 (11%)	8 (89%)	NS
Localization of infarction			
anterior	20 (38%)	32 (62%)	
inferior	10 (18%)	47 (82%)	< .02
Infarction type			
Q wave	30 (27%)	80 (73%)	
non Q wave	4 (36%)	7 (64%)	NS
Heart failure	10 (45%)	12 (55%)	< .05
Hospital mortality	6 (35%)	11 (65%)	NS
Late mortality	2 (33%)	4 (67%)	NS

Effusion was not associated with more extensive infarction assessed by enzyme release, or with procedures involving possible cardiac trauma, such as the insertion of pacing electrodes or cardiopulmonary ressuscitation. In contrast, pericardial effusion was associated with cardiac failure ($p < 0.05$); the incidence being higher in more advanced Killip classes. This is not a surprising finding, as heart failure is well established cause of pericardial effusion in other types of heart disease (24). Pericardial effusion was significantly more common ($p < 0.02$) in anterior infarctions. We do not have an apparent explanation for this finding; however, it might well be that pericardial effusion was more difficult to detect in inferior infactions because posterior wall hypokinesis could obscure the separation between epicardium and pericardium, in contrast to anterior infarction where the posterior wall has a vigorous compensatory contraction. If this explanation were true, there might have been some underestimation of the prevalence of effusion in inferior infarction. On the other hand, there were no differences in the incidence of effusion among Q wave and non Q wave infarctions; however, this might be due at least in part to the low specificity of this electrocardiographic classification regarding the transmural or non transmural nature of an infarction (25, 26).

The differences found between the incidence of pericardial effusion in patients with acute myocardial infarction and those with unstable angina or healthy individuals, as well as its changing prevalence throughout the evolution of infarction, leave no doubt about the existence of a pathogenetic relation between events in the acute phase of infarction and the development of effusion. However, of all possible mechanisms, we have only identified heart failure as clearly associated, and even then only in 10 patients of the 34 with pericardial effusion were signs of heart failure present. Thus, there are two possibilities: either the remaining 24 patients had subclinical heart failure, which is highly unlikely, or they had pericardial effusion of a different or multifactorial origin. We are inclined to accept this latter explanation. It has been suggested that effusion might be caused by edema and inflammation of the infarcted myocardium (27), but this hypothesis, like others regarding this point, is difficult to prove.

Early postinfarction pericarditis and pericardial effusion

A particularly interesting aspect of our investigation was to establish the possible association between effusion and early postinfarction pericarditis. As definite criteria for the definition of early postinfarction pericarditis are not well established in the literature (28–35), we therefore adopted specific criteria. We defined early postinfarction pericarditis in three different successively less stringent ways. First (definition A), all patients with a pericardial friction rub during the initial days. Second (definition B), all patients with pericardial rub plus those without rub and at least two of the following: fever, chest pain suggestive of pericarditis or consistent ECG changes. Finally (defi-

Table 8.3.   Correlation between pericardial effusion and early postinfarction pericarditis.

Definition	Patients (n)	Pericardial effusion		p
		Present	Absent	
A	14	6 (42%)	8 (58%)	NS
B	21	8 (38%)	13 (62%)	NS
C	30	9 (30%)	21 (70%)	NS

A: all patients with pericardial rub; B: all patients with pericardial rub plus those patients without a rub and at least two of the following: fever, chest pain suggestive of pericarditis or consistent ECG changes; C: all patients with at least one of the following: pericardial rub, chest pain suggestive of pericarditis or consistent ECG changes.

nition C), all patients with at least one of the following: pericardial rub, chest pain suggestive of pericarditis or consistent ECG changes. We found no correlation between post infarction pericarditis, defined by any of these criteria, and the development of pericardial effusion (Table 8.3). We can conclude, therefore, that early postinfarction pericarditis is not responsible, at least in a significant way, for the development of pericardial effusion. This is a surprising finding, as any type of pericarditis can be associated with pericardial effusion. However, our finding has been confirmed by other authors (17). It might be that early postinfarction pericarditis possibly is a phenomenon localized over the necrosis area rather than a diffuse pericarditis; thus, the exudative area might be much smaller.

Use of anticoagulants

The use of anticoagulants in the presence of pericardial effusion has long been a cause for concern, particularly if effusion is a component of pericarditis. In the course of myocardial infarction, instances of hemopericardium have been reported in association with cardiac rupture (36, 37) or anticoagulant therapy (38, 39). If, as we have shown, pericardial effusion is quite common in myocardial infarction, it is important to establish whether anticoagulants can be safely used. The present series did not evaluate the association between pericardial effusion and fibrinolytic drugs, as these were not used in our institution at the time of the study. However, heparin was routinely used in our Coronary Care Unit for infarction, and we did not feel justified in depriving patients of its potential benefit. Thus, we did not compare the prevalence of pericardial effusion with and without heparin therapy; rather, we compared two different administration regimens: low dose, 5000 U/12 hours, which does not modify partial thromboplastin time, and full dose, 2500 U/10 kg/12 hours subcutaneously, adjusted to prolong the partial thromboplastin time 1.7–2.5 times control. The results are shown in Table

Table 8.4. Relation between pericardial effusion (PE) and the level of anticoagulation in acute myocardial infarction.

	Patients	PE	no PE	p
Full dose heparin	50	16 (32%)	34 (68%)	NS
Low dose heparin	71	18 (25%)	53 (75%)	

8.4, from which it can be seen that there was no significant difference between the two regimens in the incidence of effusion.

In view of these results, and considering that no patient in the whole series developed severe effusion or tamponade in spite of our administering heparin to all of them, we feel that heparin administration does not involve a significant risk of intrapericardial bleeding in the presence of effusion. Our results are in agreement with a recent report (40) in which the risk of anticoagulation was evaluated in patients with infarction who also had pericardial effusion and mural thrombus: no patient developed progressive pericardial effusion or tamponade in spite of heparin and subsequent oral anticoagulant therapy.

Mortality and pericardial effusion

Figure 8.3 shows the 6 month survival curves of the patients with myocardial infarction, comparing those with and without pericardial effusion. Although the mortality rate at the end of that period was higher in those patients who had developed pericardial effusion at some time in their course, the differ-

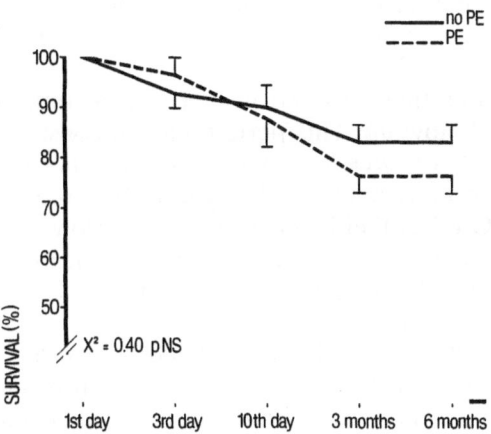

Fig. 8.3. Actuarial survival curves of the patients with and without pericardial effusion (PE). Each point on the curves indicates the probability of surviving to that time period. Vertical bars indicate the standard deviation. As shown, the occurrence of effusion was not associated with a significantly increased mortality rate.

ence was not significant. Therefore, in our experience the development of pericardial effusion does not indicate a worse prognosis.

It has been suggested (13) that pericardial effusion might be a harbinger of cardiac rupture, and therefore predict the likelihood of this devastating complication. In our series there were two cases of acute cardiac rupture in autopsied patients. In one of them pericardial effusion was demonstrated by the last echocardiographic evaluation before death. Because of the high incidence of pericardial effusion in acute myocardial infarction, it is our contention that the simple finding of pericardial effusion is not a predictor of cardiac rupture, particularly when the effusion is found on a routine echocardiogram in a clinically stable patient. Another study (41) suggests that two dimensional echocardiography may be useful for the identification of subacute rupture. The relevant data include a large effusion, intrapericardial high density images, and right atrial and ventricular collapse, none of which were found in our patients.

Clinical implications

Pericardial effusion is a common occurrence during the acute phase of myocardial infarction, but is basically benign and does not predict specific complications. Therefore, the main clinical implication for management is that the finding of pericardial effusion, particularly when it is not large and in the absence of cardiac tamponade or rupture, does not justify any change in the therapeutic approach or the performance of serial evaluations, which would not be cost effective.

Another clinical implication is related to early postinfarction pericarditis. Echocardiography is not adequate to confirm the diagnosis of pericarditis in a patient who develops atypical chest pain in the early days after acute infarction.

In the present series there was no instance of postinfarction syndrome during the 6-month follow up. This period may be considered adequate to rule out a first episode of Dressler's syndrome. This lack of incidence is in agreement with the recently noted tendency towards a reduced frequence of this syndrome (42). On the other hand, in view of the slow reabsorption of the effusion that we found in our series, finding a small pericardial effusion in the first months after acute infarction does not suggest Dressler's syndrome in the absence of additional findings.

The present study also shows that an isolated pericardial effusion during acute myocardial infarction does not mean that heparin therapy has to be modified. Although our study was primarily directed to the evaluation of pericardial effusion, our results with heparin therapy in the presence of early postinfarction pericarditis also suggest that heparin is not contraindicated in these patients; however, this particular group requires a closer clinical surveillance, as isolated instances of hemopericardium have been reported.

References

1. Parkinson J, Bedford E. Cardiac infarction and coronary thrombosis. Lancet 1928; 1: 4–11.
2. Master AM, Jaffe HL. Coronary artery thrombosis with pericardial effusion. JAMA 1935; 104: 1212–1214.
3. Wolff L. Diagnostic implications of pericardial, pleural and pulmonary involvement in cardiovascular disease. N Engl J Med 1951; 244: 965–970.
4. Feigenbaum H. Echocardiographic diagnosis of pericardial effusion. Am J Cardiol 1970; 26: 475–479.
5. Gibson AT, Segal MB. A study of the composition of pericardial fluid, with special reference to the probable mechanism of fluid formation. J Physiol (Lond) 1978; 277: 367–377.
6. Thadani U, Chopra MP, Aber CP, Portal RW. Pericarditis after acute myocardial infarction. Br Med J 1971; 2: 135–137.
7. Toole JC, Silverman ME. Pericarditis of acute myocardial infarction. Chest 1975; 67: 647–653.
8. Lichstein E, Liu HM, Gupta P. Pericarditis complicating acute myocardial infarction. Incidence and complications and significance of electrocardiogram on admission. Am Heart J 1974; 87: 242–252.
9. Dressler W. The post-myocardial infarction syndrome. A report of forty four cases. Arch Int Med 1959; 103: 28–42.
10. Goldberg RJ, Gore JM, Dalen JE. The role of anticoagulant therapy in acute myocardial infarction. Am Heart J 1984; 108: 387–393.
11. Chesebro JH, Fuster V. Antithrombotic therapy for acute myocardial infarction: mechanisms and prevention of deep venous, left ventricular, and coronary artery thromboembolism. Circulation 1986; 74 (suppl III): 1–10.
12. Bates RJ, Beutler S, Resnekov L, Anagnostooulos CE. Cardiac rupture-challenge in diagnosis and management. Am J Cardiol 1977: 40: 429–437.
13. Norris RM, Sammel NL. Predictors of late hospital death in acute myocardial infarction. Prog Cardiovasc Dis 1980; 23: 129–140.
14. Galve E, García-del-Castillo H, Evangelista A, Batlle J, Permanyer-Miralda G, Soler-Soler J. Pericardial effusion in the course of acute myocardial infarction: incidence, natural history, and clinical relevance. Circulation 1986; 73: 294–299.
15. Horowitz MS, Schultz CS, Stinson EB, Harrison DC, Popp PL. Sensitivity and specificity of echocardiographic diagnosis of pericardial effusion. Circulation 1974; 50: 239–247.
16. Weitzman LB, Tinker WP, Kronzon I, Cohen ML, Glassman E, Spencer FC. The incidence and natural history of pericardial effusion after cardiac surgery. An echocardiographic study. Circulation 1984; 69: 506–511.
17. Kaplan K, Davidson R, Parker M, Przybylek J, Light A, Bresnahan D, Ribner H, Talano JV. Frequency of pericardial effusion as determined by M mode echocardiography in acute myocardial infarction. Am J Cardiol 1985; 55: 335–337.
18. Somolinos M, Violán S, Sanz R, Marrero P. Early pericarditis after acute myocardial infarction: A clinical echocardiographic study. Crit Care Med 1987; 15: 648–651.
19. Pierard LA, Albert A, Henrard L, Lempereur P, Sprynger M, Carlier J, Kulbertus HE. Incidence and significance of pericardial effusion in acute myocardial infarction as determined by two-dimensional echocardiography. J Am Coll Cardiol 1986; 8: 517–520.
20. Wunderink RG. Incidence of pericardial effusions in acute myocardial infarctions. Chest 1984; 85: 494–496.
21. Savage DD, Garrison RJ, Brand F, Anderson SJ, Castelli WP, Kannel WB, Feinleib M. Prevalance and correlates of posterior extra echocardiographic spaces in a free-living population based sample (The Framingham Study). Am J Cardiol 1983; 51: 1207–1212.
22. Rhode EA. Physiology of the normal pericardium in pericardial disease. In: Reddy PS, Leon DF, Shaver JA. eds. New York: Raven Press, 1982: 33.

152   ENRIQUE GALVE

23. Rifkin RD, Isner JM, Carter BL, Bankoff MS. Combined posteroanterior subepicardial fat simulating the echocardiographic diagnosis of pericardial effusion. J Am Coll Cardiol 1984; 3: 1333–1339.
24. Berger M, Bobak L, Jelveh M, Goldberg E. Pericardial effusion diagnosed by echocardiography. Clinical and electrocardiographic findings in 171 patients. Chest 1978; 74: 724–729.
25. Phibbs B. "Transmural" versus "subendocardial" myocardial infarction: an electrocardiographic myth J Am Coll Cardiol 1983; 1: 561–564.
26. Spodick DH Q-wave infarction versus ST infarction. Nonspecificity of electrocardiographic criteria for differentiating transmural and non-transmural lesions. Am J Cardiol 1983; 51: 913–915.
27. Editorial Pericardial effusion after acute myocardial infarction. Lancet 1986; 1: 1015–1016.
28. Rosenbaum FF, Levine SA. Prognostic value of various clinical and electrocardiographic features of acute myocardial infarction. Arch Int Med 1941; 68: 913–917.
29. Mintz SS, Katz LN. Recent myocardial infarction. An analysis of five hundred and seventy-two cases. Arch Int Med 1947; 80: 205–236.
30. Niarchos AP, McKendrick CS. Prognosis of pericarditis after acute myocardial infarction. Br Heart J 1973; 35: 49–54.
31. Liem KL, Durrer D, Lie KI, Wellens HJJ. Pericarditis of acute myocardial infarction. Lancet 1975; 2: 1004–1006.
32. Guillevin L, Valere PE. Pericarditis in acute myocardial infarction. Lancet 1976; 1: 429.
33. Sawaya JI, Mujais SK, Armenian HK. Early diagnosis of pericarditis in acute myocardial infarction. Am Heart J 1980; 100: 144–151.
34. Krainin FM, Flessas AP, Spodick DH. Infarction associated pericarditis. Rarity of diagnostic electrocardiogram. N Engl J Med 1984; 311: 1211–1214.
35. Tofler GH, Muller JE, Stone PH, Willich SN, Davis VG, Poole K, Robertson T, Braunwald E, MILIS study group. Pericarditis in acute myocardial infarction: Characterization and clinical significance. Am Heart J 1989; 117: 86–92.
36. Aarseth S, Lange HF. The influence of anticoagulant therapy on the occurrence of cardiac rupture and hemopericardium following heart infarction. I. A study of 89 cases of hemopericardium (81 of them cardiac ruptures). Am Heart J 1958; 56: 250–256.
37. Waldrom BR, Fennell RH Jr, Castleman B, Bland EF. Myocardial rupture and hemopericardium associated with anticoagulant therapy; a post-mortem study. N Engl J Med 1954; 251: 892–894.
38. Goldstein R, Wolff L. Haemorrhagic pericarditis in acute myocardial infarction treated with bis hydroxicumarin. JAMA 1951; 146: 616–621.
39. Rose OA, Ott RH Jr, Maier HC. Hemopericardium with tamponade during anticoagulant therapy of myocardial infarction: report of case with recovery following pericardiotomy. JAMA 1953; 152: 1221–1223.
40. Khanderia BK, Shub C, Nishimura RA, Miller FA Jr., Seward JB, Tajik AJ. To anticoagulate or not: implications for the management of patients with acute myocardial infarction complicated by both left ventricular thrombus and pericardial effusion. Can J Cardiol 1987; 3: 173–176.
41. López-Sendón J, González A, Sotillo J. Diagnostic approach to subacute ventricular rupture following acute myocardial infarction. X World Congress of Cardiology, Washington (Abstract Book) 1986; 100.
42. Lichstein E, Arsura E, Hollander G, Greengart A, Sanders M. Current incidence of post-myocardial infarction (Dressler's) syndrome. Am J Cardiol 1982; 50: 1269–1271.

9. Massive chronic idiopathic pericardial effusion

J. SOLER-SOLER, M.D.

Pericardial effusion is a common clinical finding now that echocardiography has become a routine tool for the study of patients with cardiac or systemic diseases. Thus, in a consecutive series (1) of 2106 patients pericardial effusion was diagnosed in 178 (8.4%), a prevalence similar to that found by other authors (2). A significant number of pericardial effusions are missed if diagnosis is based on clinical grounds alone (41% and 61% in the two series), as either they are small or do not give rise to clinical suspicion of pericardial disease. By contrast, in some patients pericardial effusion may be the dominant finding because of its great size (massive pericardial effusion), whether or not clinical findings suggesting pericardial disease are present. Occasionally, pericardial effusion persists over years or even decades, thereby constituting the syndrome of chronic pericardial effusion (3–5). This clinical syndrome has multiple etiologies (6–8); in fact, it can be caused by a great number of the disorders that may involve the pericardium.

The present chapter is devoted to the most dramatic and puzzling form of chronic pericardial effusion: massive chronic idiopathic pericardial effusion. This syndrome has not received a lot of attention in the literature; the currently available information is based on reports of isolated cases, short series (3, 9–14) and in three reviews (6, 7, 15) which unfortunately include many instances of effusion of known etiology. Altogether, these features explain why an adequate study algorithm has not been developed, and why these patients are even today treated in a random fashion (corticosteroid therapy, antituberculous chemotherapy, repeated pericardiocenteses, pericardiectomy, or even drainage of the pericardial effusion to the gastrointestinal tract). In

J. Soler-Soler et al. (Eds.), Pericardial Disease, pp. 153–165.
© 1990 Kluwer Academic Publishers

this chapter we analyze a consecutive series of 14 patients who were prospectively studied by our group.

Definition

The lack of a precise definition of this syndrome, together with its low incidence, is one of the major reasons for its being poorly appreciated and understood. For inclusion in our series, the following requirements had to be fulfilled: a) The pericardial effusion as assessed by echocardiographic criteria must be large. We use the sum of anterior and posterior echo-free spaces greater than 20 mm at end-diastole (Fig. 9.1). In our series, all patients presented with a great increase in the cardiac size on the chest radiogram (Fig. 9.2). b) The amount of the effusion should be stable over the observation period. c) The effusion should be present for at least three months to be considered chronic. d) The patient should be free from systemic disease, even if the latter has no known association with pericardial effusion. e) Finally, a

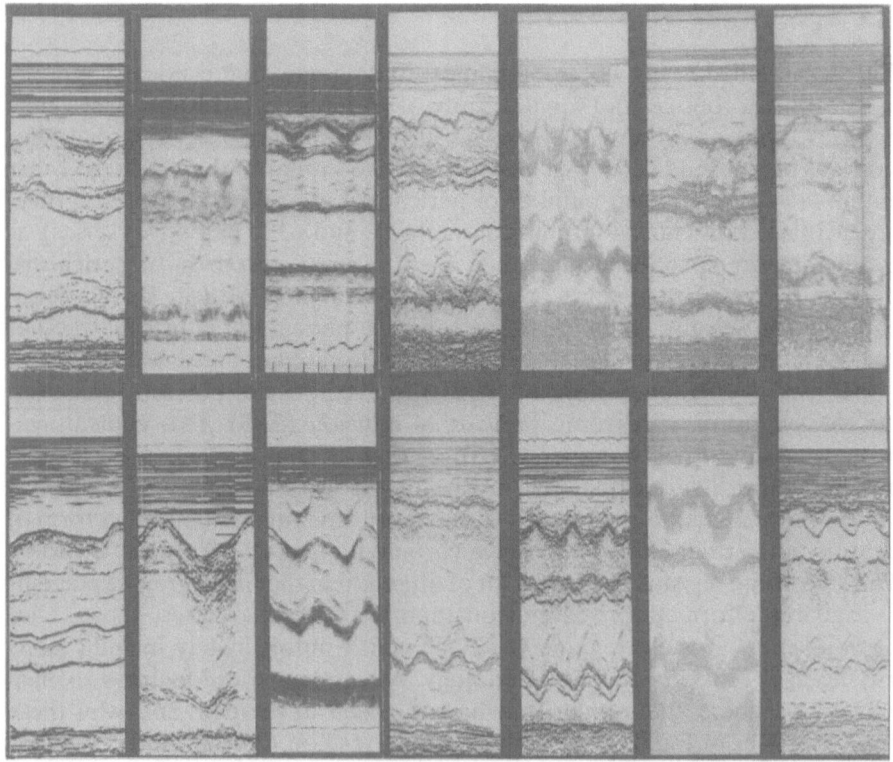

Fig. 9.1. Echocardiograms of the 14 patients before pericardiectomy.

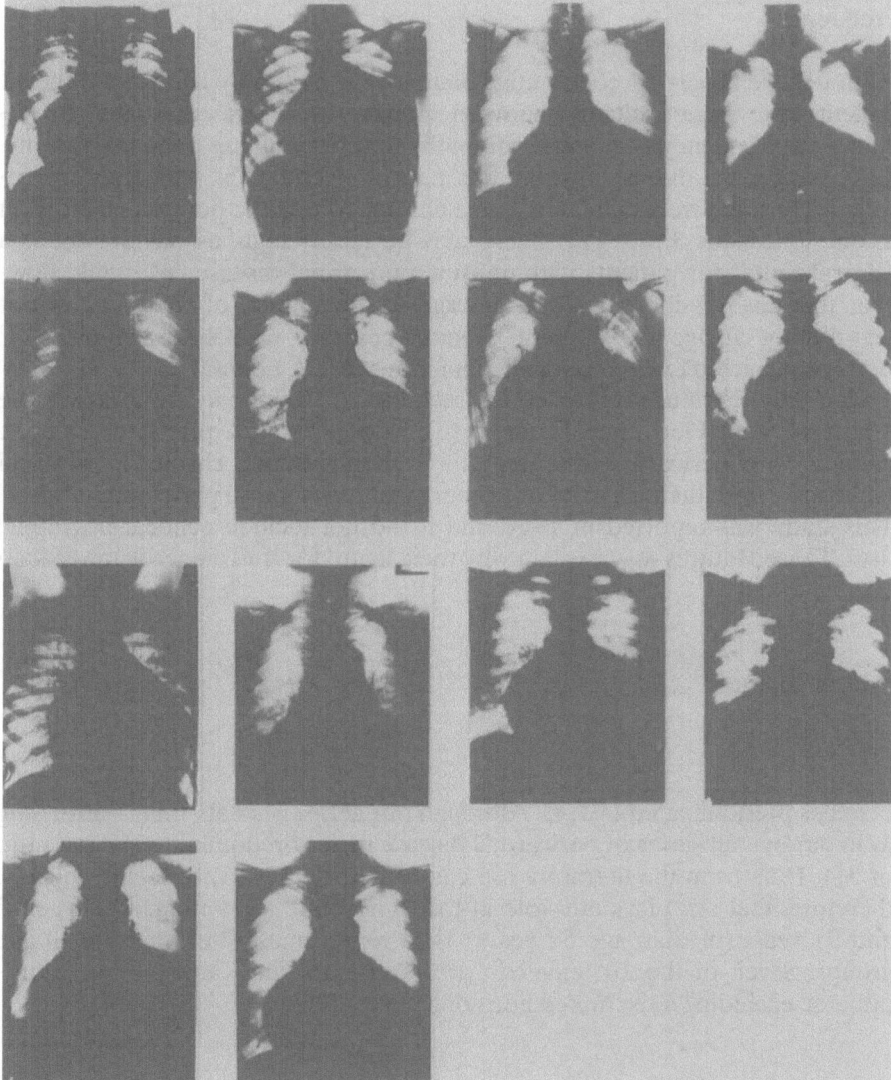

Fig. 9.2. Chest radiograms of the 14 patients before pericardiectomy. Most of them show the classical bottle-shaped silhouette.

thorough systematic etiologic study should be negative, thus allowing the effusion to be labelled as idiopathic.

Some authors (16) have called this syndrome "chronic effusive pericarditis", but we prefer to avoid this name because these patients do not usually report symptoms suggesting pericarditis.

Frequency

Although we report 14 consecutive patients, we have only considered the 11 patients who were evaluated between January 1977 and June 1986 to calculate the frequency of massive idiopathic effusion among patients with primary pericardial disease. During this period, overall 309 patients were enrolled. Thus, the frequency of massive chronic idiopathic pericardial effusion in our series was 3.5%. This figure may be falsely high, as our Service is a referral center for patients with unusual pericardial disease. We think, however, that this possible bias was not large, as the number of patients seen per year did not change (1–2 patients). On the contrary, we believe that our high index of suspicion exerted a significant influence (see below).

The only literature reference to frequency of which we are aware is the report by Saint-Pierre and Froment (6), who gave a 2% prevalence among patients with pericardial disease. They did not define chronic pericardial effusion or state their criteria for primary ("autonomous") pericardial disease. This study was reported in 1966 and it did not include echocardiographic data. These features may explain why their figure for prevalence is lower than ours.

Clinical features

Patients

Females predominated (10:4). Although our series is small, this is surprising as in our overall series of pericardial disease males predominated with a ratio of 3:1. Data from the literature are contradictory (10, 15); it seems unlikely, therefore, that sex plays any role in this syndrome. Ages ranged between 7 and 91 years (median age 54 years), with representation of virtually all age groups. Seven of the 10 females were postmenopausal and two were prepuberal, excluding a sex linked hormonal factor (10).

Duration of pericardial effusion

The duration of the effusion, as evidenced in the echocardiogram or chest radiogram, ranged between 10 months and 17 years, with a mean value of 5.5 years. It had been present for longer than 10 years in four patients. In a woman aged 91 years pericardial effusion persisted until her death, and its presence was traced to a chest radiogram that we had the chance to examine taken 17 years previously. The long duration of these effusions is one of their most puzzling features; a case from the report by Connolly et al. (10) probably persisted for 29 years.

Hospital admission

Table 9.1 shows the reasons for admission. In one half, the admission was scheduled for evaluation of a large cardiac silhouette in an asymptomatic patient discovered on routine chest radiography. Four other patients were admitted because of mild dyspnea and or nonspecific chest pain. Finally, three patients were admitted for severe cardiac tamponade; all had clinical features consistent with acute pericarditis in the days preceding admission.

Table 9.1. Cause of hospital admission.

Evaluation (asymptomatic patients)	7
Dyspnea or atypical chest pain	4
Severe tamponade	3

Suspicion of the diagnosis

We feel that our high index of suspicion of this syndrome played an important role in disclosing its true prevalence. Thus, none of the seven patients admitted for symptoms were aware that they had pericardial disease; at most, some of them reported that they knew they had "a cardiac disorder". Our approach to any patient with large pericardial effusion is a tenacious search for previous chest radiograms or echocardiograms, dating from as long as possible, that we can personally examine. This approach enabled us to adequately identify the three patients who were admitted with tamponade and the four in whom dyspnea or chest pain were the cause for admission; otherwise they might have been categorized as acute pericardits or unqualified pericardial effusion. It is quite likely that the true prevalence of chronic idiopathic pericardial effusion is really about 3.5% of primary pericardial disease, suggesting that this syndrome is more common than apparent from monographs on pericardial diseases (17, 18) or comprehensive cardiology textbooks (19). We believe, therefore, that a sound clinical rule is to suspect this syndrome in all patients with large pericardial effusions, independently from the symptoms at presentation.

Etiologic study

Once the diagnosis was established, the study was oriented towards etiologic diagnosis. To this end, all the steps of stage I of our protocol for the study and treatment of pericardial disease were carried out, supplemented by a thyroid function study. The latter should be carried out in all cases, even in the absence of clinical features of hypothyroidism, as we have seen, in agreement with others (20), symptomless hypothyroidism with massive chronic pericar-

Table 9.2. Cardiac catheterization.

	Patient 13		Patient 14	
	Baseline	P-centesis 900 ml	Baseline	P-centesis 700 ml
RA	5	1	4	0
RV	30/7	22/4	25/15	30/6
LV	148/12	132/10	155/12	145/9
Per	+5	−3	+4	−5
HR	93	95	61	60
CI	2.7	3.2	3.0	3.5

P-centesis: pericardiocentesis; RA: mean right atrial pressure; RV: right ventricular pressure; Per: intrapericardial pressure; HR: heart rate; CI: cardiac index.

dial effusion as the only clinical feature. If all these studies did not disclose the etiology, pericardiocentesis was undertaken. Pericardial fluid was analyzed following stage II of our protocol. Pericardiocentesis was not carried out in the 91-year-old patient as she did not consent. In the two last patients of the series pericardiocentesis was combined with the recording of intracardiac and intrapericardial pressures. These were two completely symptom free patients (aged 60 and 64 years), whose effusion had been discovered nine months and eight years before. Their hemodynamic data are shown in Table 9.2. Remarkably, intrapericardial pressure was somewhat high in both patients (mean values of +5 and +4 mmHg), and equal to right atrial pressure. The study protocol did not include surgical pericardial drainage with biopsy.

In the 13 patients who underwent pericardiocentesis, variable amounts of fluid were removed (250–2700 ml, mean 1165 ml), depending on the improvement in hemodynamic state (in patients with tamponade) or, simply, on the operator's judgement. The fluid appearance was serofibrinous in eight patients and serosanguineous in five, with a protein content from 3.5 to 5.2 g/100 ml and scanty cells. There were no complications.

Our patients had the following nonpericardial diseases: stable angina (one), congenital facial lymphangioma (one), and moderate hypertension (two). Even though some authors (12) have discussed a possible relationship between hypertension and chronic pericardial effusion, we think the association is coincident.

Only patients in whom the systematic workup was negative were included; that is, those in whom effusion could be considered idiopathic. Our protocol is not exhaustive; however, as discussed elsewhere (21), its cost effectiveness certainly is adequate for practical ends. Subsequent histological study of the pericardium (see below) confirmed the absence of specific abnormalities or active pericardial disease in the 12 patients who underwent pericardiectomy, thus confirming the adequacy of the diagnostic approach.

Natural history

Most studies (4–6, 9, 11, 12, 16) stress that one of the remarkable features of this syndrome is its good long term hemodynamic tolerance. Fowler (22) mentioned that tamponade is virtually never seen in those patients, and, if it develops, it does so gradually. Likewise, Shabetai (16) stated that "in some cases, signs of tamponade can be seen in the initial stages, but they subside and eventually disappear in the subsequent months". Our experience shows that this benign character is far from universal in massive chronic idiopathic pericardial effusion. Thus, in our series, five of the 14 patients (36%) developed severe or fatal (one patient) tamponade, which was therefore present in more than one third of them; however, this high frequency was influenced by a selection bias. There are reported patients (3–5, 23, 24) in whom tamponade developed with varying severity and in a recent series of 8 patients with large idiopathic pericardial effusion (8) tamponade was demonstrated in 3 (37%).

The only patient who died of pericardial disease was a 91-year-old woman whom we admitted for evaluation when she had no signs of tamponade. Her pericardial effusion had lasted at least 17 years, but she refused all invasive procedures. Three months after discharge she was seen in routine follow up in our outpatient clinic, and was stable. However, four months afterwards she was admitted to another institution with low cardiac output state and died in 36 hours. The final illness was strongly suggestive of cardiac tamponade (markedly distended neck veins, severe hypotension, persistence of large effusion and absence of other cardiac abnormalities), as reflected in the clinical record personally reviewed by us.

The pericardial effusions of the five patients who developed tamponade had persisted for at least 1, 4, 4, 5, and 17 years, respectively, and had not previously caused any symptoms. The only episodes clinically consistent with acute pericarditis (pain and/or friction rub, with fever) developed 7–20 days before admission in three of the patients who had tamponade. Adequate information to assess whether the 91-year-old patient also had previous pericarditis was not available. In the remaining patient there were no clinical features of acute pericarditis.

It is highly likely that, in these patients, clinical stability need not mean normal hemodynamics. Isolated observations (16) show that at least some of these patients have high intrapericardial pressures. In two of our asymptomatic patients, catheterization disclosed mild tamponade (Table 9.2), as baseline pericardial pressures were definitely abnormal (+4 and +5 mmHg, respectively) and became −5 mmHg and −3 mmHg, respectively, after removal of 900 and 700 ml of effusion (Fig. 9.3). In these patients pericardial effusion probably develops gradually, with adaptation of the pericardial volume to the increasing amount of fluid. This mechanism allows huge volumes to accumulate with only a small increase in intrapericardial pressure. The state of clinically silent mild tamponade could persist until a subsequent rise

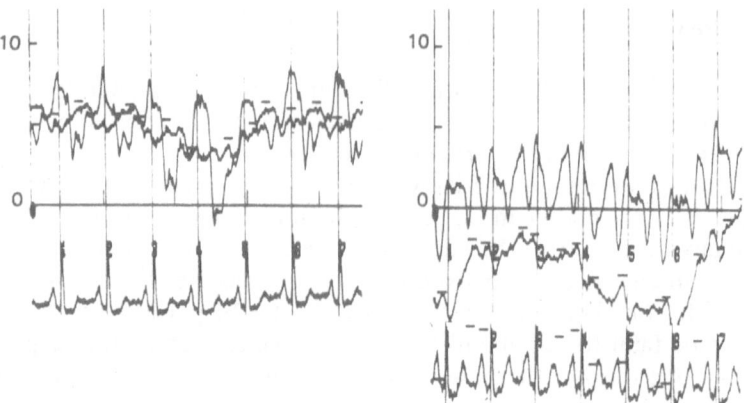

Fig. 9.3. Chronic pericardial effusion in an asymptomatic patient. Left panel shows an increased intrapericardial pressure (+5 mmHg), equal to the right atrial pressure. In the right panel, intrapericardial pressure has become normal (−3 mmHg) after the removal of 700 ml by pericardiocentesis. These data indicate that the patient, in her baseline state, had a mild, clinically silent tamponade.

in pericardial fluid volume, either spontaneous or after an intercurrent illness (for instance, acute pericarditis), exceeded the pericardial capacity for distension, resulting in severe tamponade with its characteristic clinical features and poor outlook if not adequately treated.

Constrictive pericarditis has been reported (3, 15, 25) as one of the possible outcomes of this syndrome. Our series could hardly be expected to show constriction, as our protocol includes pericardiectomy six months after the diagnosis is established and thus constrictive pericarditis is prevented.

Spontaneous disappearance of a huge apparently idiopathic pericardial effusion was recorded in two patients of Bedford's series (4) and one in the series by Connolly et al. (10). Our protocol prevented us from observing this pattern of evolution. However, in a 62-year-old woman, not included in the present series because of an antinuclear antibody titer of 1/800, disappearance of the effusion was documented. This observation and the presence of concomitant diseases in the three mentioned cases from the literature (probable cardiomyopathy and acromegaly (4), and polycythemia secondary to iron and cobalt intake (10)), raise doubts about whether spontaneous remissions really occur in massive chronic idiopathic pericardial effusion.

Therapy

There is no consensus on the therapy. The available information suggests that patients are treated in an empirical fashion. Most reports state that treatment with corticosteroids or other antiinflammatory drugs, antituberculous chemotheraphy and repeated pericardiocentesis result, at their best, in a transient improvement, but do not modify the outcome of the disease. Lorell and Braunwald recommend against treating these patients if they are symptom free (26). On the other hand, some authors (4, 7, 10, 12, 15, 16, 22, 23) recommend pericardiectomy if tamponade develops, the effusion persists for a long time or the condition is not well tolerated. However, the last two circumstances are not defined. We agree with Silber (27) that the presumed benefits of pericardiectomy in the absence of tamponade have not hitherto been validated.

Before we designed a protocol for the study of this syndrome, our limited experience suggested that, at least in some patients, the outcome was not so favorable as a prolonged symptom free course might lead one to believe. Thus, one patient with a stable massive chronic idiopathic pericardial effusion, whom we had followed irregularly for several years (not included in the present series as she had been seen before January 1977), died in another hospital with an illness strongly suggestive of acute cardiac tamponade. This observation and the previous considerations prompted us to recommend elective pericardiectomy in patients with massive chronic idiopathic pericardial effusion even in the absence of tamponade. Our protocol indication reads as follows: "In case of optimal tolerance and absence of etiologic diagnosis, the patient will be followed up without therapy, and pericardiectomy will be indicated when stable effusion has persisted for at least six months" (p. 221).

In accord with our protocol, pericardiectomy was carried out in 12 out of our 14 patients; the 91-year-old patient refused surgery, and the last patient included in the series is awaiting operation. The indication was elective in eight patients and emergent (owing to severe tamponade) in four. There were no operative deaths. Postoperatively, pleural effusion was occasionally seen and cleared up spontaneously; this complication did not eventually result in a clinical problem in any case.

Pericardial resection was carried out by several surgeons. In all cases, it was supposedly as extensive as possible. However, pericardial effusion recurred in two. In both of these cases the pericardial resection turned out to have been incomplete. This was demonstrated in the first patient, who underwent a second pericardiectomy indicated 4.5 years after the first owing to persistence of massive pericardial efusion. Three years later pericardial effusion remains absent. This case confirms that pericardiectomy must be extensive (28). In the second patient, in whom the extent of pericardial resection had been only 4 × 5 cm, a second pericardiectomy was contraindicated by a cerebral tumor.

The pericardium was macroscopically normal in seven patients and slightly thickened (2–3 mm) in the remaining five; the histology was chronic nonspecific pericarditis in all 11 cases where it was carried out.

Table 9.3. Pericardiectomy. Outcome.

Asymptomatic without evidence of pericardial disease	10
Dead	2
Cerebral tumor 16 months after pericardiectomy	
Stroke 24 months after pericardiectomy	
Awaiting pericardiectomy	1
Refused pericardiectomy	1*

* Subsequently died from cardiac tamponade.

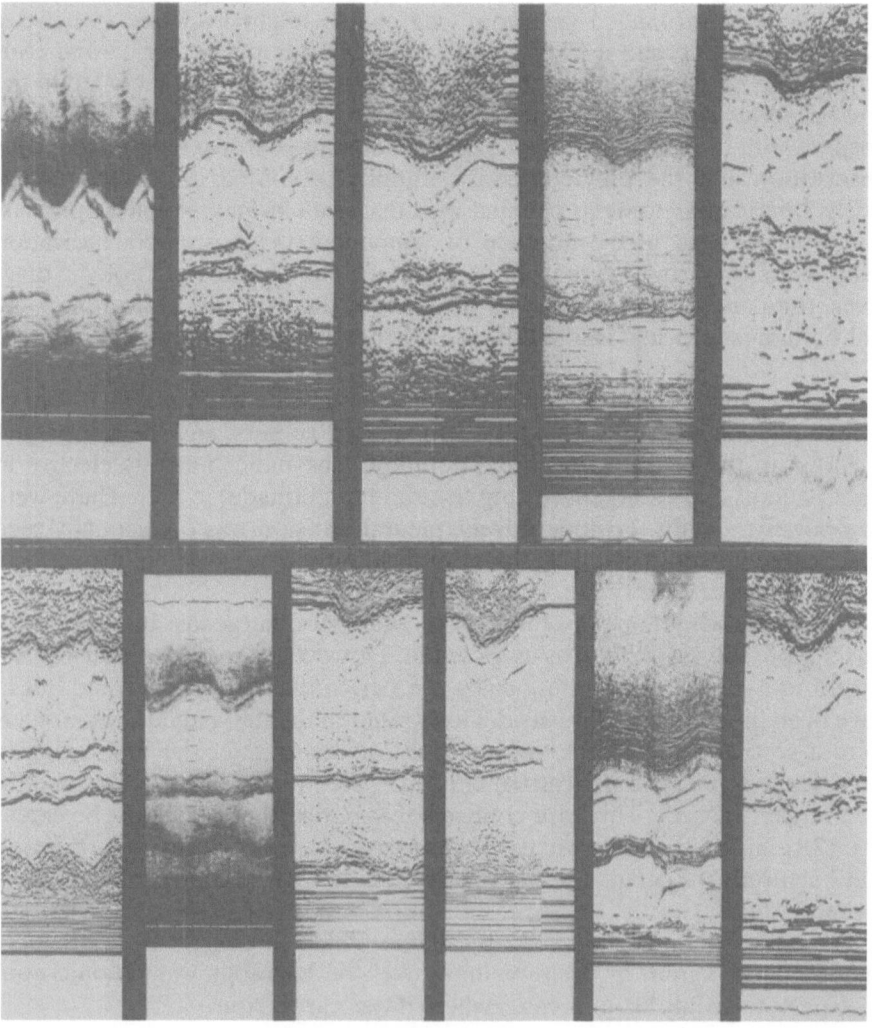

Fig. 9.4. Echocardiograms at the last follow up after pericardiectomy. Note the absence of pericardial effusion. The recording of one patient is not shown because of a poor acoustic window.

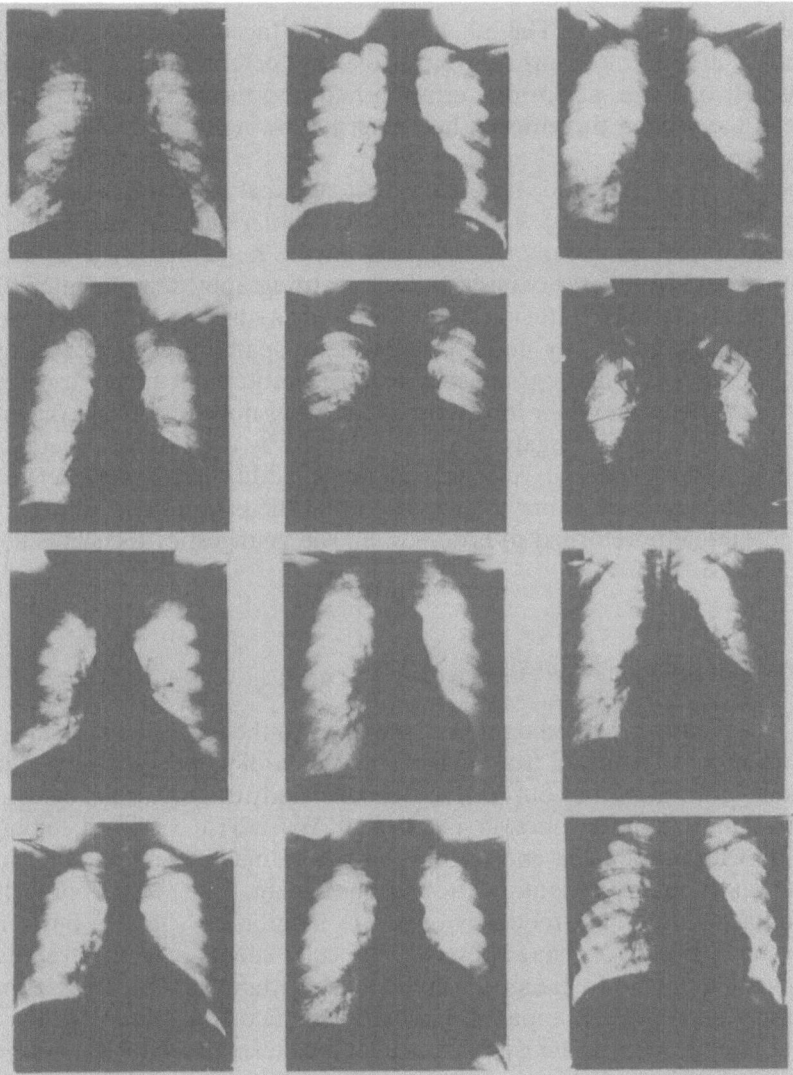

Fig. 9.5. Chest radiograms of all patients after pericardiectomy. Note that the cardiac silhouette has become smaller, but, except in two cases, it has not returned to normal. The fact that these radiograms were simultaneous with the echocardiograms rules out pericardial effusion as the cause of cardiomegaly.

Follow up

No patient has been lost to follow up (16 months–10.4 years; mean 5.1 years). All survivors are symptom free (four of them more than six years after peri-cardiectomy) (Table 9.3). Three patients have died; of them, only the 91-year-old female died of pericardial disease and she was the only patient who had refused pericardiectomy. The other two patients (aged 66 and 57 years) died 24 and 16 months after surgery from stroke and cerebral tumor, respectively. In the first of these, pericardial effusion had disappeared after pericardiectomy; in the second the effusion had persisted owing to incomplete pericardial resection.

The last follow up echocardiogram disclosed that pericardial effusion was absent in all patients (Fig. 9.4). In contrast, the cardiac silhouette (Fig. 9.5) returned to normal in only two patients. In the remaining patients cardiomegaly of variable degree persists, but echocardiography demonstrated that it cannot be attributed to effusion. Shabetai (16) has suggested that such cardiomegaly may be caused by underlying cardiomyopathy; we are not in agreement, because echocardiographically assessed ventricular function was normal in all patients and their long term course does not support this diagnosis. We believe that cardiomegaly may be explained by the extensive pericardial resection, but we cannot rule out unknown additional factors related to chronic effusion itself. It may be pertinent that the two patients in whom the cardiac silhouette returned to normal were the youngest of the series (7 and 11 years, respectively).

Present approach to diagnosis and therapy

We have recently modified our initial protocol on the basis of our results. The main change is to refrain from diagnostic pericardiocentesis if all the investigations in the stage I of our protocol for the study of pericardial disease are negative and thyroid function is normal. We advise pericardiectomy in patients with tamponade and in those in whom massive chronic effusion is stable longer than six months. The reasons for this aggressive approach are the following: the high frequency of severe tamponade (36% in our series), the state of mild tamponade (even if clinically silent) present in an as yet undefined number of patients, the absence of mortality and the low morbidity of pericardiectomy, the apparent lack of spontaneous resolution of the syndrome, and, most importantly, the excellent long term outcome after surgery.

Following this approach, some exceptional diseases (such as chylous (29, 30) or cholesterol (31, 32) effusions) will be initially missed until pericardiectomy is performed; however, in view of their rarity, we feel that the risk/benefit ratio justifies not to carry out pericardiocentesis.

References

1. Berger M, Bobak K, Jelveh M, Goldberg E. Pericardial effusion diagnosed by echo cardiography. Clinical and electrocardiographic findings. Chest 1978; 74: 174–179.
2. Riba AKK, Morganroth J. Unsuspected pericardial effusion detected by echocardiography. JAMA 1976; 236: 2623–2625.
3. Barker PS, Johnston FD. Chronic pericarditis with effusion. Circulation 1950; 2: 134–138.

4. Bedford DE. Chronic effusive pericarditis. Br Heart J 1964; 26: 499–512.
5. Brown AK. Chronic idiopathic pericardial effusion. Br Heart J 1966; 28: 609–614.
6. Saint-Pierre A, Froment R. Epanchements péricardiques chroniques. Diagnostic étiologique. Conduite thérapeutique. In: Froment R, Gonin A, Michaud P, eds. Pathologie péricardique. Paris, Masson & Cie, 1966; 300–320.
7. Marion MML, Le Gall F, Baille Y, Chagnon A, Pierron JR. Les épanchements péricardiques chroniques. Revue générale a propos de 2 observations. Bordeaux Medical 1979; 23: 1449–1456.
8. Colombo A, Olson HG, Egan J, Gardin JM. Etiology and prognostic implications of a large pericardial effusion in men. Clin Cardiol 1988; 11: 389–394.
9. Contro S, De Giuli G, Ragazzini F. Chronic effusive pericarditis. Circulation 1955; 11: 844–848.
10. Connolly DC, Dry TJ, Good CA, Clagett OT, Burchell HB. Chronic idiopathic pericardial effusion without tamponade. Circulation 1959; 20: 1095–1105.
11. Soulié P, Vernant P, Corone P, Georges R. Epanchement péricardique chronique idiopathique chez des şujets jeunes. Arch Mal Coeur 1960; 53: 1248–1256.
12. Wood P. Diseases of the heart and circulation. London, Eyre & Spottiswoode, 1968; 784.
13. Dressler W, Levin EJ, Axelrod M. Huge chronic pericardial effusion of 15 years's duration. JAMA 1966; 195: 188–190.
14. Gómez Sánchez MA, Fernández Yáñez J, López Gil M, García Martínez J, Saenz de la Calzada C. Derrame pericárdico crónico. Monocardio 1982; 3: 24–44.
15. Scheuer J. Chronic idiopathic pericardial effusion. Circulation 1960; 21: 41–48.
16. Shabetai R. The pericardium. New York, Grune and Stratton, 1981; 147.
17. Spodick DH. Pericardial diseases. Philadelphia, F.A. Davis Company, 1976.
18. Reddy PA, Leon DF, Shaver JA. Pericardial disease. New York, Raven Press, 1982.
19. Hurst JW. The heart. New York, McGraw-Hill Book Co., 1986.
20. Zimmerman J, Yahalon J, Bar-On, H. Clinical spectrum of pericardial effusion as the presenting feature of hypothyroidism. Am Heart J 1983; 106: 770–771.
21. Permanyer-Miralda G, Sagristà-Sauleda J, Soler-Soler J. Primary acute pericardial diseases: a prospective series of 231 consecutive patients. Am J Cardiol 1985; 56: 623–630.
22. Fowler NO. Chronic pericarditis. In: Fowler NO, ed. The pericardium in health and disease. Mount Kisco, Futura Publishing Company, 1985; 231.
23. Mannix EP, Dennis C. The surgical treatment of chronic pericardial effusion and cardiac tamponade. J Thorac Cardiovasc Surg 1955; 29: 381–397.
24. Markiewicz W, Borovik R, Ecker S. Cardiac tamponade in medical patients: treatment and prognosis in the echocardiographic era. Am Heart J 1986; 111: 1138–1142.
25. Spodick DH. The pericardium: structure, function, and disease spectrum. In: Spodick DH, ed. Pericardial disease. Philadelphia, F. A. Davis Company, 1976; 7.
26. Lorell BH, Braunwald E. Pericardial disease. In: Braunwald E, ed. Heart disease. Philadelphia, W. B. Saunders Company, 1988; 1492.
27. Silber EN. Heart disease. New York, MacMillan Publishing Copany, 1987; 1342.
28. Pielher JM, Pluth JR, Schaff HV, Danielson GK, Orszulak TA, Puga FJ. Surgical management of effusive pericardial disease: influence of extent of pericardial resection on clinical course. J Thorac Cardiovasc Surg 1985; 90: 506–516.
29. Dunn RP. Primary chylopericardium: a review of the literature and an illustrated case. Am Heart J 1975; 89: 369–377.
30. Alvarado F, López-Herce J, Matamoros M, Borches D, Castro MC, Ruza F. Quilopericardio idiopático en el niño: presentación de un caso y revisión de la literatura. Rev Esp Cardiol 1986; 39 (suppl I): 81–84.
31. Rosenbaum DL, Yu PN. Idiopathic cholesterol pericarditis with effusion. Am Heart J 1965; 70: 515–520.
32. Brawley RK, Vasko JS, Morrow AG. Cholesterol pericarditis: considerations of its pathogenesis and treatment. Am J Med 1966; 41: 235–248.

10. Indications for pericardiectomy in the absence of constriction

G. PERMANYER-MIRALDA, M.D.

The indication for pericardiectomy is unequivocal in moderate or severe chronic constrictive pericarditis. Constrictive pericarditis has been the basic indication for pericardiectomy for more than fifty years. However, constrictive pericarditis is the common end stage of a variety of pericardial diseases and, in many cases, it implies a course of many years. As in other heart diseases in which early operation has gained ground, one might wonder whether in pericardial diseases resection of the pericardium would not be indicated before constriction develops or becomes severe. One might also wonder whether pericardiectomy might not also be indicated to treat non constrictive cases with an unfavorable course such as severe tamponade, bacterial pericarditis or recurrent pericarditis. A critical assessment of these types of indication is made in the present chapter.

Aims of pericardiectomy in the absence of constriction: historical overview

On theoretical grounds, pericardiectomy might be indicated not only to prevent constriction, but also as radical therapy in a variety of conditions where a better outcome could be predicted with surgical treatment. The major indications for pericardiectomy in the absence of constriction up to the present

J. Soler-Soler et al. (Eds.), Pericardial Disease, pp. 167–181.
© 1990 Kluwer Academic Publishers

have been the prevention of constriction (1, 2), persistent or recurrent cardiac tamponade (2), the suppression or the control of severe recurrent acute idiopathic pericarditis (1, 3, 4), and the control of life threatening infective pericarditis, such as the purulent and tuberculous types (5).

These aims of pericardiectomy in the absence of constriction have given rise to several reports from the literature, all of them published several years ago, and which may be taken as representative of the opinions favoring this indication. We will now review the most outstanding among these reports, with an analysis of the clinical experience on which their authors' opinions are based.

In 1951, Holman and Willett (5), on the basis of their experience in five patients, recommended pericardiectomy to treat *tuberculous pericarditis*, not only when a diagnosis of constrictive pericarditis was made, but also when hemodynamic compromise by tamponade was detected. These authors considered that surgical therapy not only relieved the hemodynamic disorder but also facilitated the cure of the infection. This latter point was more relevant at a time when antituberculous chemotherapy was only in its beginning.

In 1959, Zinsser et al. (3), in a classical report of eight patients, advised pericardiectomy for *recurrent acute idiopathic pericarditis*. It is well known that, in this condition, the development of repetitive episodes may be a real challenge both for symptomatic therapy and prevention. We will discuss another classical report in more detail later. Here we will only mention that, despite initial hopes (1, 3, 4), experience has not been uniform.

In 1963, Iturrino and Holland (2) introduced the concept of emergency pericardiectomy, which was recommended as a radical therapy for all cases of *cardiac tamponade* of any etiology not readily responsive to medical therapy. Their report consisted of six cases, two idiopathic, one tuberculous, one purulent, one neoplastic and one traumatic. They considered that, in spite of their small series and the variety of diseases, pericardiectomy offered a greater likelihood of a good outcome in view of the unpredictable outcome of untreated tamponade. They even suggested that pericardiectomy could, as an additional advantage, prevent constrictive pericarditis, which they seemed to consider a frequent late complication of tamponade.

Some years later (1971), Wychulis, Connolly and McGoon (1) reviewed the whole experience of the Mayo Clinic with pericardiectomy, numbering 191 operations. Only 13 of the 191 were wide resections for conditions other than constriction. The remaining instances were for constrictive pericarditis or were so limited that they may scarcely be considered as pericardiectomies in the usual sense of the word. In spite of these limitations, the authors concluded that pericardiectomy is a safe and effective therapy for severe pericardial disease, although they did not provide definite indications.

Our analysis of the literature underlines two features. First, semantic confusion, as the term pericardiectomy covers a variety of procedures. Unless specified otherwise, all patients reported in the present chapter underwent a wide resection of the anterior and left posterior pericardium through median sternotomy. Second, the initial recommendations of the different authors are based on a limited material, and the surgical indications have not been based on systematic study of a large varied population.

Although the rationale appears unclear, pericardiectomy in the absence of constriction has been widely recommended in some institutions. For instance, in a recent Cardiology textbook (6) early pericardiectomy is advocated for most types of severe pericardial disease of any etiology. The authors report that the number of cases in which pericardiectomy was indicated in the absence of constriction was 98 during the last ten years which was more than twice the number indicated for constrictive pericarditis (42 cases). Undoubtedly, this could reflect the referral pattern to their institution. However, the recommendation of the authors is that pericardiectomy should be carried out in all severe cases of exudative pericarditis of any etiology that do not respond promptly to medical therapy (6, 7).

The indications for pericardiectomy in the absence of constriction do not appear so clear cut to other authors (8). One wonders to what extent it is based on the natural history of the different types of pericardial diseases or if it is an intuitive recommendation.

Indications for pericardiectomy in the absence of constriction based on the natural history of the different subsets of pericardial disease

To attempt to answer the question in the preceding paragraph we will review our data from the series of patients with primary acute pericardial disease (9, 10) prospectively seen in our Service. They were distributed in several groups depending on etiology. We remind the reader that, in our protocol for the study and management of pericardial diseases (9), pericardiectomy is not as precisely indicated as other invasive procedures (pericardiocentesis and pericardial biopsy), being left more to the clinician's judgement.

Acute idiopathic pericarditis

In the 221 patients with acute idiopathic pericarditis from our series (Table 10.1), the following observations are relevant to the present discussion. The 32 instances of tamponade that occurred were satisfactorily treated with pericardiocentesis or surgical drainage; in no case did tamponade recur after hospital discharge. In the eight patients who developed constrictive pericarditis, constriction was transient in six (11), and pericardiectomy was required in only the other two patients. An additional six pericardiectomies were carried out for miscellaneous indications, discussed below (recurrent pericarditis, iatrogenic hematoma or associated cardiac operation), but none of them

Table 10.1. Acute idiopathic pericarditis.

221	patients	
	cardiac tamponade	32
	recurrent course	44
8	pericardiectomies	
	constrictive pericarditis	2
	other indications	6

was based on poor hemodynamic evolution or on severe clinical features. In a subsequent paragraph the 44 patients with recurrent evolution will be discussed.

Reviewing these results it becomes evident that pericardiectomy would have not resulted in an improved course compared with conservative treatment. This consideration also applied to patients in whom a modest or moderate effusion persists after clinical resolution as, in our experience, they recover spontaneously as a rule.

Recurrent acute idiopathic pericarditis

Recurrent acute idiopathic pericarditis has been one of the more frequent indications of pericardiectomy in the absence of constriction since it was first recommended by Zinsser et al. in 1959 (3). In our series of 44 patients we only indicated pericardiectomy in two (Table 10.2). However, both patients continued to experience recurrent episodes after the operation. It is beyond the scope of the present chapter to discuss the whole topic of therapy for relapsing pericarditis including the possible harmful effect of corticosteroids. Nevertheless, it is remarkable that our two patients, whom we saw early in our experience, had previously been treated with prednisone. Subsequently, we have not administered corticosteroids to any other patient with this condition and, despite the 20% frequency of recurrences, the disease has been self limited in most patients. Even in the three of five patients with more than five episodes, the disease was not considered incapacitating owing to the short duration of the recurrences, and pericardiectomy has not been carried out.

Table 10.2. Recurrent acute idiopathic pericarditis.

44	patients among 221 (20%)	
	patients with 2 episodes	20
	patients with 3–5 episodes	19
	patients with >5 episodes	5
2	pericardiectomies	

As our own data are insufficient to evaluate the usefulness of pericardiectomy in treating recurrent idiopathic pericarditis, it is necessary also to review
data from the literature. We consider it remarkable that, since 1971, no series
as large or as successful as that of Hatcher et al. (4), where 24 patients
underwent pericardiectomy with 22 successes and only 2 recurrences, has
been reported. On the other hand, many isolated instances of failure of pericardiectomy to prevent recurrences have been described (1, 12, 13). In a
recent series (14) only two of nine pericardiectomies were successful.
Moreover, in the series by Hatcher et al. (4), which is often quoted as an
example of the success of pericardiectomy, the number, duration and severity
of recurrences required to indicate surgery was not stated, and surgery seems
to have even been indicated because of relapse of effusion without other clinical features, including pain.

It appears that, although some isolated patients with recurrent idiopathic
pericarditis unresponsive to other therapy have been successfully managed
with pericardiectomy, this indication is not solid enough to recommend it on
a systematic basis. On the other hand, it appears that only rarely will pericardiectomy have to be considered if medical therapy is prudent, as in most
cases the disease is self-limited in the long run.

Massive chronic pericardial effusion

The decision raised by huge chronic pericardial effusion is somewhat different. Sixteen cases of this syndrome have been observed on our Service (14
idiopathic and two toxoplasmosis (15)) (Table 10.3). The idiopathic cases are
analyzed in detail in chapter 9. It is pertinent to mention here that 6 (38%) of
the 16 patients (five with idiopathic disease and one with toxoplasmosis)
developed severe cardiac tamponade late in the clinical course, and, in several
of these, tamponade was sudden and unexpected. On the other hand, in the
14 patients who underwent pericardiectomy, recurrence of the effusion has
not been noted. Accordingly, we routinely recommend pericardiectomy for
stable massive chronic pericardial effusion. The reason for this recommendation is the unfavorable spontaneous long term outcome in a high proportion
of patients, characterized by acute, life threatening complications such as
cardiac tamponade in a previously asymptomatic individual. On the other
hand, pericardiectomy has been safe and effective and there are no alternative
therapies. The literature on this topic is surprisingly scanty, and does not

Table 10.3. Massive chronic pericardial effusion.

16	patients	
	cardiac tamponade	6 (38%)
14	pericardiectomies	

allow consistent conclusions about the need for pericardiectomy, which we routinely advocate on the basis of our experience. Chronic pericardial effusion of known etiology that responds to specific therapy, such as hypothyroidism (16), should initially receive medical therapy even if the effusion is massive. The chronic pericardial effusion that is occasionally associated with atrial septal defect (17, 18) should be surgically managed at the time of closure of the defect.

Tuberculous and purulent pericarditis

Our series of tuberculous pericarditis is the topic of chapter 6. Here the discussion is limited to those patients seen up to January 1985 (Table 10.4), even though after this date our findings have been similar. The possible benefits of pericardiectomy in non constricting tuberculous pericarditis differ from those previously considered for pericardial disorders of other etiology. For the first time we have a specific pericardial disease that often evolves to constriction (five of eleven of our patients). In these patients, moreover, constriction was severe and progressive, requiring prompt pericardiectomy. This clinical course raises the consideration of early routine pericardiectomy. In our part of the world, such an approach is not warranted because about one half of our patients and those of others (19, 19a) recovered with medical therapy and did not develop constriction.

Can evolution to constrictive pericarditis be predicted in tuberculous pericarditis? The answer appears to be that we often cannot, although three of the four patients who developed tamponade went on to constriction, suggesting the possibility that both of these hemodynamic complications depended on related factors. However, this is not always the case. Cases of tuberculous pericarditis may develop constriction without previous tamponade while the reverse is also true; therefore, it is not possible to predict the patients who will develop constriction.

Another shortcoming is that when a patient with cardiac tamponade is first evaluated, the diagnosis of tuberculosis has usually not yet been made. This was indeed the case with the four patients in our series who developed tamponade due to tuberculous pericarditis; at the time of pericardial subxiphoid drainage, tuberculosis had not yet been identified.

In view of the course of non constricting tuberculous pericarditis with

Table 10.4. Tuberculous pericarditis.

11	patients	
	cardiac tamponade	4
	evolution to constriction	5
5	pericardiectomies	

medical therapy, we believe that pericardiectomy in the absence of constriction should be reserved for those few patients with known tuberculous pericarditis in whom, at the time of surgical pericardial drainage to treat tamponade, the surgeon finds a thickened pericardium with adhesions, and patients in whom tamponade persists or recurs in spite of adequate medical therapy and pericardial drainage. In the first situation, which should be rare, pericardiectomy could be performed during the same operative procedure as pericardial drainage.

Similar considerations to those made for tuberculous pericarditis may be pertinent to purulent pericarditis (20, 20a), because this condition is also known to result in constrictive pericarditis. We are not reporting our own experience as only three patients with this diagnosis are included in our series.

Neoplastic pericarditis

A systematic approach to the treatment of non constricting neoplastic disease cannot be drawn from the literature, because the reported series tend to be small and heterogeneous. Many authors (8, 21–25b) favor a conservative approach using pericardiocentesis or surgical drainage and reserving pericardiectomy for established constriction. Others (6, 7) advocate pericardiectomy whenever the general condition of the patient and the stage of the underlying neoplastic disease allow.

Our series (Table 10.5) suffers from the same problem and therefore does not solve the dilemma. However, our results tend to favor a conservative approach. Seven of the ten patients in our series who developed tamponade were discharged from hospital in a satisfactory hemodynamic state; although six of the seven died before one year. Death was not cardiovascular but was related to dissemination of underlying neoplasia. In our series of 12 patients three pericardiectomies were performed, two for constriction (one classic and one effusive constrictive) and one for cardiac angiosarcoma. The first two patients died from dissemination of neoplasia within a few months, and the third is discussed below ("Diagnostic" pericardiectomy).

Our overall results do not permit us to state categorically whether pericardiectomy has any definite place in the treatment of neoplastic pericarditis in the absence of constriction, but they point in the conservative direction which

Table 10.5. Neoplastic pericarditis.

12 patients	
tamponade	10 (7*)
constrictive pericarditis	2

* Cases with initial resolution after pericardiocentesis or pericardial drainage.

is in accord with much of the literature. A systematic approach to this difficult problem may eventually establish which patients, if any, with non constrictive neoplastic pericarditis may benefit from pericardiectomy.

Pericarditis associated with renal failure

Pericarditis associated with renal failure has received a variety of contrasting approaches (26). Several authors (27–30) have recommended pericardiectomy for all types of pericardial disease associated with renal failure when complications develop or effusion accumulates progressively. The justification is that the hemodynamic outcome of these patients is poor and the risk of more conservative measures, especially pericardiocentesis, is high. An extensive discussion of this as yet unresolved dilemma can be found in chapter 7, where the less aggressive approach adopted by the Nephrology Service of our institution is outlined. Following this approach, pericardiectomy is indicated only for patients with constrictive pericarditis or when tamponade or large effusion persist or recur after adequate pericardiocentesis. In the series reported in that chapter (as in the series from the Cardiology Service (9) constrictive pericarditis is excluded), seven pericardiectomies were carried out in patients with pericardial involvement due to renal failure or hemodialysis (Table 10.6). It should be noted, however, that in these patients pericardiectomy was partial rather than extensive as in the rest of patients reported in the present chapter. In none of them constrictive pericarditis was the indication; three patients had tamponade and four had persisting effusion. All seven patients had undergone unsuccessful pericardiocentesis. Most authors agree that in the patients with these characteristics the prognosis is poor (26, 29). Accordingly, early pericardiectomy seems justified in them, as it provides an adequate management with a reasonable risk. This is an instance of pericardiectomy indicated in the absence of constriction in an etiologic subset of patients with known poor outcome without operation.

Table 10.6. Renal failure. Pericardial disease.

85	patients	
	pericardial effusion	71
	cardiac tamponade	18
7	partial pericardiectomies	
	tamponade	3
	persisting effusion	4

"Diagnostic" pericardiectomy

In rare instances in which there is evidence of clinical activity without systemic involvement, the etiology of pericardial disease remains elusive even after following a strict systematic protocol. This situation arises most often when a pericardial tumor is suspected; for instance, because of deformation of the cardiac silhouette on the chest radiogram or other imaging modality. In such circumstances, consideration of pericardiectomy may be justified despite the absence of an etiologic diagnosis. We have indicated pericardiectomy in two instances of this kind: in one patient (Fig. 10.1) from our prospective series (31), in whom pericardiectomy disclosed cardiac angiosarcoma which had escaped detection by pericardial biopsy and cytological examination of pericardial fluid. In the other (Fig. 10.2), whom we saw prior to our series, pericardial mesothelioma was demonstrated. Both patients had developed large asymmetric cardiomegaly that raised the suspicion of the tumor.

It should be recalled, however, that diagnostic pericardiectomy should not be considered without sound evidence of severe disease and without having ruled out systemic disorders. Specifically, persistence of a moderate pericardial effusion after acute pericarditis is not an indication for pericardiectomy,

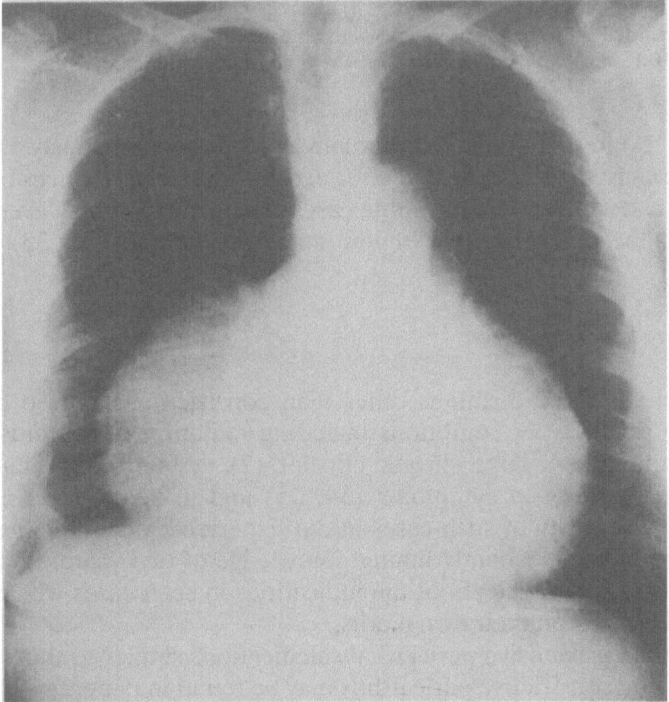

Fig. 10.1. Cardiac angiosarcoma, diagnosed after pericardiectomy with previously negative diagnostic evaluation including pericardial biopsy. The remarkably asymmetric cardiomegaly had developed within three months.

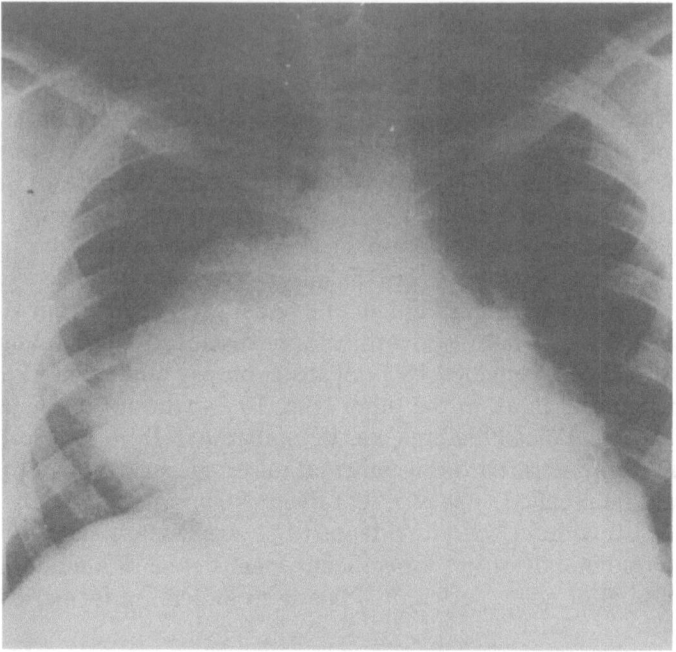

Fig. 10.2. Pericardial mesothelioma. Patient with similar clinical features to the patient illustrated in Fig. 10.1., in whom the diagnosis was also established by pericardiectomy.

because as a rule such patients eventually recover spontaneously. Diagnostic pericardiectomy should be reserved for exceptional circumstances but is fully justified in a few otherwise insoluble cases. Their number may even become smaller with the widespread use of new imaging techniques (32, 33).

Miscellaneous indications

Pericardiectomy for indications other than constriction has also been performed for a variety of conditions including radiation pericarditis with relapsing tamponade or large chronic effusion (7), cysts or congenital pericardial defects resulting in symptoms (34, 35) and in some cases of cardiac trauma (7). The rarity of such cases in our experience, as in the literature in general, and the consequently limited knowledge of their natural history, do not allow us to generalize about the indications in such cases which must be judged individually on their own merits.

Uncommonly, extensive pericardial calcifications similar to those found in chronic calcific constrictive pericarditis may be found in patients without constrictive pericarditis (Fig. 10.3). In these cases, the clinician may feel compelled to indicate pericardiectomy, but although the long term natural history of this condition is not known for certain, we recommend careful follow up

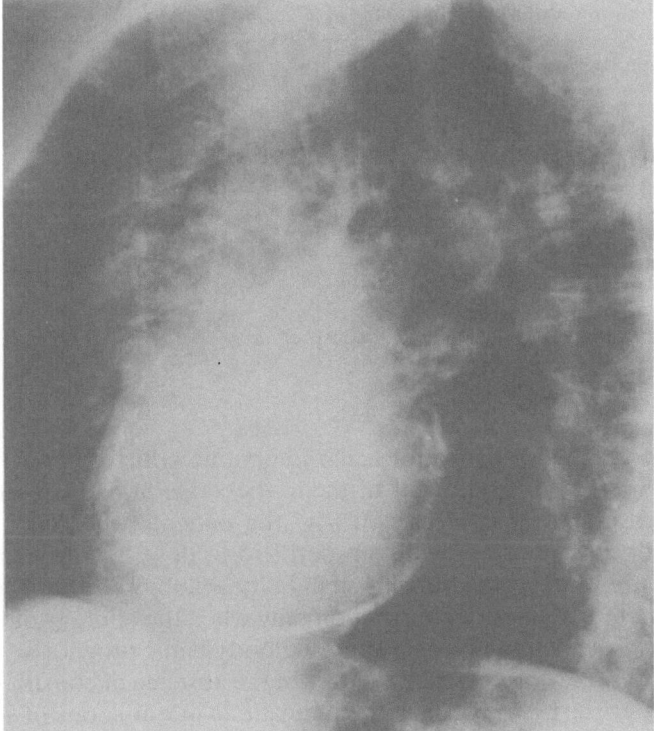

Fig. 10.3. Lateral chest radiogram of a patient with extensive pericardial calcification, with no previous history of pericarditis, and without features of cardiac constriction.

including serial noninvasive tests, and that pericardiectomy should not be carried out unless unequivocal features of constriction appear, as in any type of constrictive pericarditis (36).

General guidelines

On the basis of the foregoing information, a general approach to the indications for pericardiectomy in the absence of constriction can be delineated. Pericardiectomy in the absence of constriction should only be considered for patients known to be at high risk for a poor hemodynamic outcome. Much of the literature on early pericardiectomy can be faulted for neglecting this principle. For instance, extensive pericardiectomy has been recommended when a thickened or adherent pericardium is found during surgical subxiphoid pericardial drainage, on the alleged basis that constriction is common in these patients. We believe that this policy may be misleading without knowledge of the etiology. In our series (10), only one of the 26 patients who underwent

Table 10.7. Indications for pericardiectomy in 272 patients.

Massive chronic pericardial effusion	14*
Primary acute pericardial disease	
Subacute constrictive pericarditis	11
Pericardial thickening	3*
Recurrent course	2*
Iatrogenic hematoma	1*
Associated cardiac surgery	1*
"Diagnostic" pericardiectomy	1*
Total	33
Total pericardiectomies in the absence of constriction	22*

* = cases without constriction.

surgical pericardial drainage for acute idiopathic effusive pericarditis developed constriction. In about half of them, the surgeon had reported a thickened pericardium. By contrast, 60% of the patients who required surgical drainage for purulent or tuberculous pericarditis developed constriction. Our approach, therefore, is to strongly weigh in the etiology and to accept pericardiectomy in the absence of constriction only when the etiology of the patient's pericarditis is known to portend a poor hemodynamic prognosis.

Our experience with pericardiectomy in the absence of constriction is summarized in Table 10.7, where all the indications in our series of 256 patients with primary acute pericardial disease and in our 16 patients with massive chronic pericardial effusion are listed (33 instances). The most common indication in the 22 patients who underwent pericardiectomy without constriction was massive chronic pericardial effusion (14 patients). The remaining 8 patients were operated on for miscellaneous reasons, discussed in preceding paragraphs. Three pericardiectomies were carried out because the pericardium was found to be thickened at the time of subxiphoid drainage. At present we would agree with the indication in one of these three, a patient with purulent pericarditis, but not in the other two, who had acute idiopathic pericarditis. The case listed in the table as "diagnostic" pericardiectomy corresponds to the patient with cardiac angiosarcoma.

Diagnostic yield of pericardiectomy

Pericardiectomy is not indicated for purely diagnostic reasons, except in very unusual circumstances as previously discussed. However it is appropriate to remember that the diagnostic yield of pericardiectomy in acute or subacute pericardial disease is not negligible. In Table 10.8 the diagnostic yield of the 19 pericardiectomies in our series of 256 patients with acute pericarditis or cardiac tamponade is shown. In 8 of the 19 patients (42%) a specific etiologic diagnosis was obtained by the investigation of the surgical specimen. As

Table 10.8. Pericardiectomy (n: 19): diagnostic yield.

Overall diagnostic yield	8 (42%)
Tuberculous pericarditis	4
Neoplastic pericarditis	3*
Purulent pericarditis	1
False positive (neoplastic pericarditis)	1
False negative (purulent pericarditis)	1

* = in two of them the diagnosis was first made by pericardiectomy.

shown in the table, there was only one false negative diagnosis among the patients with specific disease. Two of the diagnoses obtained by pericardiectomy were new, justifying the rare indication of pericardiectomy in selected patients with persistent severe pericardial disease and negative results of local and general investigation. Against this, it should be borne in mind that a histologic diagnosis of neoplasia may be falsely positive, as occurred in one of our patients in whom severe inflammatory changes in the surgical specimen were interpreted as neoplasia. This error, which we have also encountered in pericardial biopsies (9, 10) also occurs in the histological study of other serous membranes (37).

References

1. Wychulis AR, Connolly DC, McGoon DC. Surgical treatment of pericarditis. J. Thorac Cardiovasc Surg 1971; 62: 608–617.
2. Iturrino JL, Holland RH. The emergency surgical management of acute pericarditis. J Thorac Cardiovasc Surg 1963; 45: 324–333.
3. Zinsser HF, Blakemore WS, Kirby CK, Johnson J. Invalidism due to recurrent idiopathic pericarditis with recovery after pericardiectomy. JAMA 1959; 171: 274–279.
4. Hatcher CR, Logue RB, Logan WD, Symbas PN, Mansour KA, Abbott OA. Pericardiectomy for recurrent pericarditis. J Thorac Cardiovasc Surg 1971; 62: 371–378.
5. Holman E, Willett F. Treatment of active tuberculous pericarditis by pericardiectomy. JAMA 1951; 146: 1–7.
6. Miller JI. Surgical management of pericardial disease. In: Hurst JW, ed. The Heart. New York, McGraw-Hill Book Co, 1986; 2.008–2.013.
7. Miller JI. Pericardiectomy. In: Hurst JW, ed. The Heart (Update III). New York, McGraw-Hill Book Co, 1980; 147–158.
8. Shabetai R. Diseases of the pericardium. In: Hurst JW, ed. The Heart, New York, McGraw-Hill Book Co, 1986; 1.249–1.275.
9. Permanyer-Miralda G, Sagristà-Sauleda J, Soler-Soler J. Primary acute pericardial disease: A prospective series of 231 consecutive patients, Am J Cardiol 1985; 56: 623–630.
10. Sagristà-Sauleda J, Permanyer-Miralda G, Soler-Soler J. Utilidad clínica de la pericardiocentesis y de la biopsia pericárdica en las enfermedades agudas del pericardio. Rev Esp Cardiol 1987; 40: 94–99.
11. Sagristà-Sauleda J, Permanyer-Miralda G, Candell-Riera J, Angel J, Soler-Soler J.Transient cardiac constriction: An unrecognized pattern of evolution in acute effusive idiopathic pericarditis. Am J Cardiol 1987; 59: 961–966.

12. Goldfarb B, Gold B, Latts E, Wexler H, Wang Y. Recurrent "pericardial pain" after pericardiectomy for recurrent acute benign pericarditis. Circulation 1966; 33: 283–286.
13. Fowler NO. Chronic pericarditis. In: Fowler NO, ed. The pericardium in health and disease. Mount Kisco, Futura Publishing Co, 1985; 217–234.
14. Fowler NO, Harbin AD. Recurrent acute pericarditis: Follow-up study of 31 patients. J Am Coll Cardiol 1986; 7: 300–305.
15. Sagristà-Sauleda J, Permanyer-Miralda G, Juste Sánchez C, de Buen Sánchez ML, Pujadas Capmany R, Arcalís Arce L, Soler-Soler J. Huge chronic pericardial effusion caused by *Toxoplasma gondii*. Circulation 1982; 66: 895–897.
16. Kerber RE, Sherman B. Echocardiographic evaluation of pericardial effusion in myxedema. Incidence and biochemical and clinical correlation. Circulation 1975; 52: 823–827.
17. Just H, Mattingly TW. Interatrial septal defect and pericardial disease. Am Heart J 1968; 76: 157–167.
18. Pietras RJ, Lam W. Large pericardial effusion associated with congenital heart disease: five-eight-year follow-up. Am Heart J 1988; 115: 1334–1336.
19. Fowler NO. Infectious pericarditis. In: Fowler NO, ed. The pericardium in health and disease. Mount Kisco, Futura Publishing Co, 1985; 195–215.
19a. Long R, Younes M, Patton N, Hershfield E. Tuberculous pericarditis: Long-term outcome in patients who received medical therapy alone. Am Heart J 1989; 117: 1133–1139.
20. Rubin RH, Moellering RC jr. Clinical, microbiologic and therapeutic aspects of purulent pericarditis. Am J Med 1975; 59: 68–78.
20a. Hall IP. Purulent pericarditis. Postgrad Med J 1989; 65: 444–448.
21. Hill GJ, Cohen BI. Pleural pericardial window form palliation of cardiac tamponade due to cancer. Cancer 1970; 26: 81–93.
22. Smith FE, Lane M, Hudgins PT. Conservative management of malignant pericardial effusion. Cancer 1974; 33: 47–57.
23. Ramakrishnan S, Marshall AJ, Pickard JG, Tyrell CJ. Pericardiocentesis and systemic chemotherapy in the management of cardiac tamponade secondary to disseminated heart carcinoma. Br Heart J 1988; 60: 162–164.
24. Press DW, Livingston R. Management of malignant pericardial effusion and tamponade. JAMA 1987; 257: 1088–1092.
25. Kralstein J, Frishman W. Malignant pericardial disease: diagnosis and treatment. Am Heart J 1987; 113: 785–790.
25a. Hawkins JW, Vacek JL. What constitutes definitive therapy of malignant pericardial effusion? "Medical" versus surgical treatment. Am Heart J 1989; 118: 428–432.
25b. Cormican MC, Nyman CR. Intrapericardial bleomycin for the management of cardiac tamponade secondary to malignant pericardial effusion. Br Heart J 1990; 63: 61–62.
26. Morlans M. Pericarditis urémica. Med Clín. (Barc) 1983; 80: 263–264.
27. Sing S, Newmark K, Ishikawa I, Mitra S, Berman LB. Pericardiectomy in uremia. The treatment of choice for cardiac tamponade in chronic renal failure. JAMA 1974; 228: 1.132–1.135.
28. Wray TM, Humphreys J, Perry JM, Stone WJ, Bender HW. Pericardiectomy for treatment of uremic pericarditis. Circulation 1974; 49–50 (Supl II): 268–271.
29. Ali-Regiaba S, Gay WA, Sullivan JF, Tapia L, David DS, White RP, Stenzel KH, Riggio RR, Cheigh JS, Rubin AL. Treatment of uraemic pericarditis by anterior pericardiectomy. Lancet 1974; 2: 12–14.
30. Comty CM, Wathen RL, Shapiro FL. Uremic pericarditis. In: Spodick DH, ed. Pericardial diseases. Philadelphia, FA Davis Co, 1976; 219–235.
31. Mayor G, Carcía del Castillo H, Sagristà-Sauleda J, Murtra-Ferré M, Soler-Soler J. Angiosarcoma de corazón. Hallazgos ecocardiográficos. Rev Esp Cardiol 1986; 39: 456–458.
32. Moncada R, Baker M, Salinas M, Demos TC, Churchill R, Love L, Reynes C, Hale D, Cardoso M, Pifarré R, Gunnar RM. Diagnostic role of computed tomography in pericardial heart disease: Congenital defects, thickening, neoplasms and effusions. Am Heart J 1982; 103: 263–282.

33. Caputo GR, Higgins ChB. Magnetic resonance imaging of the heart. In: Partain CL, Price RR, Paton JA, Kulkarni MV, James AE jr, eds. Magnetic resonance imaging. Philadelphia, WB Saunders Company, 1988; 414–417.
34. Nasser WK. Congenital defects of the pericardium. In: Fowler NO, ed. The pericardium in health and disease. Mount Kisco, Futura Publishing Co, 1985; 51–78.
35. Muñoz Gil J, Chorro FJ, Martínez León J, Losada A, Carbonell C, Llopis R, López-Merino V. La ecocardiografía en el diagnóstico del quiste pericárdico. Presentación de un caso. Rev Esp Cardiol 1985; 38: 298–299.
36. Kirklin J, Barrat-Boyes BG. Cardiac surgery. New York, John Wiley & Sons 1986; 1440.
37. Rosai J, Dehner LP. Nodular mesothelial hyperplasia in hernia sacs. A benign reactive condition simulating a neoplastic process. Cancer 1975; 35: 165–175.

11. Limitations of surgery for constrictive pericarditis

MARCOS MURTRA, M.D.

General considerations

Constrictive pericarditis was one of the first cardiac diseases to be surgically treated. As early as 1649 Riolan (1) predicted that one day the surgeon would be able to free the heart from strangulation. Weill (2), in 1895, and Delorme (3), in 1898, proposed removal of the thickened, fibrous pericardium as the treatment of choice for constrictive pericarditis. The first successful pericardiectomies were carried out simultaneously in Germany by Rehn (4, 5) and by Sauerbruck (6), in 1913. Subsequently, several series of operations were reported, and pericardiectomy was established as the correct treatment for chronic constrictive pericarditis (7–11). In 1941, Blalock and Burwell (12) emphasized the importance of resecting not only the thickened pericardium, but also the residual fibrous epicardium. Likewise, in 1944, Harrington (13) insisted on the need for epicardiolysis in cases of constrictive fibrous epicardium.

The natural history of chronic constrictive pericarditis is not well known. The development of pericardial constriction can occur long after the beginning of pericardial involvement, which may have been clinically unnoticed. In addition, the factors that determine the progression of the disease are not well established. However, when the signs and symptoms of constrictive pericarditis are fully developed, prognosis and quality of life are poor, particularly when ascites and edema develop (14). The diagnosis of chronic constrictive pericarditis is, therefore, an indication for operation in virtually all cases. Only in those instances where the pathophysiologic disorder resulting from the pericardial compression is minimal can the indication for surgery be

J. Soler-Soler et al. (Eds.), Pericardial Disease, pp. 183–192.
© 1990 Kluwer Academic Publishers

delayed until clinical features or hemodynamic changes become more apparent (15).

The problem

The object of surgery for constrictive pericarditis is to free the heart from constriction so as to allow normal diastolic filling before secondary myocardial damage develops; this latter occurrence might hamper both short and long term results (15–17). This aim is met in most cases, as pericardiectomy offers a good outcome to the majority of patients. Nevertheless, despite this clear cut rationale and the major developments in cardiac surgery during the last years, the mortality of surgery in constrictive pericarditis is still reported as 5–15% (15). Also, its results are not satisfactory in some patients. This is the reason why in the present chapter the limitations of surgical therapy are reviewed. Such limitations can be related to the operative technique or to other factors such as the stage of the disease, the previous functional status, the timing of operation, the etiology of constrictive pericarditis, and the occurrence of associated diseases.

Limitations arising from the surgical technique

Surgical approach

The initial approach was a curved parasternal incision, with resection of the anterior costal portions, including costal carthilages from the third to the seventh (8). This procedure resulted in a wide pericardial exposure, but the approach was highly aggressive and is currently obsolete. Subsequently, several approaches have been used: left anterolateral or posterolateral thoracotomy, bilateral anterior thoracotomy, and median sternotomy (11, 18–23). Left anterolateral thoracotomy is still the preferred approach of several surgical groups (24, 25), as it provides access to the anterolateral and inferior aspects of the left ventricle, with little mobilization of the heart and, if necessary, thoracotomy may be widened through the sternum to the right side of the thorax. Bilateral anterior thoracotomy facilitates the exposure of both sides of the heart, but, as a rule, it is less well tolerated than the left or the median approaches. Median sternotomy allows complete exposure of the heart, but requires greater mobilization of the heart when attempting to reach the anterolateral and diaphragmatic aspects. It has the major advantage of facilitating dissection of the right atrium and both venae cavae, and permitting a convenient access for cardiopulmonary bypass (19). Median sternotomy is currently preferred by most surgeons, as, being routinely used for most cardiac operations, it offers the advantages of experience and thus safety. There has been no demonstration of any relationship between the surgical approach and the operative mortality or the late results (24).

Extent of the pericardial resection

Many terms have been used to describe the type of pericardial resection; all of them may be misleading: partial, limited, wide, adequate, radical, total, etc. (24). It should be remembered that, although constriction involves all four cardiac chambers and the intrapericardial portions of the venae cavae, pulmonary veins and great arteries, impairment of the ventricular diastolic filling is the major hemodynamic abnormality in constrictive pericarditis (24, 26–29). Therefore, excision wide enough to liberate the anterior and posterior aspects of the right ventricle and the anterolateral, apical and inferior aspects of the left should be carried out. Dissection should extend beyond the right and left atrioventricular grooves (18, 19, 24). It is wise to liberate the left ventricle first and then the right to prevent possible pulmonary congestion. The right atrium and the venae cavae may also be liberated. In my experience their involvement is not often significant, and many surgeons believe that their liberation does not alter the surgical results (24, 25, 27). The phrenic nerves must be spared, and the surgeon has two options for accomplishing this: either to identify and isolate the phrenic nerves to allow resection of the posterior pericardium or to perform only a wide anterophrenic pericardiectomy. Nevertheless, resection must be as complete as possible.

Depth of pericardial resection

Sometimes, constrictive epicarditis may persist after the resection of the parietal pericardium (12, 13, 24); this can be suspected when heart size does not increase, cardiac contraction does not become more vigorous or the right atrial pressure does not fall. In these cases, the widest possible visceral resection should be carried out over both ventricles. This is critically important, as the residual epicardial fibrosis will likely result in persisting hemodynamic abnormalities and a poor clinical result (22). Epicardial liberation should be meticulous, avoiding injury to coronary vessels and penetrating the myocardium. It is sometimes a wise precaution to leave unresected small isolated islands of thickened pericardium which do not appear to be causing cardiac compression.

Use of cardiopulmonary bypass

In some patients, resection of either the parietal or visceral layers of the pericardium may be difficult, specially in reoperations or when there is extensive penetrating calcification. In these cases total cardiopulmonary bypass can be very helpful (19, 21). The resulting decompression of cardiac chambers facilitates the dissection and identification of anatomical planes allowing the surgeon to reach the lateral and posterior aspects of the heart more easily and safely. Some surgical groups recommend the routine use of cardiopulmonary bypass, so as to be able to perform more complete resection (19, 21); however, there is no evidence that this policy has resulted in better early or late postoperative results, whereas cost is increased (24, 30). We believe that cardiopulmonary bypass is unnecessary in many cases, but it must always be immediately available in case the dissection proves difficult, the heart does not tolerate the procedure, or in case of an operative accident. It has been speculated that cardiopulmonary bypass may increase the incidence of postoperative bleeding, with resulting increase in the number of reoperations. However, it should be remembered that cardiopulmonary bypass is commonly used only in the technically more difficult cases or in those with complications, and therefore the bleeding may not be attributed to bypass by itself. No significant differences have been found in the incidence of hemorrhagic complications and reoperation whether or not cardiopulmonary bypass was used (30).

In summary, it should be considered that the limitations of pericardiectomy arising from the surgical technique itself are currently minimal and virtually reduced to operative or postoperative bleeding. The reported incidence of reoperation is less than 2%, and generally related to incomplete resection or unrecognized constriction by the visceral pericardium (22). In the present day, these are exceptional occurrences.

Limitations arising from the stage of the disease

When adequate freeing from pericardial constriction is achieved, the heart clearly increases in size and contractility, while right atrial and pulmonary wedge pressure decrease (24). However, in some patients cardiac dilatation with poor contractility develops in spite of adequate pericardiectomy. The result is low cardiac output that may continue after the operation, requiring pharmacologic therapy for the first 24–48 or more postoperative hours. Eventually the patient's status usually improves, with progressive resolution of heart failure. This low cardiac output syndrome is more common when the preoperative functional class is advanced (with ascites and significant edema), and is still the most frequent cause or operative morbidity and mortality (24, 25, 30). About 5% of patients, despite satisfactory pericardiectomy, remain in heart failure and die from it. In these patients a more or less pronounced degree of myocardial atrophy is present. Clinical, operative, hemodynamic and pathologic data indicate that, in most such cases, heart failure is secondary to myocardial dysfunction rather than to pericardial constriction

(16, 18, 27, 31, 32). McCaughan et al. (24) reviewed 231 patients with constrictive pericarditis operated on between 1936 and 1982 at the Mayo Clinic, and found low cardiac output of varying severity in 65 patients free from clinical or hemodynamic evidence of persisting constriction. Low cardiac output significantly correlated with hospital mortality and the preoperative functional class. Thus, the risk of operative death from low cardiac output syndrome was 1% in patients with functional classes I and II (72 patients), increasing to 10% with functional class III (146 patients) and to 46% with functional class IV (13 patients). Surprisingly, low cardiac output did not influence the late postoperative outcome. Seifert et al. (30) also found a good correlation between functional class and the development of low cardiac output, but not with hospital or late mortality. The actuarial curves reported by these authors showed a lower survival rate for patients in class IV, but no significant difference when operative mortality was excluded. They found, like McCaughan et al. (24), that hospital mortality rate was significantly associated with increased right, but not with left, ventricular end diastolic pressure. Univariate analysis showed that renal failure significantly correlated with hospital mortality. Regarding late results, in the series by McCaughan et al. (24) 199 patients survived after the operation and were followed for up to 43 years (median 9 years). The probability of survival, excluding hospital mortality, was 84% at 5 years, 71% at 15 years, and 52% at 30 years. During the initial five years, survival was higher in patients in preoperative functional classes I and II than in those in classes III and IV, but this difference did not

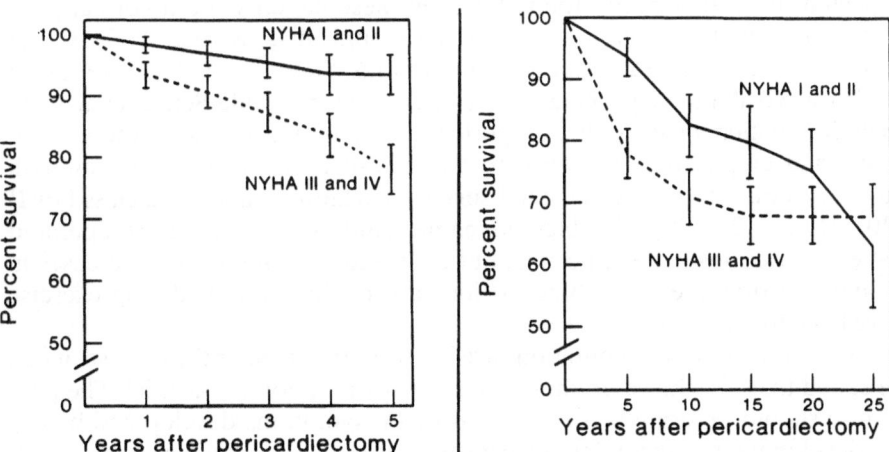

Fig. 11.1. Left panel. 5-year survival curves (excluding operative mortality) after pericardiectomy for constrictive pericarditis, showing a worse prognosis for patients with advanced preoperative NYHA functional class. *Right panel.* The long term differences are small. NHYA: New York Heart Association. (Reproduced, with permission, from: McCaughan BC, Schaff HV, Piehler JM, Danielson GK, Orszulak TA, Puga FJ, Pluth JR, Connolly DC, McGoon DC. Early and late results of pericardiectomy for constrictive pericarditis. J Thorac Cardiovasc Surg 1985; 89: 340–350).

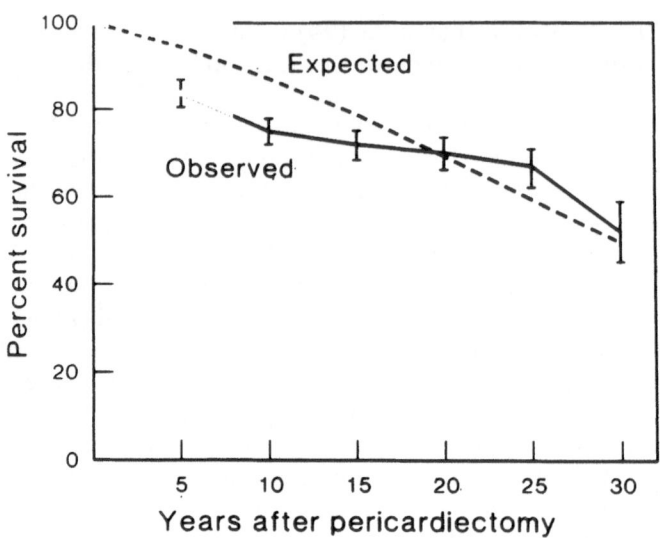

Fig. 11.2. Comparative survival curves (excluding operative mortality) between patients after pericardiectomy for constrictive pericarditis and a normal age and sex matched population. (Reproduced, with permission, from: McCaughan BC, Schaff HV, Piehler JM, Danielson GK, Orszulak TA, Puga FJ, Pluth JR, Connolly DC, McGoon DC. Early and late results of pericardiectomy for constrictive pericarditis. J Thorac Cardiovasc Surg 1985; 89: 340–350).

persist later into the follow up period (Fig. 11.1). Significant differences in expected survival were not found between these patients and a normal population matched for age, sex, and demographical data (Fig. 11.2). Other authors report comparable survival curves; thus, Stalpaert et al. (33) reported a 73% survival after 5 years and 68% after 10 years, while Seifert et al. (30), excluding patients with radiation pericarditis, found a 83% survival after 10 years, and emphasized the need to distinguish between high and low risk groups. About 80–90% of hospital survivors achieve a functional class I or II (20, 21, 24, 25, 30, 32). Hemodynamic studies carried out in operated patients have mostly been normal, but in 10–20% of them small increases in pulmonary pressure or inability to increase cardiac output during exercise have been found (27).

As a summary of the limitations arising from the stage of the disease, it can be stated that to achieve optimal results early operation is essential. The procedure should be done before class III or IV symptoms develop and before the development of secondary myocardial damage, both of which could result in worsened immediate and late outcome.

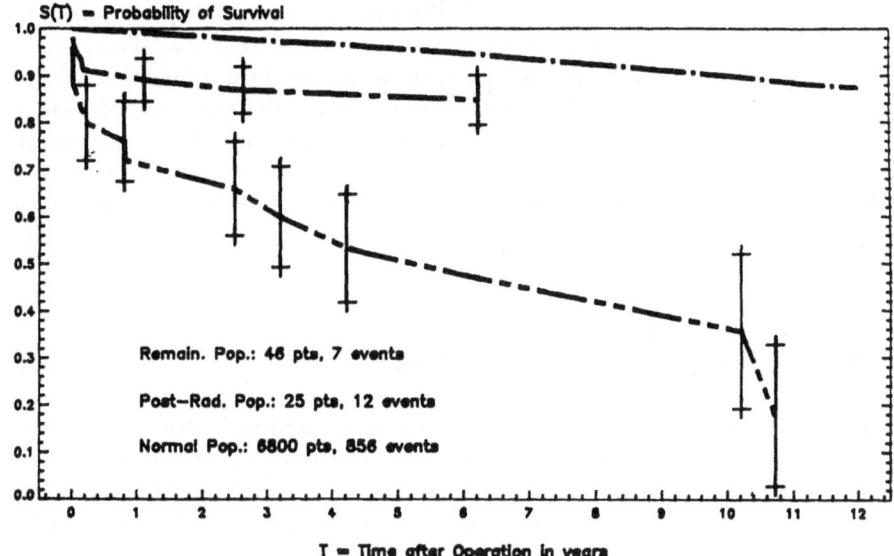

Fig. 11.3. Actuarial survival curves after pericardiectomy for constrictive pericarditis (Kaplan-Meier method). Lower curve: radiation induced constrictive pericarditis. Middle curve: remaining patients. The survival in the radiation group was significantly worse (Gehan p = 0.005) than a computer simulated normal population (upper curve), but there was no significant difference (Gehan p = 0.1551) between the normal population and the remaining patients. The survival curves from radiation patients and the other pericardiectomy patients were significantly different (Gehan p = 0.0168). The vertical bars indicate ± 1 standard error. Hospital mortality has been included. (Reproduced from: Seifert FC, Miller DC, Oesterle SN, Oyer PE, Stinson EB, Shumway NE. Surgical treatment of constrictive pericarditis: analysis of outcome and diagnostic error. Circulation 1985; 72 (suppl II) I: 264–273. With authorization of the American Heart Association, Inc.).

Limitations arising from the etiology

Some cases of constrictive pericarditis may be the result of a previous non-identified episode of viral pericarditis (18, 20). In recent years, the incidence of tuberculous pericarditis has dramatically decreased in developed countries (33–38) but it remains as high as 61% in some series from the Third World (25). By way of contrast, other causes have been increasingly recognized. These include ionizing radiation (18, 20, 22, 33, 39–41), connective tissue diseases (18, 33, 42–46), infiltrative diseases (31), Dressler's syndrome (47), hemopericardium (18, 20, 48) and cardiac operation (20, 49–55a). Furthermore, the etiology of many cases of constrictive pericarditis is unknown (24, 30, 56); in the series by Seifert et al. (30), 45% of cases were idiopathic, and McCaughan et al. (24) reported the even higher figure of 73%. It is difficult, therefore, to compare the results from different etiologic groups. However, Seifert et al. (30) in a series of 81 patients with constrictive pericarditis operated on between 1970 and 1981, identified 25 patients (35%) with radiation induced constrictive pericarditis. Within this group the hospital mortality was higher (16%). Late mortality rate was also increased (32%). The probability of survival was $51 \pm 12\%$ for patients with radiation induced constrictive pericarditis, as compared to $83 \pm 7\%$ in the remaining patients (Fig. 11.3). Radiation affects the mediastinum, the pericardium and the heart itself. Radiation doses of or above than 4000 rads cause ventricular function abnormalities in 95% of patients. Some develop myocardial disease, independent of constrictive pericarditis, that may influence the outcome, particularly at long term.

Limitations arising from associated conditions

In addition to the problems of myocardial atrophy and radiation cardiomyopathy, similar problems arise in patients with constrictive pericarditis and co-existent myocardial disease (such as ischemic or idiopathic). The results of pericardiectomy will also be influenced by the severity of the myocardial disease.

Finally, it should be recalled that the results of pericardiectomy in patients with malignant pericardial disease are poor, despite relief of constriction.

References

1. Riolan J. Encheiridium Anatomicum et Pathologicum Lugduni Batavorum. Ex Officina Adriani Wyngaerden, 1649; 206.
2. Weill E. Traité Clinique des Maladies du Coeur chez les Enfants. Paris, O. Doin Co, 1895.
3. Delorme E. Sur un traitement chirurgical de la symphyse cadio-pericardique. Gaz Hop 1898; 71: 1.150.
4. Rehn L. Zurexperimentellen Pathologie des Herzbeutels. Verth Dtsch Ges Chir 1913; 42: 339.
5. Rehn L. Die perikardialen Verwachsungen im Kindesalter. Arch Klin Chir 1920; 68: 179.
6. Sauerbruck F. Die Chirurgie der Brustorgame. Berlin, Julius Springer, 1925; 1.075.
7. Schmieden V, Fischer H. Die Herzbeutelentzundung und ihre Folgezustande. Ergebnisse des Chirurgie u Orthopädie 1926; 19: 98.
8. Churchill ED. Decortication of the heart (Delorme) for adhesive pericarditis. Arch Surg 1929; 19: 1.457.
9. Beck CS. The surgical treatment of pericardial scar. J Am Med Assoc 1931; 97: 824.
10. Heuer GJ, Stewart HJ. The surgical treatment of chronic pericarditis. Surg Gynecol Obstet 1939; 68: 979.
11. Harrington SW, Barnes AR. Diagnosis and surgical treatment of chronic constructive pericarditis. The Southern Surgeon 1940; 9: 459.
12. Blalock A, Burwell CS. Chronic pericardial disease. Surg Gynecol Obstet 1941; 73: 433.
13. Harrington SW. Chronic constrictive pericarditis. Partial pericardiectomy and epicardiolysis in twenty-four cases. Ann Surg 1944; 120: 468–485.
14. Somerville W. Constrictive pericarditis with special reference to the change in natural history brought about by surgical intervention. Circulation 1969; 38 (supl V): 102–111.
15. Kirklin J, Barrat Boyes BG. Cardiac Surgery. New York, John Wiley & Sons, 1986; 1.433–1.447.

16. Dines DE, Edwards JE, Burchell HB. Myocardial atrophy in constrictive pericarditis. Mayo Clin Proc 1958; 33: 93–99.
17. Roberts JT, Beck CS. The effect of chronic cardiac compression on the size of the heart mucle fibers. Am Heart J 1941; 22: 314–320.
18. Wychulis AR, Connolly DC, McGoon DC. Surgical treatment of pericarditis. J Thorac Cardiovasc Surg 1971; 62: 608–617.
19. Copeland JC, Stinson EB, Griepp RB, Shumway NE. Surgical treatment of chronic constrictive pericarditis using cardiopulmonary bypass. J Thorac Cardiovasc Surg 1975; 69: 236–238.
20. Kilman JW, Bush CA, Wooley CF, Stang JM, Teply J, Baba N. The changing spectrum of pericardiectomy for chronic pericarditis. Occult constrictive pericarditis. J Thorac Cardiovasc Surg 1977; 74: 668–673.
21. Culliford AT, Lipton M, Spencer FC. Operation for chronic constrictive pericarditis. Do the surgical approach and degree of pericardial resection influence the outcome significantly? Ann Thorac Surg 1980; 29: 146–152.
22. Walsh TJ, Baughman KL, Gardner TJ, Bulkley BH. Constrictive epicarditis as a cause of delayed or absent response to pericardiectomy. A clinicopathological study. J Thorac Cardiovasc Surg 1982; 83: 126–132.
23. Miller JI, Mansour KA, Hatcher CR Jr. Pericardiectomy. Current indications, concepts, and results in a university center. Ann Thorac Surg 1982; 34: 40–45.
24. McCaughan BC, Schaff HV, Piehler JM, Danielson GK, Orszulak TA, Puga FJ, Pluth JR, Connolly DC, McGoon DC. Early and late results of pericardiectomy for constrictive pericarditis. J Thorac Cardiovasc Surg 1985; 89: 340–350.
25. Bashi VV, John S, Ravikumar E, Jairaj PS, Shyamsunder PS, Krishnaswani S. Early and late results of pericardiectomy in 118 cases of constrictive pericarditis. Thorax 1988; 43: 637–641.
26. Shabetai R, Fowler NO, Guntheroth WG. The hemodynamics of cardiac tamponade and constrictive pericarditis. Am J Cardiol 1970; 26: 480–489.
27. Kloster FE, Crislip RL, Bristow JD, Herr RH, Ritzmann LW, Griswold HE. Hemodynamic studies following pericardiectomy for constrictive pericarditis. Circulation 1965; 32: 415–424.
28. Harrison EC, Crawford DW, Lau FYK. Sequential left ventricular function studies before and after pericardiectomy for constrictive pericarditis. Delayed resolution of residual restriction. Am J Cardiol 1970; 26: 319–323.
29. Viola AR. The influence of pericardiectomy on the hemodynamics of chronic constrictive pericarditis. Circulation 1973; 48: 1.038–1.042.
30. Seifert FC, Miller DC, Oesterle SN, Oyer PE, Stinson EB, Shumway NE. Surgical treatment of constrictive pericarditis: analysis of outcome and diagnostic error. Circulation 1985; 72 (supl II): II-264–273.
31. Meany E, Shabetai R, Bhargava V, Shearer M, Weidner C, Mangiardi LM, Smalling R, Peterson K. Cardiac amyloidosis, constrictive pericarditis and restrictive cardiomyopathy. Am J Cardiol 1976; 38: 547–556.
32. Harrison EC, Crawford DW, Lau FYK. Sequential left ventricular function studies before and after pericardiectomy for constrictive pericarditis. Delayed resolution of residual restriction. Am J Cardiol 1970; 26: 319–323.
33. Stalpaert G, Suy R, Daenen W, Nevelsteen A. Total pericardiectomy for chronic constrictive pericarditis. Early and late results. Acta Chir Belg 1981; 80; 262–277.
34. Gooi HC, Morrison Smith J. Tuberculous pericarditis in Birmingham. Thorax 1978; 33: 94–96.
35. Desai HN. Tuberculous pericarditis. A review of 100 cases. S Afr Med J 1979; 55: 877–880.
36. Ortbals DW, Avioli LV. Tuberculous pericarditis. Arch Intern Med 1979; 139: 231–234.
37. Pitt Fennell WM. Surgical treatment of constrictive tuberculous pericarditis. S Afr Med J 1982; 62: 353–355.

38. Sagristà-Sauleda J, Permanyer-Miralda G, Soler-Soler J. Tuberculous pericarditis: ten year experience with a prospective protocol for diagnosis and treatment. J Am Coll Cardiol 1988; 11: 724–728.

39. Westerhof PW, van der Putte SCJ. Radiation pericarditis and myocardial fibrosis. Eur J Cardiol 1976; 4: 213–218.

40. Watson PT, Havelda CJ, Sorosky J, Kochenour NK, Sohi GS, Gray L Jr. Irradiation-induced constrictive pericarditis requiring pericardiectomy during pregnancy. J Reprod Med 1980; 24: 127-130.

41. Applefeld MM, Slawson RG, Hall-Craig M, Gren DC, Singleton RT, Wiernik PH. Delayed pericardial disease after radiotherapy. Am J Cardiol 1981; 47: 210–213.

42. Cooper DKC, Cleland WP, Bentall HH. Collagen diseases as a cause of constrictive pericarditis. Thorax 1978; 33: 368–371.

43. Sunder SK, Shah A. Constrictive pericarditis in procainamide-induced lupus erythematosus syndrome. Am J Cardiol 1975; ;36: 960-962.

44. John JT Jr, Hough A, Sergent JS. Pericardial disease in rheumatoid arthritis. Am J Med 1979; 66: 385–390.

45. Burney DP, Martin CE, Thomas CS, Fisher RD, Bender HW Jr. Rheumatoid pericarditis. Clinical significance and operative management. J Thorac Cardiovasc Surg 1979; 77: 511–514.

46. Stevens MB. Lupus carditis. N Engl J Med 1988; 319: 861–862.

47. Goldhaber SZ, Lorell BH, Green LH. Constrictive pericarditis. A case requiring pericardiectomy following Dressler's postmyocardial infarction syndrome. J Thorac Cardiovasc Surg 1981; 81: 793–796.

48. Ehrenhaft JL, Taber RE. Hemopericardium and constrictive pericarditis. J Thorac Surg 1952; 24: 355–366.

49. Kendall ME, Rhodes GR, Wolfe W. Cardiac constriction following aorta-to-coronary bypass surgery. J Thorac Cardiovasc Surg 1972; 64: 142–153.

50. Simon JS, Pluth JR. Constrictive pericarditis. Ann Thorac Surg 1976; 21: 440–441.

51. Brown DF, Older T. Pericardial constriction as a late complication of coronary bypass surgery. J Thorac Cardiovasc Surg 1977; 74: 61–64.

52. Marsa R, Mehta S, Willis W, Bailey L. Constrictive pericarditis after myocardial revascularization. Report of three cases. Am J Cardiol 1979; 44: 177–183.

53. Kanakis C, Skeikh AI, Rosen KM. Constrictive pericardial disease following mitral valve replacement. Chest 1981; 79: 593–594.

54. Rice PL, Pifarré R, Montoya A. Constrictive pericarditis following cardiac surgery. Ann Thorac Surg 1981; 31: 450–453.

55. Kutcher MA, King SB III, Alimurung BN, Craver JM, Logue RB. Constrictive pericarditis as a complication of cardiac surgery. Recognition of an entity. Am J Cardiol 1982; 50: 742–748.

55a. Cimino JJ, Kogan AD. Constrictive pericarditis after cardiac surgery: report of three cases and review of the literature. Am Heart J 1989; 118: 1292–1301.

56. Cameron J, Oesterle SN, Baldwin JC, Hancock EW. The ethiologic spectrum of constrictive pericarditis. Am Heart J 1987; 113: 354–360.

12. Acute pericardial disease: an approach to etiologic diagnosis and treatment

G. PERMANYER-MIRALDA, M.D., J. SAGRISTÀ–SAULEDA, M.D., R. SHABETAI, M.D., J. SOLER-SOLER, M.D., AND D. H. SPODICK, M.D.

Dr. Permanyer: Despite long decades of research and clinical experience, the pericardium still holds mysteries for the clinician. The present Round Table is dedicated to some of them.

I must emphasize at this point that the topic of the present discussion will be not only acute pericarditis, but what we have called "primary" acute pericardial disease. We include in this designation cases of acute pericarditis and/or cardiac tamponade of unknown cause at the initial evaluation. We define acute pericarditis as the occurrence of two or more of the following: suggestive chest pain, pericardial friction rub, and ECG showing characteristic ST segment elevation. We define cardiac tamponade as venous hypertension and/or paradoxical pulse associated with proof of pericardial effusion in the absence of other features that could account for these findings. By definition, then, the clinical history and routine studies at the time of hospital admission do not point to a probable etiologic diagnosis. We appreciate that this definition lacks precision; nevertheless, its clinical meaning is evident, in that most of those pericardial syndromes that raise etiologic dilemmas fall within it. Accordingly, conditions such as uremic pericarditis, postinfarction pericarditis, and pericardial involvement in the course of proven neoplastic or other systemic disorders of known etiology will not be covered in this discussion.

We will confine our discussion to two aspects of primary acute pericardial disease: the etiologic diagnosis (to which the initial and longest part of the discussion will be devoted), and controversial aspects of therapy.

Etiology of primary acute pericardial disease

I wish to remind that there are three diagnostic approaches commonly used by the clinician when faced with a case of primary acute pericardial disease (Table 12.1); each of them will be dealt with in the present discussion. The

J. Soler-Soler et al. (Eds.), Pericardial Disease, pp. 193–214.

Table 12.1. Primary acute pericardial disease: possible diagnostic approaches.

1. Demonstration of associated disease
2. Specificity of the clinical findings
3. Direct investigation of the pericardial fluid and tissue

first is the search for associated diseases; the second is based on the possible specificity of clinical findings for the etiologic diagnosis, and the third consists of the direct investigation into the nature of pericardial fluid or tissue.

Demonstration of associated diseases

At first sight, this approach may seem to be contradictory, as we have defined primary pericardial diseases as those where etiology is not readily apparent at the initial clinical investigation. However, there are many disorders (bacterial and nonbacterial infections, systemic diseases, etc.) that may be clinically occult when pericardial disease presents and which should be specifically sought by the clinician. Identification of a condition commonly associated with pericardial involvement may make the pericardium "guilty by association" (1); however, the coexistence of two diseases does not necessarily establish a causal relationship between them. The first question I will ask the panel is whether any of the diseases frequently associated with pericardial disease, such as infection by viruses and other nonbacterial organisms, should be systematically and objectively ruled out. Specifically, when are systematic virologic studies and investigation of other nonbacterial infections warranted in primary acute pericardial disease? Which of these studies are being carried out at your institution, and what are the results?

Dr. Spodick: In most cases of acute pericarditis special studies for etiologic agents are not necessary, because there are no specific treatments for viral disease, and because by the time clinical pericarditis exists the usual serologic changes may be present but non-specific. Furthermore, specific therapy for viral disease is seldom available. Pericardial fluid and tissue may not contain retrievable viruses. On the other hand, when a non-bacterial infection appears to be caused by more or less exotic organisms including parasites or fungi, the appropriate test should be done based upon the clinical picture, the appearance of pericardial fluid and the geographic area (certain parasites, for example, like amebae, being endemic in certain parts of the world). In the United States, local areas of endemicity exist for histoplasmosis and coccidiodomycosis and in those areas at least serologic tests or skin tests can be done. However, these would be relatively non-specific, with a need for tissue and fluid as superior material for identifying precisely causative organisms.

Dr. Permanyer: Can you comment on this point, Dr. Shabetai?

Dr. Shabetai: By and large, I agree with Dr. Spodick's answer. Even though at my institution we have an outstanding laboratory for the study of viral diseases and expert virologists, I seldom find viral studies helpful. Perhaps this is to some extent a matter of timing, because by the time that results of viral titres become available, the clinical problem has been solved one way or the other. Indeed, in a teaching hospital with constantly rotating housestaff, it is difficult to keep track of convalescent serum studies. I doubt whether it would be very cost-effective to undertake extensive serological tests for other non-bacterial infections causing acute pericarditis. Before we undertake such tests, we require some clue suggesting the possibility of infection with such an agent. Thus, if there has been an epidemic of infectious mononucleosis we would search for evidence of infection with the Epstein-Barr virus. Exposure to other infections, or other clinical findings pointing to the possibility of such infection, would lead to the appropriate tests. They are not, however, done on a routine basis in our institution. In general, when we have done these tests, the yield has been disappointingly small.

Dr. Permanyer: Tuberculosis is another important though not very common cause of pericarditis. Characteristically, it may be present even in the absence of suggestive clinical signs at the initial examination. When is the search for tubercle bacilli in sputum or gastric aspirate warranted?

Dr. Soler: Considering that tuberculosis is still quite prevalent in our area, we perform screening studies to rule out tuberculous pericarditis. This is the reason why our present study protocol includes, in its stage I, the culture of three samples of sputum for tubercle bacilli in specific media. In our first protocol (1977) (2) we systematically carried out three gastric aspirations in the patients who did not produce sputum. This study, owing to the low incidence of tuberculous pericarditis (13 cases in 10 years (3, 4)), had a low diagnostic yield; in addition, it is cumbersome and sometimes poorly tolerated. Therefore, in our current protocol, when the patient cannot produce sputum, gastric aspirates are recommended only for patients in whom pericardial effusion lasts for longer than one week, patients with clinically severe disease, and patients with a history of tuberculosis or who are suspected of active tuberculous infection. I have mentioned the low diagnostic yield of the search for tubercle bacilli in the sputum or gastric aspirate, but strong emphasis should nevertheless be placed on our observation that this was the investigation most often leading to the correct diagnosis in our patients with tuberculous pericarditis. Thus, in the 11 of 13 patients with tuberculous pericarditis in whom this study was performed, tubercle bacilli were isolated in six (four in sputum, one in gastric aspirate, and one in both). Finally, I wish to mention the new observation that the measurement of adenosine deaminase activity in the pleural (5) and pericardial (6) fluids has a high diagnostic yield for tuberculosis. This point, however, will be later on discussed in greater detail by Dr. Sagristà.

Dr. Permanyer: Just as an extensive search for tuberculosis is not warranted in all patients, it would also be wise to limit the search for antinuclear or anti-DNA antibodies to those patients whose disease is not rapidly self-limited, except in individual patients in whom there are clinical grounds to suspect a systemic disease in which these abnormalities are frequent.

Up to this point we have discussed laboratory investigation of cases in which there is no clue to the etiology. Even in cases of primary acute pericarditis, the clinician may suspect a specific cause and wish to address it more specifically. I will ask Dr. Sagristà to discuss his approach to this kind of case.

Dr. Sagristà: If we remember that the major problem for the clinician faced with primary pericarditis is often to identify or rule out tuberculous and neoplastic disease, it seems apparent that the question boils down to the appropriate studies that might lead to these diagnoses. The most common studies to this end are bronchoscopy, lymph node biopsy and pleural biopsy. Bronchoscopy should, obviously, be carried out in all patients with radiological images consistent with neoplasia. In patients with pericarditis without evidence of this etiology we have performed bronchoscopy in those with relapsing cardiac tamponade, particularly if they are male smokers, and in those in whom clinical activity persisted for three or more weeks after admission. Bronchoscopy has not, on the whole, been very useful for the etiologic diagnosis in our series, as even though it confirmed the bronchial origin in five cases of neoplastic pericardial disease, in none of them it was the first or only study to demonstrate the correct diagnosis. Lymph node biopsy had a high diagnostic yield in the four patients in which it was carried out, as it was the first study to yield the diagnosis in two patients with tuberculous pericarditis and in one patient with neoplastic pericarditis. Pleural biopsy was the first study to yield the diagnosis in one patient with tuberculous pericarditis. In five patients of our series, therefore, the etiologic diagnosis of pericarditis was achieved by means of specific noncardiovascular studies. Accordingly, the clinician ought not to overlook their possible indication in patients with lymphadenopathy, pleural effusion, etc.

Dr. Permanyer: What has been discussed until now could be summarized in the following way: the search for tuberculosis (sputum or gastric aspirate examination and culture, adenosine deaminase in pleural fluid) should be carried out in all patients in whom acute pericarditis is not quickly self-limited, or when there is any clinical finding consistent with severe disease, or when the patient has a history of tuberculosis or suspected tuberculous infection. A similar policy might be adopted to rule out systemic conditions such as collagen vascular disease. The routine investigation of nonbacterial infections (viruses, mycoplasma, toxoplasma, chlamydia, etc.) would slightly increase the diagnostic yield but would not be cost effective. On the other hand, following a clue to an associated disease suggested by epidemiological or clinical findings in particular patients usually has a high diagnostic yield.

Specificity for etiology of the clinical findings

The leading motive of this second approach to the etiological diagnosis may be summarized in the following questions: are there clinical findings that may allow us to suspect with reasonable accuracy that a patient has idiopathic or viral pericarditis versus a specific type of pericardial disease? Does the classical picture of acute, dry, self-limited pericarditis always suggest viral or idiopathic pericarditis?

Dr. Spodick: There are no absolute clinical features that will definitely differentiate between specific rather than idiopathic pericarditis. However, a severe constitutional reaction with high fever and a prolonged course should induce a search for specific agents rather than the classical "acute, dry, benign pericarditis". This becomes even more important when in addition to the constitutional reaction there is a great deal of pericardial fluid, and especially if pericarditis is recognized in the presence of minimal symptoms and a nonspecific electrocardiographic change.

Dr. Permanyer: A relatively common clinical feature of idiopathic pericarditis is its relapsing character, present in up to 20% of patients. Is idiopathic pericarditis the only type that relapses? Are there special etiologic studies warranted in relapsing pericarditis?

Dr. Shabetai: First, I would say that one can never be certain whether a given patient has idiopathic pericarditis or unrecognized viral pericarditis. One strongly suspects that many of the cases of idiopathic pericarditis are in fact owing to viral infection. Viral and idiopathic pericarditis are certainly the forms most commonly associated with relapse. Dressler's syndrome may certainly relapse on several occassions and must therefore be included among causes of relapsing pericarditis. Likewise, the postcardiotomy syndrome may also recur on several occasions before it finally disappears, and is yet another instance of relapsing pericarditis. Finally, both blunt and sharp trauma causing pericarditis may be followed by several relapses. Accordingly, idiopathic pericarditis is not the only cause of the relapsing pericarditis syndrome. Acute viral or idopathic pericarditis, Dressler's syndrome, trauma, and the postcardiotomy syndrome have in common mesothelial cell injury together with blood, sometimes only in small quantity, in the pericardial space. This combination appears to be capable of setting up an immune reaction that may continue off and on over a period of many years. Thus, I believe that relapsing pericarditis should be investigated in a similar way to any other case of acute pericarditis, although once the clinician is reasonably satisfied with the etiology, a full workup is not justified or cost effective with each relapse.

Dr. Permanyer: I would like to know what Dr. Spodick and Dr. Soler think about this point.

Dr. Spodick: Idiopathic (presumably viral) pericarditis appears to be the main kind of relapsing pericarditis when we eliminate conditions such as post-myocardial injury syndromes (for which viral complicity has not been ruled out). Relapsing pericarditis should always call for a search for diseases in the vasculitis-connective tissue disease group and, of course, tuberculosis. Even malignancy may be involved in relapsing pericardial disease since, despite its usual relentless course, occasionally there are remissions.

Dr. Soler: One should differentiate between relapsing pericarditis and pericarditis with an undulating course. In the latter the disease remains clinically active with varying degrees of severity in the course of time. In this form, specific etiologies are more common than in the total population with acute pericarditis. On the contrary, genuine relapsing pericarditis is usually idiopathic; in our series (2), all 45 relapsing cases were idiopathic except one with lupus erythematosus.

Dr. Permanyer: It has been stated that the occurrence of hemodynamic complications in acute pericarditis is unusual in idiopathic or viral forms (7). Does the development of cardiac tamponade point to a specific etiology?

Dr. Shabetai: Without doubt there are causes of pericarditis with effusion that are more commonly associated with cardiac tamponade than other causes of pericardial effusion. Thus, for example, cardiac tamponade is a relatively frequent and important complication of pericarditis in patients undergoing chronic hemodialysis and in any patient with malignant pericardial effusion; even the so called acute benign pericarditis may present with severe cardiac tamponade. Postoperative pericardial effusion is an important cause of cardiac tamponade. On the other hand, uremic pericarditis (in patients not undergoing hemodialysis), pericardial effusion associated with fluid overload and heart failure, cholesterol pericarditis, and chylous pericarditis are among examples in which cardiac tamponade is rare or does not occur. Tuberculous and pyogenic infections, on the other hand, can lead to the rapid development of cardiac tamponade. Thus, the answer to your question is in the affirmative. Although the list of conditions that should be considered is quite long, it mostly depends upon the patient population in question. Patients exposed to tuberculosis and with evidence suggesting that this disease may be present pose a real question concerning the possibility of tuberculous pericarditis when they present with cardiac tamponade. Similarly, while other causes of cardiac tamponade may occur in patients undergoing dialysis, the most usual cause of cardiac tamponade in such patients is the dialysis process itself. These are good examples of Bayes' theorem. Your own protocol approach strengthens this argument, because you have shown that so called diagnostic pericardiocentesis had a low diagnostic yield, whereas the so called therapeutic pericardiocentesis, paradoxically, has a high diagnostic yield.

Dr. Sagristà: It is widely held that the development of cardiac tamponade points to a specific etiology of pericarditis, usually tuberculosis, neoplasia or purulent pericarditis. While we agree that in these conditions the development of tamponade is more common than in idiopathic pericarditis, it is also

Table 12.2. Cardiac tamponade. Etiology.

	Patients n: 256	Tamponade n: 49
Neoplastic pericarditis ⎫ Tuberculous pericarditis ⎬ Purulent pericarditis ⎭	26	16 (61%)
Idiopathic pericarditis	221	32 (14%)
Hypereosinophilic syndrome	1	1
Viral pericarditis (proven)	3	0
Toxoplasmic pericarditis	2	0
Rheumatic pericarditis	2	0
Lupus erythematosus	1	0

true that the most common cause of tamponade, in primary acute pericardial disease, is acute idiopathic pericarditis. Thus, Table 12.2 shows that, in our series, of the 26 patients with neoplastic, tuberculous and purulent pericarditis, 16 (61%) had tamponade, while out of the 221 with idiopathic pericarditis only 32 (14%) had tamponade. Therefore, specific pericarditis is complicated by tamponade more often than is acute idiopathic pericarditis. Nevertheless, in 32 (65%) of our 49 patients with tamponade pericarditis was idiopathic, and it was neoplastic in 10, tuberculous in four and purulent in two; one patient had the hypereosinophilic syndrome. Thus, even though an individual patient with specific pericarditis is at greater risk of tamponade, the most common cause of tamponade in our series of primary acute pericardial disease was idiopathic pericarditis owing to its much higher prevalence.

Among patients with tamponade are those who have other features of pericarditis and those who develop tamponade without other features of pericarditis. Of the 49 patients with tamponade in our series, 27 fulfilled our criteria for acute pericarditis, while 22 did not. Among the latter patients, 60% had specific pericarditis, mostly neoplastic, while most (85%) of the 27 patients with tamponade who did have clinical features of acute pericarditis were of unknown etiology.

Dr. Permanyer: It has also been stated (7) that a prolonged or insidious course of pericarditis suggests a specific etiology, whereas abrupt onset and short duration favor idiopathic pericarditis. Do you agree?

Dr. Spodick: A course longer than three weeks can occur in any kind of pericarditis, although it is quite unusual for viral or idiopathic pericarditis syndromes to last that long. Therefore, the sustained continuous clinical course (as opposed to a relapsing course) should call for investigations for immunopathies, agents such as tuberculosis, and other causes.

Dr. Soler: I agree that a prolonged course has classically been considered more characteristic of some specific diseases (particularly tuberculous peri-carditis). Our series generally supports this idea. However, considering that idiopathic pericarditis is much more common than specific pericarditis (9 : 1 in our series), an individual patient with a prolonged course is more likely to have idiopathic pericarditis. Thus, in our series, only one of 25 patients with clinical activity lasting three weeks after admission had tuberculous pericar-ditis and another had neoplastic pericarditis. The remaining 23 had idio-pathic pericarditis.

Dr. Permanyer: In the absence of objective demonstration of tuberculous infection, one wonders whether indirect evidence is helpful. What is the value of tuberculin skin testing?

Dr. Soler: Your question seems very pertinent in an area where this test is widely performed and where a strongly positive result is usually considered sufficient evidence to start antituberculous chemotherapy, even on question-able clinical grounds. In our area, tuberculin skin testing has no diagnostic value for the individual patient, as it was negative in 25% of our cases with demonstrated tuberculous pericarditis and positive in 41% of cases of idio-pathic pericarditis. This figure is similar to the prevalence of a positive reac-tion in the healthy population from Catalonia (40%) (8). Our data may well not be valid for other geographical areas where tuberculosis is less prevalent, as the value of skin testing is highly dependent on the prevalence of the dis-ease one is testing for. We debated whether or not to include tuberculin testing in the present version of our protocol, but it was finally included. In view of the outcome I think that this illustrates the difficulty doctors have in discarding old obsolete routines.

Dr. Permanyer: Does the presence of pleural effusions keep in the etiologic diagnosis? When and how should pleural fluid be examined?

Dr. Sagristà: The presence of pleural effusion, either unilateral or bilateral, is helpful in population studies but not when considering individuals. The question is similar to the one raised previously about tamponade. In our series of 256 consecutive patients, there was radiological evidence of pleural effusion in 7 (64%) of 11 patients with tuberculous pericarditis, in 5 (41%) of 12 patients with neoplastic pericarditis, and in 54 (24%) of 221 patients with idiopathic pericardits. Thus, although pleural effusion is more common in specific pericarditis, it is present in one fourth of all idiopathic cases, and therefore it is not useful for the etiologic diagnosis in the individual patient.

The other question you asked concerns the diagnostic yield of pleural fluid investigation. In some series, the sensitivity and specificity of cytologic exam-ination of pleural fluid for neoplasia are 66% and 100%, respectively (9). The sensitivity of pleural fluid investigation for identifications of tubercle bacilli is only about 20%, and it requires culture in specific media, with its inherent delay. That is why I want to discuss the possible role of measuring adenosine deaminase activity in pleural fluid. This is a quick and easy technique of potential importance. There is evidence suggesting that an adenosine deaminase value higher than 45 U/1 in pleural fluid has a 100% sensitivity and a 97% specificity for tuberculosis (5), although not so clear cut results have been reported by other authors (10) and high values have also been found in empyema (11), rheumatoid arthritis (11, 12) and lymphoma (13). In spite of these shortcomings, the possible usefulness of this measurement is apparent and, accordingly, it should be recommended in all patients with pericarditis and pleural effusion.

Dr. Permanyer: In summary, only the acute, rapidly self-limited form of primary acute pericarditis and to a lesser extent relapsing pericarditis suggest that a specific etiology is unlikely. In other presentations (tamponade, sustained effusion, prolonged course, etc.) clinical features alone, although more common in specific diseases, are not useful as evidence of any particular condition in the individual patient, owing to the high prevalence of idiopathic pericarditis.

Direct investigation of pericardial fluid and tissue

Dr. Permanyer: This third approach is indicated for cardiac tamponade, suspicion of purulent pericarditis, and when other means fail to establish the diagnosis.

There is no general agreement on the indications and timing for pericardiocentesis and pericardial biopsy for diagnosis as opposed to therapy; thus, we will now discuss the indications for the study of pericardial fluid or tissue. The indications for pericardiocentesis are inequivocal when cardiac tamponade is present ("therapeutic" pericardiocentesis) but are far from clear in its absence ("diagnostic" pericardiocentesis). When should diagnostic pericardiocentesis be performed? I would like to have an answer from the three groups of investigators present at this Round Table.

Dr. Shabetai: Without being unduly modest, I would prefer to defer that question to my hosts, since they have over the last decade evolved an excellent protocol for the management of pericarditis and pericardial effusion. I find myself very much persuaded by their arguments, backed as they are by careful study and substantial numbers of patients. Thinking of my own clinical experience in the light of your protocol approach, I recognize that my experience has been similar to yours; it is from the therapeutic pericardiocentesis that I have derived diagnostic information.

Let me point out an example or two when pericardiocentesis need not be carried out. One example is mild cardiac tamponade with evidence pointing to acute idiopathic or viral pericarditis. Here, in my experience, it is prudent to monitor the patient carefully while administering anti-inflammatory treatment. If the venous pressure falls, hypotension and pulsus paradoxus do not make their appearance, fever, pericardial friction rub and ECG signs subside, and the patient's well being improves, pericardiocentesis is meddlesome at best and dangerous at worst.

Some patients with pericardial effusion and early cardiac tamponade who are undergoing chronic hemodialysis require only a tightening of their dialysis regimen for the pericardial effusion and thus the tamponade to disappear. In end stage malignant disease, when the status of the malignant disease is well known to the physicians, and the patient and the family are resigned to early death, it is sometimes not justified to prolong suffering by performing pericardiocentesis. This is particularly important in patients who are suffering severe pain as a result of the neoplasm.

Aside from cardiac tamponade, it is extremely important to perform pericardiocentesis any time that one has strong grounds to suspect the possibility of infection of the pericardial fluid. Untreated pericarditis, in these cases, can lead to severe complications or death. Regarding pericardiocentesis for tuberculosis, I would support the position of the protocol from the Hospital General Vall d'Hebron.

In bizarre cases, one occasionally resorts to pericardial fluid aspiration and perhaps pericardial biopsy for tissue diagnosis, but, as has been pointed out by the Vall d'Hebron group, the yield, when the procedure is not therapeutically indicated, is low. Recently, we have been interested in performing pericardiocentesis in patients with acquired immunodeficiency syndrome and pericardial effusion.

Dr. Spodick: Pericardiocentesis should only be performed in the absence of cardiac tamponade when it is definitely necessary to identify an etiology, particularly in patients with repetitive and sustained clinical courses. Other times a chronic pericardial effusion will require drainage, sometimes with surprising results like the typical fluid of cholesterol pericarditis or the presence of chyle (chylopericardium). Sometimes this is necessary to relieve symptoms due to pulmonary functional reserve by massive effusions.

Dr. Sagristà: In our original protocol, diagnostic pericardiocentesis was indicated when purulent pericarditis was suspected and in patients with persistent clinical activity one week after admission. We performed only one pericardiocentesis for suspected purulent effusion, and the diagnosis was confirmed. Of the other 36 diagnostic pericardiocenteses only one was positive (tuberculous pericarditis). Therefore, diagnostic pericardiocentesis, performed in 37 patients, yielded the diagnosis only on two occasions. This yield was very low (5%), in contrast to that of therapeutic pericardiocentesis (29%) (Fig. 12.1). Moreover, diagnostic pericardiocentesis included 11 non-productive procedures (30%), one false negative diagnosis of tuberculous pericarditis, and one false positive diagnosis of neoplasm. To conclude, diagnostic pericardiocentesis should be limited to the suspicion of purulent pericarditis.

Dr. Permanyer: Surgical biopsy of the pericardium has been advocated as an alternative procedure, safer than pericardiocentesis (14); however, its diagnostic yield has not been fully evaluated. When should diagnositc drainage

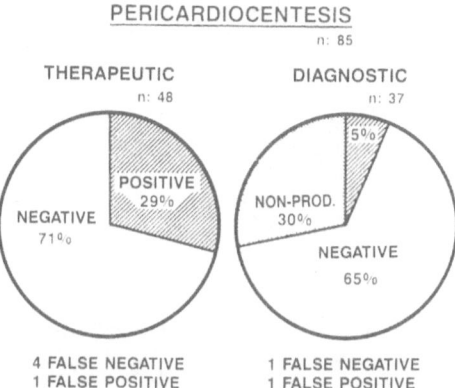

Fig. 12.1. Diagnostic yield of pericardiocentesis. Non-prod.: non-productive pericardiocentesis.

and biopsy in the absence of tamponade ("diagnostic" biopsy) be performed? When is pericardiocentesis the preferred procedure? Here again, I wish to know the opinions of several members of this Round Table.

Dr. Spodick: Surgical drainage and biopsy are seldom indicated for purely diagnostic reasons. When drainage is carried out through a subxiphoid incision, biopsy should always be done with it, because the fluid may frequently be "negative". However, the results of the group at the Hospital General Vall d'Hebron indicate that purely diagnostic drainage has very poor results and I consider this to be the most important study in that regard.

Dr. Shabetai: I am in agreement with Dr. Spodick. Most of the pericardial biopsies that we have done have been in patients who had cardiac tamponade, or in those in whom there was strong reason to believe that tuberculosis was the cause of the pericardial disease. To some extent, the question of pericardiocentesis versus open drainage is one of local preference and custom. In the case of very large pericardial effusions, needle biopsy is acceptable, but this should never be done for small or moderate size pericardial effusions. Recently, interest has developed in pericardioscopy (15, 16) for direct inspection of the pericardium. This would provide the ideal tool for safe biopsy under vision without surgical incision.

Dr. Soler: Our series shows that the routine performance of biopsy only for diagnosis has practically no justification. The yield was only 4% (one case of tuberculosis in 25 procedures) (Fig. 12.2). Even if the only false negative in a patient with neoplastic pericardial involvement had been positive the yield would still be too low (8%) to justify such an aggressive procedure on a routine basis.

Dr. Permanyer: May I now ask Dr. Sagristà to give us a comprehensive view of the overall diagnostic yield of both these invasive pericardial studies.

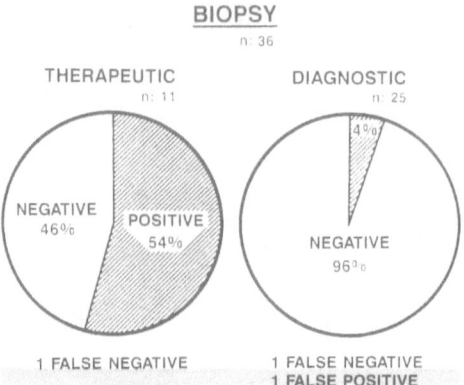

Fig. 12.2. Diagnostic yield of pericardial biopsy.

Dr. Sagristà: I will begin by discussing pericardiocentesis. The shortcomings of this procedure for the diagnosis of specific pericardial diseases have been known for many years. Regarding tuberculous pericarditis, review of the literature clearly indicates that pericardiocentesis has a low sensitivity (about 50%) (17, 18). In addition, the diagnosis depends on culture in virtually all cases rather than on direct examination of smears and this results in a significant delay. Although our series differs from others in that it is prospective and with predefined indications for pericardiocentesis, the diagnostic yield was not improved; it remained 57%. Pericardiocentesis was the first procedure to disclose the diagnosis in only three patients. This situation may in the future be improved by the measurement of adenosine deaminase, if its value for the diagnosis of tuberculous pericarditis is confirmed. Although our experience is limited, it is worth reporting that in the three cases of tuberculous pericarditis in which this measurement was carried out, adenosine deaminase values were high (92, 94 and 152 U/1), whereas they were lower than 30 U/1 in 53 patients with pericarditis of other etiologies (6).

The limitations of pericardiocentesis for the diagnosis of neoplastic pericarditis are also well known. The reported series are heterogeneous and most of them are retrospective. These limitations account for their variable diagnostic yield (from 18% (19) to 87% (20, 20a)). Nevertheless, improvements in cytological techniques can attain a 90% sensitivity for metastatic carcinoma (21), the most common malignant pericardial disease, but values are lower for lymphoma, sarcoma and mesothelioma; the latter fact is due to the lesser degree of cellular desquamation of these tumors.

In our series, pericardiocentesis was more useful in neoplastic than tuberculous pericarditis. In the former, it led to the cytological diagnosis in eight of the 10 patients with available pericardial fluid. However, cytological study of the effusion was falsely negative in one case of metastatic carcinoma and in one case of cardiac angiosarcoma. The possibility of false positive cytologic diagnosis also exists and was the case in two of our patients with idiopathic pericarditis.

To summarize, in our series the sensitivity and specificity of pericardiocentesis were 76% and 96%, respectively, for the diagnosis of tuberculous, neoplastic and purulent pericarditis considered together. There were two false positive diagnoses of neoplasia, three false negative diagnoses of tuberculosis, and two false negative diagnoses of neoplasia. The overall diagnostic yield of pericardiocentesis was 19%, but, as we shall see later, was very different when the procedure was carried out with a diagnostic (5%) or a therapeutic (29%) indication (Fig. 12.1).

I will now turn to pericardial biopsy. Most series in the literature have an insufficient size (17, 18) for calculations of sensitivity and specificity of pericardial biopsy. In the longest series (from a Third World population) (22), biopsy was positive in 27 of 32 patients (84%) with positive tubercle bacilli culture in pericardial fluid. In our series, pericardial biopsy was undertaken in three patients with tuberculous pericarditis, and it confirmed the diagnosis in all three. In addition, in five other cases the pericardiectomy specimen confirmed the diagnosis. The sensitivity of histological pericardial study for the diagnosis of tuberculosis was thus high. In neoplastic pericarditis, biopsy is considered a good diagnostic procedure (23), but it is not devoid of false negatives owing to the patchy distribution of the disease (24). We have carried out pericardial biopsy in six patients with neoplastic pericarditis, and it was negative in two (one case of angiosarcoma subsequently diagnosed from the pericardiectomy specimen, and one case of gastric adenocarcinoma). There are, in addition, other shortcomings of the histological study of the pericardium. We have seen two patients with a diagnosis of neoplasia made from biopsy or pericardiectomy specimens, which was subsequently disproved by long term follow up.

In our series the overall sensitivity and specificity of pericardial biopsy were 77% and 96%, respectively, for the diagnostic of tuberculous, neoplastic and purulent pericarditis. The overall diagnostic yield was 19%, but it was much lower when biopsy was carried out with diagnostic (4%) than with therapeutic (54%) indication (Fig. 12.2).

To summarize, the overall diagnostic yield of biopsy (19%) was the same as that of pericardiocentesis, but both procedures had a much higher diagnostic yield in therapeutic (34%) than in diagnostic (5%) indications (Fig. 12.3). We will take up this topic later in this Round Table.

Dr. Permanyer: It seems well established, therefore, that the diagnostic yield of pericardiocentesis and pericardial biopsy is low in the absence of tamponade; however, in particular patients these are the only procedures to achieve the diagnosis. Do the speakers feel that there is any method to identify those patients in whom invasive pericardial studies are more likely to have a higher diagnostic yield?

Dr. Spodick: I agree that invasive diagnostic studies are sometimes the only way to reach a diagnosis. The yield of diagnostic pericardial studies is probably much greater if a surgical approach is made so that the pericardium can

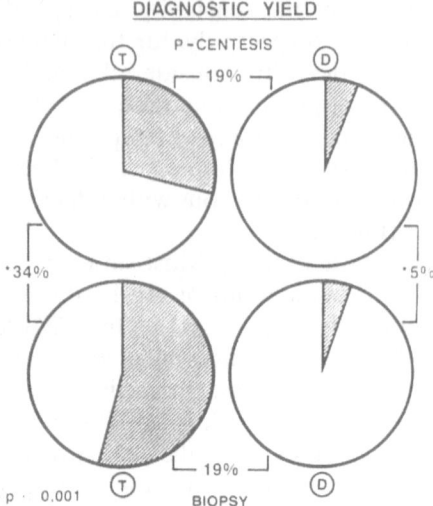

Fig. 12.3. Diagnostic yield of pericardiocentesis (P-CENTESIS) and pericardial biopsy. Shaded areas represent the rate of positive diagnostic data. The diagnostic yield of both procedures is identical (19%), but there is a significant difference (p<0.001) when therapeutic (Ⓣ) and diagnostic (Ⓓ) procedures are compared (34% and 5%, respectively).

be examined and biopsies taken as well as quantitative removal of fluid. It is important that the subxiphoid approach permits the introduction of a scope (either rigid or flexible) with which the pericardium can be examined and through biopsies can be obtained of areas which are likely to give a higher diagnostic yield (15, 16). The surgical approach has been shown, in the series from the Hospital General Vall d'Hebron, to be much more valuable when carried out for a therapeutic indication, although pericardioscopy was not used.

Dr. Shabetai: In general, a sound clinical approach is to avoid invasion of the pericardium if some other study has a good chance of yielding the correct diagnosis. For example, if a patient has pleural effusion as well as pericardial effusion, it is wise to obtain samples of pleural fluid and pleural tissue before attempting to get equivalent information from the pericardium itself. I lay great store by alerting both the bacteriology laboratory and the pathology laboratory before carrying out these procedures. Thus I ensure that anaerobic and fungal cultures are obtained as well as the routine culture studies. I make sure that a good blood free sample is sent to the virology laboratory. I discuss the diagnostic possibilities with the pathologist in some detail, and look at the specimen with him. By these means, I avoid a valuable specimen being examined in a purely routine way. I also think it is mandatory to obtain the services of a good exfoliative cytologist, since pathologists who deal mainly with solid tissue are not expert at detecting malignant cells in fluids. These are some of the steps that I would take to increase the diagnostic yield.

Dr. Soler: As discussed before, in our series diagnostic pericardiocentesis and pericardial biopsy had a poor diagnostic yield, and I do not think that there exist clinical features that may reliably identify the new cases with a specific diagnosis. It should be reemphasized, however, that our protocol was applied quite strictly, and in some of the patients who had biopsy performed three weeks after admission, the clinical features were not pronounced. Therefore, the possibility exists that, if biopsy had been limited to patients with more serious disease, the yield would have been different. The sole persistence of effusion without associated clinical manifestations is not by itself an indication for biopsy.

Dr. Permanyer: Obviously, the complexity of this situation lends itself to a systematic approach. This is one of the reasons why, in 1977, a protocol for the systematic study and management of pericardial disease was set up in our Service. I would now like Dr. Sagristà to comment on the overall results of our protocol.

Dr. Sagristà: The diagnostic yield of our initial protocol (2) has been as follows:

Stage I was limited to investigations that did not involve the heart and pericardium. It disclosed the etiologic diagnosis in 19 patients: seven with tuberculous pericarditis, three with probably viral pericarditis (Coxsackie B virus isolated from pharynx and feces), three with neoplastic pericarditis (diagnosed by the examination of peripheral blood in a patient with lymphoma, and by gastrointestinal study and lymph node biopsy in the remaining two), two with rheumatic pericarditis, two with toxoplasma pericarditis, one with systemic lupus erythematosus and one with hypereosinophilic syndrome.

Pericardiocentesis, representing the stage II of our protocol, was performed in 85 patients, and 16 diagnoses were obtained. Forty-eight of the 85 procedures were therapeutic; in this subgroup, 14 diagnoses were achieved. By contrast, only two diagnoses were made out of 37 diagnostic pericardiocenteses. The 16 diagnoses made by pericardiocentesis were: nine neoplastic, three purulent and three tuberculous pericarditis, and one hypereosinophilic syndrome. However, two of the 16 diagnoses had already been made in the stage I of the protocol; accordingly, stage II established 14 new diagnoses.

Stage III consisted of pericardial biopsy. It was carried in 36 patients, and in seven a tissue diagnosis was obtained. However, it was in six of the 11 therapeutic procedures that a positive tissue diagnosis was obtained, whereas only one of 25 diagnostic biopsies was positive. Pericardial biopsy yielded diagnostic material in three cases of neoplastic, two of purulent and two of tuberculous pericarditis. However, six out of these seven diagnoses were also made in studies from earlier stages of the protocol; thus, only one truly new diagnosis was made by pericardial biopsy. This finding clearly indicates the need to limit diagnostic invasive studies.

Stage IV of our protocol contemplated the possibility of blind antituberculous chemotherapy in those patients with persistent clinical activity in whom 5–6 weeks after admission etiologic diagnosis had not been achieved despite extensive workup. The fact that no single patient in our series reached this stage is to be emphasized.

Eighteen pericardiectomies were carried out (11 for constrictive pericarditis, two for recurrent pericarditis and for miscellaneous reasons in the rest, as discussed in chapter 10). Tissue diagnosis was obtained in seven patients (four tuberculosis, two neoplasm, and one purulent). In two of these patients the diagnosis had not been made previously (one cardiac angiosarcoma and one neoplastic pericarditis).

The final diagnosis in our 256 patients is shown in Table 12.3. The possibility that some of the cases finally diagnosed as idiopathic had specific disease should obviously be considered, but it is unlikely in view of the absence of major clinical events or late constriction in a mean prospective follow up of 38 months (2).

Dr. Permanyer: We modified the initial protocol after the analysis of the results that Dr. Sagristà has just presented. In the current version (p. 217) the investigations are conducted stepwise as in the preceding one, but invasive diagnostic studies have been limited. We still advise pericardiocentesis whenever we strongly suspect purulent pericarditis, and pericardial biopsy when, three weeks after admission, definite clinical manifestations persist. This algorithm leaves, at worst, the possibility of missing a few specific causes (e.g. early tuberculosis), but prevents a large number of unnecessary invasive procedures. In this regard, it may be pertinent to add that all the considerations of the present discussion apply to immunologically competent patients. The patients with AIDS and related syndromes may require a different approach (p. 221). Although several specific pericardial diseases (such as bacterial (25, 26) and nonbacterial infections (27, 28) or Kaposi's sarcoma (29, 30)) have been reported in these patients, their relative prevalence as compared with nonspecific pericardial disease is not yet well established (30–33). Also, the values of adenosine deaminase may have a different meaning in these patients. Thus, the yield of diagnostic procedures is not well delineated in this context and the issue awaits further clarification.

Table 12.3. Final etiologic diagnosis.

	n: 256
Acute idiopathic pericarditis	221 (86%)
Neoplastic pericarditis	12 (5%)
Tuberculous pericarditis	11 (4%)
Purulent pericarditis	3 (1%)
Viral pericarditis (proven)	3 (1%)
Toxoplasmic pericarditis	2 (1%)
Rheumatic pericarditis	2 (1%)
Hypereosinophilic syndrome	1 (0.5%)
Lupus erythematosus	1 (0.5%)

I would now like to ask Dr. Spodick and Dr. Shabetai to give us a critical overview of our diagnostic protocol.

Dr. Spodick: I do not believe there are important pitfalls in this protocol. Indeed, it is the first time that a systematic approach has been reported on a very large group of patients evaluated prospectively. For the time being, this protocol is a model for any clinical investigation on the pericardium. However, it is possible that with that protocol diagnostic material might not be obtained because the studies indicated by the protocol were either too early or too late. My own view is that, as opposed to pericardiocentesis, the subxiphoid surgical approach would be ideal in serious cases, especially in constitutionally ill patients. This has the advantage of being extrapleural and extraperitoneal and permits direct view as well as palpation of the pericardial cavity and the heart (scopes have already been mentioned) and can be done, in urgent situations, even in bed and with local anesthesia.

Dr. Shabetai: Dr. Spodick's comments are well taken. A protocol, like most things in medicine, has power for good and power for evil. Its power for good is obvious; it forces us to think in an organized methodical systematic fashion. This organization helps insure that we do not omit important diagnostic considerations when seeing patients with acute pericarditis, but go through a systematic careful routine which enables us to sort patients into categories and sub-categories in a reliable way. The potential evil of a protocol is that it may become too rigid. The protocol is made for the physicians; the physicians are not made for the protocol. Thus, properly applied, but allowing for individual judgement and assessment of individual patients on an individual basis, this protocol approach is outstanding, and it does not have major pitfalls in the hands of intelligent clinically experienced physicians. I would like to emphasize the importance of clinical experience. A protocol such as this one, in the hands of individuals who have not seen many patients, can be misused. Like all protocols, this one must be applied in the light of clinical experience and judgement.

Dr. Permanyer: It appears that a systematic approach to the etiologic diagnosis of patients with acute pericardial disease is useful. No matter whether the selected protocol is the one discussed here or another, it seems unquestionable that the selection of any investigation should be based upon its own diagnostic yield. In addition, protocols should be adapted to the prevalence of certain diseases in particular geographical areas and patient populations.

Particular aspects of therapy

Dr. Permanyer: In this section we will concentrate in some debatable aspects, as we think that the basic guidelines for the therapy of acute pericarditis are well established and accepted.

Corticosteroids are often given for acute idiopathic pericarditis when the disease does not subside rapidly; this therapy has even been recommended in some textbooks (7, 34). However, corticosteroids may be unnecessary and even dangerous. Is there any indication for corticosteroids in acute nonre-lapsing idiopathic pericarditis?

Dr. Spodick: I strongly oppose using corticosteroid agents in the therapy of acute nonrelapsing pericarditis (and also for relapsing pericarditis). There is such a number of agents now available, particularly in the "non-steroidal anti-inflammatory" group that corticosteroid therapy should be used only as a last resort and after every possible other therapy could be used (during acute pain I even use an ice bag over the precordium – excepting for coronary patients). The reason for this is that too many patients ultimately become "hooked" and it is very difficult to take them off corticosteroid therapy even though they may have complications. Indeed, there is some reason to believe that cortico-steroid therapy may, perhaps by incomplete immunosuppression while sup-pressing the inflammation, set the stage for ultimate relapsing pericarditis and steroid dependence. Actually, in a situation like systemic lupus erythematosus with pericarditis, particularly in the presence of lupus nephritis, cortico-steroids are probably the best agents to use. I would strongly emphasize that corticosteroid therapy has never been known to prevent constrictive pericar-ditis and, in fact, in the one controlled observation of 240 patients with tuber-culous pericarditis, half of them receiving corticosteroids, a similar number in both groups developed constrictive pericarditis despite concomitant anti-tuberculous therapy (22).

Dr. Permanyer: In areas where tuberculosis is frequent, it is not uncommon to give blind antituberculous therapy in the cases of acute pericarditis that do not rapidly subside. As in the case of corticosteroid therapy, there are reports in the literature favoring this policy (35). Is there any place for antituber-culous therapy in the absence of objective confirmation of the diagnosis of tuberculous pericarditis?

Dr. Soler: One of the reasons why we set up our prospective study of primary acute pericardial disease was to establish whether blind antituberculous therapy could be justified. This possibility formed the basis of stage IV of our initial protocol. In view of our results, I feel that, as a rule, when an extensive etiologic workup such as that comprising stages I through III of our protocol fails to yield a diagnosis, there is no justification for starting antituberculous treatment. Blind antituberculous therapy was not given to any patient in our series. The clinical manifestation of pericardial diseases are far too nonspeci-fic to point to any particular etiology. The results of our study suggest that, if blind antituberculous therapy were prescribed because of an indolent or pro-longed course the instances of unnecessary therapy would clearly outnumber the rare cases of tuberculous pericarditis overlooked after a systematic study. On the other hand, and contrary to what is frequently thought, less than half of our patients with tuberculous pericarditis had persistent effusion with general symptoms but no hemodynamic complications. When the latter are absent, it is even harder to justify blind antituberculous therapy. Exceptions may be considered, particularly wherever the available health care facilities do not permit a systematic study protocol such as ours, in a few patients where the suspicion of tuberculous pericarditis is based on an unquestionable past history of tuberculosis or a clearly abnormal value of adenosine deaminase in a concomitant pleural exudate.

Dr. Permanyer: Acute idiopathic relapsing pericarditis can still be a nightmare to the patient and a challenge to the physician, as well defined and effective therapeutic guidelines are not available. What is the rationale for the therapy of idiopathic relapsing pericarditis? When should corticosteroids, immunosuppressants or pericardiectomy be advocated?

Dr. Shabetai: Here I beg your leave to differ somewhat from Dr. Spodick. I fully appreciate the reasons that he gives for withholding steroidal treatment and prefering nonsteroidal antiinflammatory agents. Unfortunately, there are a number of patients with relapsing pericarditis in whom nothing short of steroid therapy, usually with prednisone in substantial dosage, will suppress the symptoms. One must remember that the pain and distress of relapsing pericarditis may be severe. After many attacks over many years the patient's morale is worn thin. The more severe attacks simply fail to yield to large doses of indomethacin or ibuprofen. In such cases I administer prednisone, usually starting at 60 mg per day for a few days and then generally tapering until I can establish the dose that just suppresses the symptoms of acute pericarditis. I maintain this dose for a month or two, and then attempt to reduce the dose toward zero. If the syndrome recurs, I raise the dose to a previous higher dose and continue this for a few weeks and then try to taper the dose again. This treatment assumes that relapsing pericarditis is some kind of an autoimmune reaction, which I believe starts when blood enters the pericardial space in which there are injured mesothelial cells. I should also mention that while I am the first to agree with Dr. Spodick that prednisone is a dangerous drug with many unwanted effects, ibuprofen, aspirin, indomethacin and the other nonsteroidal antiinflammatory agents are far from benign. They affect the platelets, they are nephrotoxic, they cause gastrointestinal bleeding, and, in patients with heart disease, by their action on prostaglandins, they cause salt and water retention. Nevertheless, I do agree with Dr. Spodick that we must make every effort to use prednisone and other steroids as sparingly as possible. For this reason, I often combine prednisone with one of the nonsteroidal antiinflammatory agents, and move when I can to a regimen which employs prednisone every other day rather than daily. The nonsteroidal drug may be given at alternate days or every day. I take a particular care to get the dose down as quickly and as low as possible. Even with this approach, the patient must know the likelihood of many setbacks in the course of this long and troublesome disease.

On the basis that relapsing pericarditis may be some kind of an autoimmune phenomenon, it has been suggested that azathioprine should be combined with prednisone (36). This combination is a potent immunosuppressive regimen and until recently it was the routine regimen for cardiac transplantation recipients. I have only treated one patient with azathioprine. The patient was already receiving this agent when I took over the care, and eventually he did well. I have no experience with cyclosporine for this indication.*

With regard to pericardiectomy, enthusiasm for this indication is declining. Pericardiectomy received a brief 10 or 15 years ago when it was proposed by several authorities (38, 39). However, recently, in a careful study, Fowler et al (40) have shown that all cases respond eventually to medical treatment. Furthermore, it is their experience and that of myself and many other investigators that the syndrome continues even after pericardiectomy. On the other hand, constrictive pericarditis is an extremely rare sequel. Thus, in almost every case, I would advise strongly against pericardiectomy.

Dr. Spodick: Relapsing pericarditis should be treated like an individual attack of acute pericarditis. Corticosteroids, if originally used, should be tapered slowly when the introduction of nonsteroidal antiinflammatory agents. I reiterate my comment above about corticosteroid therapy in general. Surgery is almost never indicated because it is nearly always a failure, possibly because one cannot remove the entire pericardium. Finally, immunosuppressants are new to the field and should be tried in appropriately designed controlled studies. They may be the final answer; however, the side effect profile is very strong and one would wish to do management with nonsteroidal agents.

Dr. Permanyer: It is very difficult to summarize in a few words the large amount of information provided by the speakers. With respect to the first part of our discussion, I reemphasize the following conclusions as the major message: first, it should never be forgotten that idiopathic pericarditis is the most common type of primary acute pericardial disease in our part of the world, no matter the clinical presentation; second, the application of a systematic paradigm to every patient with acute pericardial disease results in a rational use of invasive studies and a better understanding of one's results, avoiding unnecessary treatment. Finally, invasive studies, when undertaken in patients with hemodynamic compromise or manifest clinical severity, have the best chance of achieving a sizeable diagnostic yield.

Although a sort comment cannot adequately summarize what has been said about therapy, I will single out the following issues: first, corticosteroid therapy should be avoided as far as possible in acute idiopathic pericarditis; second, antituberculous chemotherapy should not be given in the absence of objective diagnostic data; and third, the therapeutic approach to severe re-

---

* After the manuscript was elaborated, a preliminary report (37) has appeared suggesting that colchicine may be a valuable therapy in relapsing pericarditis. (Eds.).

lapsing idiopathic pericarditis remains unsatisfactory in spite of having been a concern of investigators and clinicians for many years.

References

1. Gleckman RA. Nonviral infectious pericarditis. In: Spodick DH, ed. Pericardial Diseases. Philadelphia, FA Davis Co., 1976; 159–176.
2. Permanyer-Miralda G, Sagristà-Sauleda J, Soler-Soler J. Primary acute pericardial disease: A prospective series of 231 consecutive patients. Am J Cardiol 1985; 56: 623–630.
3. Sagristà-Sauleda J, Permanyer-Miralda G, Soler-Soler J. Tuberculous pericarditis: Ten year experience with a prospective protocol for diagnosis and treatment. J Am Coll Cardiol 1988; 11: 724–728.
4. Sagristà-Sauleda J, Permanyer-Miralda G, Soler-Soler J. Tuberculous pericarditis. Cardiol Board Rev 1989; 6: 114–120.
5. Ocaña I, Martínez-Vázquez JM, Segura RM, Fernández-de-Sevilla T, Capdevila JA. Adenosine deaminase in pleural fluids. A test for the diagnosis of tuberculous pleural effusion. Chest 1983; 84: 51–53.
6. Martínez-Vázquez JM, Ribera E, Ocaña I, Segura RM, Serrat R, Sagristà J. Adenosine deaminase activity in tuberculous pericarditis. Thorax 1986; 41: 888–889.
7. Braunwald E. Pericardial disease. In: Harrison's Principles of Internal Medicine. McGraw-Hill, Schwabe and Company Ltd, 1983; 1458–1465.
8. March P, Alcaide V, Salleras LI, Gili M. Anàlisi epidemiològica de la infecciò i malaltia tuberculosa a Catalunya. In: La tuberculosi a Catalunya. Generalitat de Catalunya. Departament de Sanitat i Seguretat Social. Barcelona, 1983; 33–85.
9. Shan SA. The pleura. Am Rev Respir Dis 1988; 138: 184–234.
10. Niwa Y, Kishimoto H, Shimokata K. Carcinomatous and tuberculous pleural effusions. Comparison of tumor markers. Chest 1985; 87: 351–355.
11. Pettersson T, Ojala K, Weber TH. Adenosine deaminase in the diagnosis of pleural effusions. Acta Med Scand 1984; 215: 299–304.
12. Pettersson T, Klockars M, Weber T. Pleural fluid adenosine deaminase in rheumatoid arthritis and systemic lupus erythematosus. Chest 1984; 86: 273.
13. Pérez Vidal R, Arán X, Broquetas J. High adenosine deaminase activity level in pleural effusion. Chest 1986; 90: 625.
14. Kossmann CE, Hancock EW. Is surgical drainage preferable to needle pericardiocentesis in patients with pericardial effusion? In: Rapaport E, ed. Current controversies in cardiovascular disease. Philadelphia, WB Saunders Company, 1980; 674–692.
15. Little AG, Ferguson MK. Pericardioscopy as adjunct to pericardial window. Chest 1986; 89: 53–55.
16. Kondos GT, Rich S, Levitsky S. Flexible fiberoptic pericardioscopy for the diagnosis of pericardial disease. J Am Coll Cardiol 1986; 7: 432–434.
17. Rooney JJ, Crocco JA, Lyons HA. Tuberculous pericarditis. Ann Intern Med 1970; 72: 73–78.
18. Fowler NO. The pericardium in health and disease. Mount Kisco, Futura Publishing Company, 1985; 195–215.
19. Flannery EP, Gregoratos G, Corder MP. Pericardial effusions in patients with malignant diseases. Arch Intern Med 1975; 135: 967–977.
20. Zipf RE, Johnston WW. The role of citology in the evaluation of pericardial effusions. Chest 1972; 62: 593–596.
20a. Meyers DG, Bouska DJ. Diagnostic usefulness of pericardial fluid cytology. Chest 1989; 95: 1142–1143.
21. Hancock EW. Management of pericardial disease. Mod Conc Cardiovasc Dis 1979; 48: 1–6.

22. Strang JIG, Gibson DG, Mitchison DA. Girling DJ, Kakaza HHS, Allen BW, Evans DJ, Nunn AJ. Controlled clinical trial of complete open surgical drainage and of prednisolone in treatment of tuberculous pericardial effusion in Transkei. The Lancet 1988; ii: 759–763.
23. Kralstein J, Frishman W. Malignant pericardial diseases: diagnosis and treatment. Am Heart J 1987; 113: 785–790.
24. Press OW, Livingston R. Management of malignant pericardial effusion and tamponade. JAMA 1987; 257: 1088–1092.
25. Foale R. Cardiac involvement with AIDS. Current Opinion in Cardiology 1988; 3: 245–248.
26. Sunderam G, McDonald RJ, Maniatis T, Oleske J, Kapila R, Reichman LB. Tuberculosis as a manifestation of the acquired immunodeficiency syndrome (AIDS). JAMA 1986; 256: 362–366.
27. Holtz HA, Lavery DP, Kapila R. Actinomycetales infection in the acquired immunodeficiency syndrome. Ann Intern Med 1985; 102: 203–205.
28. Zuger A, Louie E, Holzman RS, Simberkoff MS, Rahal JJ. Cryptococcal disease in patients with the acquired immunodeficiency syndrome. Diagnostic features and outcome of treatment. Ann Intern Med 1986; 104: 234–240.
29. Silver MA, Matcher AM, Reichert CM, Levens DL, Parrillo JF, Longo DL, Roberts WC. Cardiac involvement by Kaposi's sarcoma in acquired immunodeficiency syndrome (AIDS). Am J Cardiol 1984; 53: 983–985.
30. Cammarosano C, Lewis W. Cardiac lesions in acquired immunodeficiency syndrome (AIDS). J Am Coll Cardiol 1985; 5: 703–706.
31. Roldan EO, Moskowitz L, Hensley GT. Pathology of the heart in acquired immunodeficiency syndrome. Arch Pathol Lab Med 1987; 111: 943–946.
32. Fink L, Reichek N, St John Sutton MG. Cardiac abnormalities in acquired immune deficiency syndrome. Am J Cardiol 1984; 54: 1161–1163.
33. Bestetti RB. Cardiac involvement in the acquired immune deficiency syndrome. Intern J Cardiol 1989; 22: 143–146.
34. Lorell BH, Braunwald E. Pericardial disease. In: Braunwald E, ed. Heart disease. A textbook of cardiovascular medicine. Philadelphia, WB Saunders 1988; 1484–1534.
35. Gooi HL, Smith JM. Tuberculous pericarditis in Birmingham. Thorax 1978; 33: 94–96.
36. Asplen CH, Levine HD. Azathioprine therapy of steroid responsive pericarditis. Am Heart J 1970; 80: 109–111.
37. Rodríguez de la Serna A, Guindo-Soldevila J, Martí-Claramunt V, Bayés de Luna A. Colchicine for recurrent pericarditis. Lancet 1987; ii: 1517.
38. Zinsser HS, Blakemore WS, Kirby CK, Johnson J. Invalidism due to recurrent idiopathic pericarditis with recovery after pericardiectomy. JAMA 1959; 171: 274–279.
39. Hatcher CR, Logue RB, Logan WD, Symbas PN, Mansour KA, Abbott OA. Pericardiectomy for recurrent pericarditis. J. Thorac Cardiovasc Surg 1971; 62: 371–378.
40. Fowler NO, Harbin AD. Recurrent pericarditis: follow-up of 31 patients. J Am Coll Cardiol 1986; 7: 300–305.

APPENDICES

Appendix 1
Protocol for the diagnosis and management of pericardial diseases

SERVICE OF CARDIOLOGY, HOSPITAL GENERAL VALL
D'HEBRON, BARCELONA

General workup for all patients

Stage 1. General investigations and echocardiogram

a) In addition to a thorough physical examination and the laboratory investigations routinely performed on the Service, the following studies will be carried out in all patients with a diagnosis of *acute pericarditis*: antistreptolysin titer and rheumatoid factor, tuberculin skin test (10 units of purified protein derivative), antitoxoplasma antibodies, and the available virologic studies. In the clinical record a specific mention will be made of any recent drug treatment, trauma, surgical operation or exposure to radiations, as well as recent respiratory or gastrointestinal diseases, possible episodes of rheumatic or ischemic heart disease, history of tuberculosis and possible exposure to such infection. A mention will also be made of concomitant pleuritis or pneumonitis by clinical or radiologic criteria, and of any other clinical finding consistent with systemic disease.

b) In all patients with acute pericarditis and cardiomegaly by chest radiogram, or with any other finding suggestive of pericardial effusion, as well as in

J. Soler-Soler et al. (Eds.), Pericardial Disease, pp. 217–222.

those in whom clinical history suggests *illness lasting for more than one week*, an echocardiogram will be performed. In addition, antinuclear and antiDNA antibodies, and agglutination titers against *brucella* will be investigated, and a search for mycobacteria will be carried out in three samples of sputum, both by examination of stained smears and by culture in the appropriate media. If the patient does not produce sputum, investigation for mycobacteria will be carried out in gastric aspirates in patients with pericardial effusion lasting longer than one week or showing other criteria of severity, or in whom there is suspicion or past history of tuberculosis.

c) Any study considered necessary for etiologic investigation on the basis of the clinical findings (e.g., lymph node biopsy) will be carried out on an individual basis.

d) In patients with evidence of pleural effusion of sufficient size, thoraco-centesis will be carried out, with eventual pleural biopsy. Pleural fluid cytology, glucose, proteins, lactic dehydrogenase and adenosine deaminase levels will be measured, and Ziehl-Neelsen stain with culture for mycobacteria will be performed.

Stage 2. Pericardiocentesis

Pericardiocentesis will be carried out in the two following circumstances:

a) *Clinical signs suggesting acute severe infection*, especially in patients with pneumonia, empyema or mediastinitis, particularly in debilitated or post-operative patients ("diagnostic" pericardiocentesis).

b) Presence of *cardiac tamponade* ("therapeutic" pericardiocentesis).

Pericardiocentesis will be carried out either by the subxiphoid or apical approach. Aseptic conditions and ECG monitoring will be employed and ressuscitation equipment will be available. If possible, an epicardial ECG lead will be used.

The following studies of pericardial aspirate will be carried out: a) packed red cell volume; b) cytology; c) stain and culture for mycobacteria, culture in ordinary media and in media for viruses, and d) proteins, glucose, lactic dehydrogenase and adenosine deaminase.

Stage 3. Pericardial biopsy

After two weeks of clinical evolution and persisting significant effusion, external jugular pulse recording and apexcardiogram will be performed.

In cases where *definite unremitting clinical features of severity persist for three weeks after hospital admission* without etiologic diagnosis, surgical pericardial biopsy will be indicated ("diagnostic" biopsy).

The following investigations will be performed on the biopsy specimen: a) histology; b) stain for mycobacteria; c) culture in ordinary media and in

Löwenstein medium; d) study of the pericardial fluid (as in stage 2).

Pericardial biopsy will be carried out after one week therapy with isoniazid 450 mg/day and streptomycin 1g/day. Antituberculous therapy will be interrupted if histology is negative for tuberculosis.

Cardiac tamponade

a) *Cardiac tamponade* will be diagnosed whenever a patient with proven pericardial effusion shows venous hypertension or pulsus paradoxus (an inspiratory fall greater than 10 mmHg in systolic blood pressure). If these findings may be due to other conditions (heart failure, overhydration, chronic obstructive lung disease, etc), the diagnosis will be made on an individual basis. Specific echocardiographic findings may be helpful.

b) *Cardiac tamponade* will be considered as *decompensated* when it is associated with shock, hypotension or low cardiac output.

c) The diagnosis of cardiac tamponade *will be an indication of pericardiocentesis*, carried out as emergency if tamponade is decompensated. In extremely ill patients, the suspicion of decompensated tamponade may allow pericardiocentesis even in the absence of echocardiography when waiting for such evidence would entail critical delay.

d) In patients with *relapse of decompensated tamponade after an adequate pericardiocentesis*, surgical drainage with pericardial biopsy ("therapeutic" biopsy) will be carried out. If a previous diagnosis of tuberculous, purulent or neoplastic pericarditis has been made, the surgical finding of a thickened or adherent pericardium may justify extensive pericardiectomy. Relapsing tamponade with hemorrhagic effusion should lead to a search for neoplastic disease.

e) *Persistence of compensated tamponade* after an adequate pericardiocentesis does not necessarily indicate surgical therapy, except with persistent clinical severity or when tamponade does not subside in 1–2 weeks.

f) If therapeutic pericardiocentesis is not productive or fails to relieve decompensated tamponade, emergency surgical drainage is indicated.

Viral pericarditis. Acute idiopathic pericarditis. Postinfarction and postpericardiotomy syndromes. Relapsing acute pericarditis

a) Whenever one of the above diagnoses is made, bed rest will be instituted while pain or fever persist. Salicylates will be given for at least two weeks. The initial dose, acetylsalicylic acid 2 g daily or more if needed, will be maintained as long as pain or fever persist and then will be progressively tapered. If the response is poor, nonsteroidal agents such as indomethacin or ibuprofen will be given. Prednisone may only be administered if severe pain or high fever persist for more than five days despite the previously mentioned regimen provided that specific pericardial infections such as tuberculosis can be ruled out. Prednisone will be administered for 2–4 weeks, depending on individual circumstances. The initial dose, 40–60 mg dayly, will be maintained as long as pain, fever or severe effusion persist, and then will be progressively tapered.

b) In case of *recurrent pericarditis* the therapeutic approach will be the same as in a). Pericardiectomy may be considered only for exceptional cases, when symptoms are intractable or when intolerable steroid side effects appear. In any case, pericardiectomy will not be considered unless the syndrome has occurred at least six times and the duration of the disease is at least one year.

The diagnosis of any type of pericarditis will determine the withdrawal or modification of any type of anticoagulant therapy, which as a rule should be considered as dangerous.

Tuberculous pericarditis

If the diagnosis of tuberculous pericarditis is confirmed, triple therapy will be instituted:

- Isoniazid: 300 mg/day, before breakfast (patients weighing more than 90 kg will receive 450 mg/day), for nine months.
- Rifampin: 600 mg/day, before breakfast (patients weighing less than 50 kg will receive 450 mg/day, and those weighing more than 90 kg will receive 750 mg/day), for nine months.
- Ethambutol: 25 mg/kg/day, with breakfast, for two months.
- Prednisone 1 mg/kg/day may be given and then progressively tapered over 6–8 weeks.

Purulent pericarditis

Whenever a purulent pericardial effusion is demonstrated by macroscopic or microscopic criteria, surgical drainage will be performed and appropriate antibiotic therapy will be administered for 4–6 weeks. If the pericardium is thickened at the time of drainage, the surgeon may carry out an extensive pericardiectomy. This procedure will be mandatory in case of constrictive pericarditis, relapsing tamponade or lack of response to medical therapy.

Radiation pericarditis

Management of the various manifestations of radiation pericarditis will be based on the guidelines for acute idiopathic pericarditis.

Pericarditis in AIDS and related syndromes

At the present moment, valid guidelines for the systematic diagnostic approach to these patients cannot be given for the following reasons: 1) The relative prevalences of specific and nonspecific pericardial diseases in these patients are not well known. 2) There are wide differences in clinical presentation and prognosis, and individualization is required. However, the general workup of the present protocol may be recommended, possibly with a more liberal indication of invasive pericardial diagnostic studies depending on individual considerations. Tissue diagnosis may have a higher diagnostic yield for the diagnosis of nonbacterial infections and Kaposi's sarcoma than pericardial fluid investigation alone, while the latter may be adequate for the diagnosis of bacterial infections including tuberculosis.

Chronic pericardial effusion

The finding of mild pericardial effusion on a routine echocardiogram (overall anterior and posterior echo free spaces measuring less than 10 mm at end-diastole on the M mode recording) does not imply by itself the need for further studies.

The finding of moderate pericardial effusion (echo free spaces 10–20 mm) in the absence of other clinical findings will justify the performance of the studies indicated in the stage I of the general workup of this protocol, supplemented by a thyroid function study. If the etiology is not discovered, periodic clinical controls will be carried out. No particular treatment will be advised if the patient's condition remains stable.

If pericardial effusion is large (echo free spaces >20 mm at end-diastole) and chronic (lasting longer than three months), the investigations of the stage I of the general workup and a thyroid function study will be carried out. If etiologic diagnosis is not demonstrated and features of tamponade are present, pericardiectomy will be advised. In case of optimal tolerance and absence of etiologic diagnosis, the patient will be followed up without therapy, and pericardiectomy will be indicated when stable effusion has persisted for at least six months. Routine studies of the pericardial fluid and tissue will be carried out.

Constrictive pericarditis

At any time during evolution of pericarditis or pericardial effusion, whenever clinical findings suggesting constriction are detected, jugular pulse recording and echocardiogram will be obtained. If these confirm constriction, a different approach will be taken in idiopathic and in tuberculous or purulent pericarditis. In idiopathic pericarditis, the patient will be observed, repeating the external recordings as needed (initially weekly). Pericardiectomy will not be advised unless moderate to severe venous congestion develops and persists for at least two weeks. Pericardiectomy will be carried out after 1–2 weeks of treatment with streptomycin and isoniazid. In cases of documented tuberculous or purulent pericarditis, pericardiectomy will be advised when unquestionable features of venous congestion develop. Adequate medical therapy will also be given.

In cases of obvious severe chronic constrictive pericarditis pericardiectomy may be advised without previous cardiac catheterization.

Appendix 2
Protocol for the diagnosis and management of pericardial disease in the patients with end stage renal disease

SERVICE OF NEPHROLOGY, HOSPITAL GENERAL VALL D'HEBRON, BARCELONA

The difficulty in defining with adequate terminology the several types of pericardial disease in patients with endstage renal disease probably reflects our inability to understand the underlying pathophysiology. Moreover, attempts to achieve a unified etiologic diagnosis have failed, while the hypothesis of a multifactorial etiology and pathogenesis of pericardial disease has gained ground. This failure prevents specific therapy from being undertaken and accounts for the wide variety of therapeutic modalities that have been tried, regarding both the optimal dialysis regimen and the aggressive or more conservative management of pericardial effusion and cardiac tamponade. Accordingly, the function of the definitions used in this protocol is to help in identifying situations where the patient may benefit from particular therapeutic approaches, rather than to establish a etiologic or pathogenetical classification.

Definitions and diagnostic criteria

1. *Pericarditis.* Pericarditis is an inflammatory disease of the pericardium frequently associated with effusion. To establish the diagnosis two of the following three criteria are required: suggestive chest pain, pericardial friction rub, and characteristic electrocardiographic changes.

    1.1. Uremic pericarditis is diagnosed when the above mentioned criteria occur in a patient with endstage renal disease who has not been dialysed or is within three months from the beginning of dialysis. Uremic pericarditis is an indication to begin dialysis without delay in the patients who are not already undergoing dialysis.

    1.2. Pericarditis associated with hemodialysis. This is the term applied to

J. Soler-Soler et al. (Eds.), Pericardial Disease, pp. 223–227.

the pericarditis occurring in patients on dialysis therapy later than three months after its institution. The term *associated with hemodialysis* is used because hemodialysis is the type of dialysis more commonly used in our area and because pericarditis is uncommon in patients receiving peritoneal dialysis. This type of pericarditis may have the following etiologies:

1.2.1. Infective. This should always be suspected in the presence of fever and toxic symptoms, and also when other cases appear in the same dialysis center. The following investigations should be performed: blood culture for bacteria and viruses, stain for mycobacteria and culture in Löwenstein medium of three samples of sputum or gastric aspirate, tuberculin skin test with 10 units of purified protein derivative, hepatitis B virus markers, and serial serologic viral and toxoplasma studies. Adenosine deaminase should be measured in pleural effusion when present.

1.2.2. Associated with inadequate dialysis. This should be suspected wherever there is clinical or biochemical evidence that the patient has not received quantitatively or qualitatively adequate dialysis in the days preceding diagnosis. This may have been for the following reasons:

a) Inadequate vascular access, resulting in suboptimal dialysis flow or in recirculation.

b) Increased dialysis requirements owing to hypercatabolism secondary to infection, multiple trauma or major surgery.

c) Dialyzer surface inadequate for the needs of the patient.

2. *Pericardial effusion.* Presence of fluid in the pericardial space, recognized by echocardiography or pericardiocentesis. According to its character it may be:

2.1. Inflammatory effusion. When it is associated with clinical features of pericarditis or when the findings of the cytological or biochemical study of the fluid obtained by pericardiocentesis are consistent with an inflammatory origin.

2.2. Transudative effusion. This is diagnosed when the investigations in the pericardial fluid show scanty cells and a low protein content. In the absence of clinical features of pericarditis, it may be assumed to be present in the following circumstances:

2.2.1. Associated with congestive heart failure or overhydration. In such cases, there may be varying degrees of edema, painful hepatomegaly, raised central venous pressure, orthopnea, pulmonary rales, gallop rhythm, pulmonary venous congestion, pleural effusion or progressive increase in the interdialysis weight.

2.2.2. Asymptomatic effusion. When the echocardiogram discloses a pericardial effusion in an asymptomatic patient, it should be assumed that it is a transudate, even in the absence of cardiomegaly.

3.1. Compensated *cardiac tamponade.* This diagnosis should be established in the presence of pericardial effusion, identified by echocardiography, associated with raised venous pressure or more than 10 mmHg pulsus paradoxus in the absence of other conditions that may account for the clinical findings. It is to be remembered that in patients with left ventricular dysfunction tamponade may occur without pulsus paradoxus. Specific echocardiographic findings may help in the diagnosis.

3.2. Decompensated cardiac tamponade. This is defined as pericardial tamponade associated with hypotension, shock or low cardiac output.

Type of dialysis regimen

The therapeutic approach has as its main target the prevention of potentially decompensated cardiac tamponade. The highest incidence of critical tamponade is during, or immediately after, the dialysis procedure.

Type of dialysis regimen. This depends on the clinical status of the patient and the availability of an adequate vascular access. The choice is made by the physician in charge, who should, if hemodialysis is selected, also decide on the type of filter and the anticoagulation schedule. However, the following guidelines should be considered depending on the type of pericardial disease.

1. Uremic pericarditis improves with dialysis. Diagnosis should be followed by the immediate institution of dialysis. If hemodialysis is chosen, double puncture is preferable to guarantee adequacy. The problem with unipuncture is that the resulting recirculation prolongs the procedure and necessitates intensification of the sessions to achieve an equivalent effectiveness of purification.

2. Pericarditis associated with inadequate dialysis caused by insufficient flow through the arteriovenous fistula. Until the latter is surgically corrected, or while a new vascular access is being created, adequate dialysis flow will be provided by catheterization of a subclavian or femoral vein as a substitute arterial channel, the return being through a peripheral vein.

3. Pericarditis associated with inadequate dialysis caused by increased needs. Increased frequency of dialysis sessions is indicated. In the most severe cases daily hemodialysis should be performed.

4. When peritoneal dialysis is selected, 24 exchanges of two litres of dialysis fluid every 48 hours should be carried out; the number of exchanges should be modified according to the weight and the body surface of the patient.

Modalities of use of dialysis regimens.

1. In all types of pericarditis not associated with congestive heart failure or overhydration, ultrafiltration should be strictly controlled to reduce interdialysis increase of weight, but avoiding reduction below the ideal weight. If elevation of the central venous pressure is detected clinically or by the monitor during dialysis, ultrafiltration should be offset by a plasma expander. Blood may be given in case of severe anemia, or seroalbumin if hypoalbuminemia is severe, so as to increase the plasma oncotic pressure. If hypotension develops hemodialysis should be interrupted and pericardiocentesis be performed as soon as the effect of anticoagulation allows.

2. Transudative effusion, whether or not associated with congestive heart failure or overhydration in the absence of signs of pericarditis. Ultrafiltration should be intensified, estimating a new ideal dry weight. Dietary salt should be rigidly restricted in the interdialysis periods.

3. Pericarditis associated with congestive heart failure or overhydration. Ultrafiltration during dialysis is indicated, together with salt and water restriction and other measures to improve left ventricular function (digitalis, oxygen, packed red cell transfusion, etc.). Pericardial effusion should be monitored by serial echocardiography and, if it increases, pericardiocentesis should be carried out.

Indications of pericardiocentesis

1. When purulent pericarditis is suspected.
2. Persistence for two weeks of large pericardial effusion by echocardiographic criteria in patients with pericarditis associated with hemodialysis.
3. Considerable increase of the size of the pericardial effusion between consecutive hemodialysis sessions.
4. Compensated cardiac tamponade. For this indication, pericardiocentesis should be performed before the next hemodialysis session.
5. Decompensated cardiac tamponade.

Accessible effusion should have been demonstrated previously by echocardiography. The procedure will be carried out aseptically (with sterile surgical material and dress); an epicardial ECG lead attached to the pericardiocentesis needle and ressuscitation equipment should be available. The following investigations of the pericardial fluid will be carried out: packed red cell volume, protein, glucose, lactic dehydrogenase, adenosine deaminase, cytology, staining for mycobacteria, cultures in aerobic, Löwenstein and viral media, and hepatitis B virus markers.

A catheter will be left in the pericardial sac, with closed drainage and under mild suction, until fluid no longer drains or until the next hemodialysis. The catheter will be removed after 48 hours, and its tip will be cultured.

Indications of pericardiectomy

1. Persistence of tamponade after pericardiocentesis.
2. Recurrence of tamponade after pericardiocentesis.
3. Development of constrictive pericarditis, confirmed by external recordings and catheterization.
4. Persistence of echocardiographically large pericardial effusion after adequate pericardiocentesis.

The technique and extension of pericardiectomy will depend on the type of indication and on the surgeon's judgement. Histological studies and cultures for bacteria, viruses and mycobacteria will be performed on the surgical specimen.

Use of analgesic and antiinflammatory drugs

As studies demonstrating the effectiveness of antiinflammatory drugs in this type of pericardial diseases are lacking, and considering that they are potentially harmful in uremic patients, the use of acetylsalicylic acid, nonsteroidal antiinflammatory agents and corticosteroids should be discouraged. Paracetamol or petidine may be useful to relieve pain.

Appendix 3
Francisco Romero: a pioneer of pericardiotomy (1801)

J. PASCUAL-RODRIGUEZ, M.D.

It has been said that it took man more than 2500 years to go the short distance from the skin to the pericardium, a distance which measures less than
three centimeters. This was the achievement of the Spanish physician Francisco Romero at the beginning of the nineteenth century. Unfortunately, the
original report by Romero was thought to be lost, and thus our knowledge of
the event derived only indirect mentions of it by Merat (1) and Hernández
Morejón (2) in the past century, and more recent references to it by López
Piñero and Peset Reig (3), Kilpatrick and Chapman (4), and Ruiz Caballero
and Quijano-Pitman (5).

My interest in the life and work of Francisco Romero grew into a true
obsession with the passage of time. In view of the limited bibliographical
information available, I decided that three key cities held the secret of the life
and works of Romero: Paris, Huesca and Almería. Thus, I determined that I
would journey to these three cities in an attempt to solve the mystery of the
"Romero case".

Paris

After several false starts, two of Romero's works finally appeared in the
archives of the Library of the School of Medicine of Paris. One of them included the report I had so eagerly been looking for: *Observatio experimentis
confirmata, pro hydrope pectoris, pulmonum anasarca, et hydropericardio
cognoscendis et nova methodus dictos morbos operandi.* ("Observations, confirmed by experiments, on the knowledge of hydrops of the chest, lung
anasarca and hydropericardium, with new methods to treat these disorders").
It had been published in Paris by Jeunehomme's widow, in 1815 (Fig. 1). The
efforts of other investigators to find these works, originally in the *Bibliothèque
Royale*, had undoubtedly failed because they had only recently been trans-
ferred to the *Bibliothèque Nationale*. We reproduce here the most significant
passages related to pericardiotomy. This important report by Romero was
originally published in Latin and was presented to the Society of the School
of Medicine, in Paris, on April 13th, 1815.

Most learned Academy:

I have been consecrated for 22 years to Apollo's art. I have cared for

J. Soler-Soler et al. (Eds.), Pericardial Disease, pp. 229–235.
© 1990 Kluwer Academic Publishers

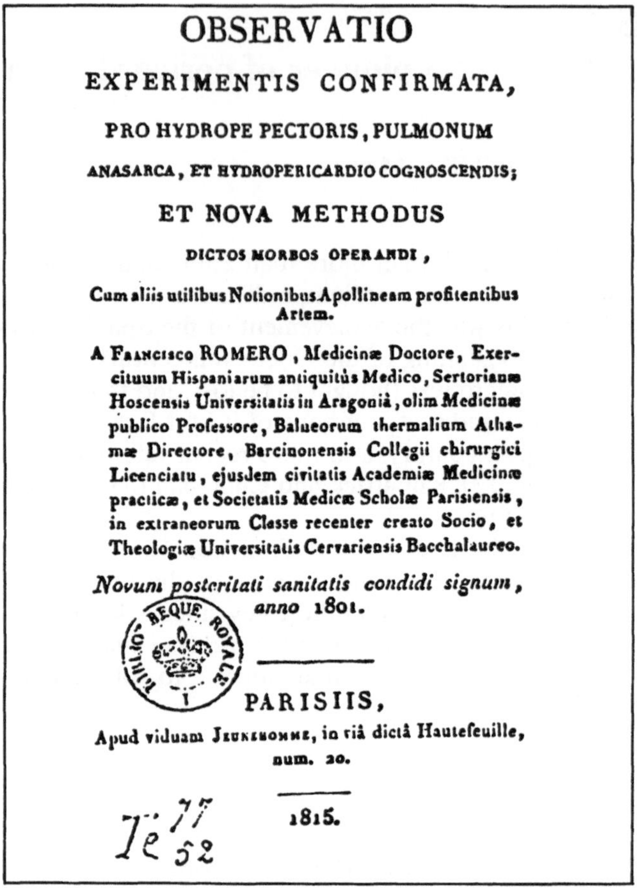

OBSERVATIO

EXPERIMENTIS CONFIRMATA,

PRO HYDROPE PECTORIS, PULMONUM

ANASARCA, ET HYDROPERICARDIO COGNOSCENDIS;

ET NOVA METHODUS

DICTOS MORBOS OPERANDI,

Cum aliis utilibus Notionibus Apollineam profitentibus
Artem.

A FRANCISCO ROMERO, Medicinæ Doctore, Exer-
cituum Hispaniarum antiquitùs Medico, Sertorianæ
Hoscensis Universitatis in Aragoniâ, olim Medicinæ
publico Professore, Balueorum thermalium Atha-
mæ Directore, Barcinonensis Collegii chirurgici
Licenciatu, ejusdem civitatis Academiæ Medicinæ
practicæ, et Societatis Medicæ Scholæ Parisiensis,
in extraneorum Classe recenter creato Socio, et
Theologiæ Universitatis Cervariensis Bacchalaureo.

Novum posteritati sanitatis condidi signum,
anno 1801.

PARISIIS,

Apud viduam JEUNEHOMME, in viâ dictâ Hautefeuille,
num. 20.

1815.

Fig. 1. Front page of Francisco Romero's report where he describes his technique for pericardiotomy.

many patients of both sexes afflicted with hydrops of the chest, as this
condition is almost endemic in villages and cities of the diocese of Almería,
near the seaside in Andalusia, and carries away men in their prime.

Insofar as the first and foremost of the physician's duties is to keep men's
present health, I tried with all my might to hinder and detain the progress
of such a disease. However, my efforts were of no avail among those people
enjoying good health, as they did not heed my advice of prevention. That is
the reason why I was compelled to carry out the second of the physician's
duties, namely, to restore lost health to the patient.

(....)

Hydrops of the chest, as far as I have seen it, kills men straight within
forty days or torments them throughout many months only to do away with
them at the end. Hydrops of the chest consists of an unnatural accumula-

tion of serous fluid within the chest; this fluid can be retained in both cavities of the chest or in the pericardium, or in the mediastinum, or it can be
deposited within the cellular meshes of the lung or its interstitium.

(....)

While the serous fluid is confined to the pericardium, the disease is so
difficult to identify that it quite often misleads the most experienced observers; this is so because, on the one hand, the tightness of the anguished
feeling in the anterior part of the chest and the patient continuously bringing his own hands to that part of the body (according to the proverb "ubi
manus, ibi dolor" – where the hands go, there the pain is –), the palpita-
tions of the heart, the irregular and often dicrotic pulse, the cough and the
faints, lead to the suspicion of hydrops of the pericardium (as these symptoms are common with those coming from the heart and the aneurysms of
the adjacent blood vessels); on the other hand, however, owing to the lack
of any pathognomonic sign, no conclusive argument demonstrating the
unnatural presence of fluid in the pericardium can be inferred.

(....)

I have thoroughly consulted the best famed authors who have discussed
hydrops of the chest, such as Morgagni, Senac, Hoffman, Van Swieten and
Lieutaud, and I have been unable to find any clue to identify with certainty
hydrops of the pericardium; and, neither the usual chest contusions, nor
the Vieussens' signs of lividness around the lips and the eyelids are of any
use to demonstrate its occurrence (as hydrops of the pericardium is sometimes present without them), the idea came to my mind, after deep consideration, to open up the thorax with a scalpel as for a paracentesis,
between the fifth and the sixth ribs (at the level of the incurvation where
the carthilage lays), and, through this opening, once the patient's body is
brought to slumber, to palpate the pericardium to make sure whether it was
filled with serous fluid or not. I did not regret having performed this experiment, as I found what I had been looking for at the first attempt.

(....)

When, owing to the findings that I have mentioned, I have convinced
myself of the occurrence of pericardial hydrops, I have carried out a small
opening in the anterior part of the chest, with a scalpel, as for a paracentesis, near the curvature of the sixth true rib where the carthilage is inserted, having placed the patient slightly on the side through which he was
to be approached; I have then introduced a small annular forceps to pull
out the pericardial layers (not forgetting the anatomical knowledge of the
region), and I have carried out a short incision of the pericardium with a
small pair of curved scissors, whereby the serous fluid has been drawn to
the cavity of the chest, and thence it has been removed, according to the
physician's wishes, after placing the patient in the most convenient posi-

tion. I have performed two pericardial paracenteses in this fashion with a successful outcome. All these steps should be speedily undertaken to prevent air from entering the cavity.

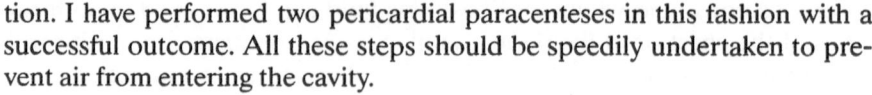

Although I have personaly discovered, performed and recommended all that I have reported here, I do not think it is so safely established as to divulge it widely. Further experiences are needed, and I will go on with them for as long as I will be able to, submitting them to your consideration.

> Paris, April 13th, 1815
> Franciso Romero
> Medicus Gotholaunicus.

In view of the difficulties in the diagnosis and the danger attendant on any maneuver near the heart, the referees of this report thought this operation to be "so important and full of risk that we cannot pronounce a judgement on its value", so they proposed it to the practitioner as a "matter for meditation". They did not agree with Romero, who advocates "opening the thorax as soon as the presence of water in the pleural and pericardial cavities is known". The report went on: "The Society proposes that more details be submitted about those patients he claims to have successfully operated on with that technique" (6).

Romero presented another report in July of the same year, in response to the Society of the School of Medicine. I was able to identify the original manuscript *Responsio a Societatis Scholae parisiensis ex me scriptis petita* ("Response requested of me by the Society of the School of Medicine of Paris regarding my reports") among bundles of as yet unclassified Academy documents. The following paragraphs are quotations from this second report.

Most learned Academy:

The name of the first patient in whom I carried out pericardial paracentesis because of pericardial hydrops, during the spring of the first year of the current century, was Francisco de Mira. He was a widowed peasant, and he lived in the Campo de Gata, near the seaside. He had been cared for during the last five months by the military surgeon Jorge Grenier, appointed to the city of Almería. I was called in consultation, and, as soon as I saw the patient, I made the diagnosis of pericardial hydrops and I decided that to confirm it, an incision should be made at the level of the incurvation of the sixth rib, to reach the pericardium. As it was evident at first sight that the pericardium was abnormally filled with fluid, straightaway I performed, with a pair of curved scissors, the second part of the operation in the presence of the above mentioned surgeon. Immediately, the patient declared that he felt better. The amount of fluid removed was about five pounds in weight and it had the color of a brick. Five hours afterwards, fever, thirst, stinging pain, troubled respiration, insommia and reddening of the jaws appeared; these symptoms gradually increased until the fifth day, and thereafter they began to subside with the help of reiterated small amounts of emulsions and with the application of emollients to the external parts of the chest.

(....)

The patient resumed his work after four months. He had a cachectic temperament. Three years after the operation I met him by chance and, when I asked him about his health, he answered that he felt well; he complained of a small fixed pain that I judged to correspond to the same spot where the inflammatory adhesion between the pericardial layers had taken place owing to the incision performed at the time of the operation.

The second patient upon whom I operated because of the same disease was thirty-seven years old, had a bilious temperament and had never married. His dwelling place was near the Armilla mount; he was a peasant, and was being cared for by the surgeon Cisneros, the second appointed surgeon of the above mentioned city. I was called in consultation, and I suspected pericardial hydrops. After the first thoracic incision and much discussion, I did not find anything; nearly despairing of discovering the hydrops, another method came to my mind: I introduced a pair of anular forceps until I touched the pericardium; I kept them at this level, and I made concussions throughout the thorax, and by this means the sound made by the serous fluid was confusely heard about the slumbering body. This difficulty, as I discovered when I evacuated the fluid, arose from the fact that hydrops was not yet complete, as the disease had not yet reached its final stage.

(....)

After he had recovered health, this patient too complained of a small fixed internal pain and of some breathing trouble. The surname of the patient was Trapat.

The third patient with the same disease lived outside the city walls, he had not married, and his temperament was melancholic; I cannot recall exactly his name, but I remember he was a craftsman and had been ill for eight months. When I was called to relieve him in some way, I suspected pericardial hydrops and I performed the first part of my operation in both parts of the chest. However, my endeavor was of no avail because of the bilateral adhesions of the lungs to the pleura. The patient, who suffered a high fever as a consequence of the surgical wound, quickly died after four days. I was denied, and was deeply sorry for it, the permission to furtively examine the corpse, although I had offered a sum of money to obtain it.

(....)

Most learned Academy: Here you have all that you have asked from me. This is all that, as far as I can remember, I can offer you regarding my experience in the observation of hydrops of the chest and the pericardium.

Paris, July 7th, 1815
Francisco Romero,
Medicus Gotholaunicus.

Romero's scientific output is not limited to these reports. Some lesser studies are described in *Observatio de croup* and in essays on venereal disease. Remarkably, in contrast with his daring approach to hydrothorax and hydropericardium, Romero was extremely cautious about the indications for tracheostomy for diphtheria.

Huesca

As the place and date of Romero's birth were unknown, I directed my subsequent research to Huesca. Here, I found that a Francisco Romero, born in Concabella (Lérida) had been graduated at Huesca University in the term 1795–96. The record is repeated for a graduation in 1798–99, which might correspond to his doctorate (7). Verification of Romero's birthplace could not be made in Concabella, because the parish archives had been destroyed during a war. In any case, a small note in the Bulletin of the School of Medicine of Paris (8) stating that he was appointed corresponding member of the Society of Medicine, confirms that he had been born in the mentioned village.

Almería

In Almería, Romero was appointed as physician of the Hospital de Santa María Magdalena on April 12, 1812, and, in the following month, as a municipal physician (9). Data about his activities in both the hospital and the town are difficult to obtain, as he probably departed with the French army in September, 1812. His professional activity there was thus limited to the interval between April and September 1812.

Not much more is known about Francisco Romero. He entertained the hope, during his exile, of returning to Spain; however, we do not know whether the changing Spanish political scene allowed him to fulfil his wish. Possibly he died in Paris, in his home at 24, rue de l'Ecole de Médecine. This address is printed at the foot of the front page of his *Essai sur les moyens de reconnaître l'existence de la maladie vénérienne*.

References

1. Mérat F. Péricardite. In: Dictionnaire des Sciences Médicales. Paris, volume XL 1819; pp. 369–75.
2. Hernández Morejón A. Historia bibliográfica de la Medicina Española. Madrid, Viuda Jordán, 1842; 52.
3. López Piñero JM, Peset Reig R. Francisco Romero y los orígenes de la cirugía cardíaca. Arbor, 206. Madrid, 1963.
4. Kilpatrick ZM, Chapman CB. On pericardiocentesis. Am J Cardiol 1965; 16: 722–8.
5. Ruiz Caballero M, Quijano-Pitman F. La primera pericardiotomía. Medicamenta 1972; 59: 498.
6. Husson HM, Mérat FV. Extrait d'une mémoire de M. le docteur F. Romero, médecin de Catalogne, sur l'hydrotorax et l'hydropéricarde. Bull Fac Méd Paris 1815; 4: 373.
7. Menéndez de la Fuente L. Graduados en medicina, cirugía y farmacia por la Facultad de Medicina de la Universidad de Huesca. IV Congreso Español de Historia de la Medicina (Granada), 1973; III: 223–225.
8. Bull Fac Méd París 1814–15; 4: 419.
9. Documentación procedente del Archivo del Municipio y del Hospital de Almería, comunicada por D. A. Ruiz, en 1980.

Index

244

Developments in Cardiovascular Medicine

43. S. Sideman and R. Beyar (eds.): [3-D] *Simulation and Imaging of the Cardiac System*. State of the Heart. Proceedings of the International Henry Goldberg Workshop, held in Haifa, Israel (1984). 1985 ISBN 0–89838–687–X
44. E. van der Wall and K.I. Lie (eds.): *Recent Views on Hypertrophic Cardiomyopathy*. Proceedings of a Symposium, held in Groningen, The Netherlands (1984). 1985
 ISBN 0–89838–694–2
45. R.E. Beamish, P.K. Singal and N.S. Dhalla (eds.), *Stress and Heart Disease*. Proceedings of a International Symposium, held in Winnipeg, Canada, 1984 (Vol. 1). 1985 ISBN 0–89838–709–4
46. R.E. Beamish, V. Panagia and N.S. Dhalla (eds.): *Pathogenesis of Stress-induced Heart Disease*. Proceedings of a International Symposium, held in Winnipeg, Canada, 1984 (Vol. 2). 1985 ISBN 0–89838–710–8
47. J. Morganroth and E.N. Moore (eds.): *Cardiac Arrhythmias*. New Therapeutic Drugs and Devices. Proceedings of the 5th Symposium on New Drugs and Devices, held in Philadelphia, Pa., U.S.A. (1984). 1985 ISBN 0–89838–716–7
48. P. Mathes (ed.): *Secondary Prevention in Coronary Artery Disease and Myocardial Infarction*. 1985 ISBN 0–89838–736–1
49. H.L. Stone and W.B. Weglicki (eds.): *Pathobiology of Cardiovascular Injury*. Proceedings of the 6th Annual Meeting of the American Section of the I.S.H.R., held in Oklahoma City, Okla., U.S.A. (1984). 1985 ISBN 0–89838–743–4
50. J. Meyer, R. Erbel and H.J. Rupprecht (eds.): *Improvement of Myocardial Perfusion*. Thrombolysis, Angioplasty, Bypass Surgery. Proceedings of a Symposium, held in Mainz, F.R.G. (1984). 1985 ISBN 0–89838–748–5
51. J.H.C. Reiber, P.W. Serruys and C.J. Slager (eds.): *Quantitative Coronary and Left Ventricular Cineangiography*. Methodology and Clinical Applications. 1986
 ISBN 0–89838–760–4
52. R.H. Fagard and I.E. Bekaert (eds.): *Sports Cardiology*. Exercise in Health and Cardiovascular Disease. Proceedings from an International Conference, held in Knokke, Belgium (1985). 1986 ISBN 0–89838–782–5
53. J.H.C. Reiber and P.W. Serruys (eds.): *State of the Art in Quantitative Cornary Arteriography*. 1986 ISBN 0–89838–804–X
54. J. Roelandt (ed.): *Color Doppler Flow Imaging and Other Advances in Doppler Echocardiography*. 1986 ISBN 0–89838–806–6
55. E.E. van der Wall (ed.): *Noninvasive Imaging of Cardiac Metabolism*. Single Photon Scintigraphy, Positron Emission Tomography and Nuclear Magnetic Resonance. 1987
 ISBN 0–89838–812–0
56. J. Liebman, R. Plonsey and Y. Rudy (eds.): *Pediatric and Fundamental Electrocardiography*. 1987 ISBN 0–89838–815–5
57. H.H. Hilger, V. Hombach and W.J. Rashkind (eds.), *Invasive Cardiovascular Therapy*. Proceedings of an International Symposium, held in Cologne, F.R.G. (1985). 1987 ISBN 0–89838–818–X
58. P.W. Serruys and G.T. Meester (eds.): *Coronary Angioplasty*. A Controlled Model for Ischemia. 1986 ISBN 0–89838–819–8
59. J.E. Tooke and L.H. Smaje (eds.): *Clinical Investigation of the Microcirculation*. Proceedings of an International Meeting, held in London, U.K. (1985). 1987
 ISBN 0–89838–833–3

Developments in Cardiovascular Medicine

Developments in Cardiovascular Medicine

78. M.M. Scheinman (ed.): *Catheter Ablation of Cardiac Arrhythmias.* Basic Bioelectrical Effects and Clinical Indications. 1988   ISBN 0–89838–967–4
79. J.A.E. Spaan, A.V.G. Bruschke and A.C. Gittenberger-De Groot (eds.): *Coronary Circulation.* From Basic Mechanisms to Clinical Implications. 1987
                                                                        ISBN 0–89838–978–X
80. C. Visser, G. Kan and R.S. Meltzer (eds.): *Echocardiography in Coronary Artery Disease.* 1988   ISBN 0–89838–979–8
81. A. Bayés de Luna, A. Betriu and G. Permanyer (eds.): *Therapeutics in Cardiology.* 1988   ISBN 0–89838–981–X
82. D.M. Mirvis (ed.): *Body Surface Electrocardiographic Mapping.* 1988
                                                                        ISBN 0–89838–983–6
83. M.A. Konstam and J.M. Isner (eds.): *The Right Ventricle.* 1988 ISBN 0–89838–987–9
84. C.T. Kappagoda and P.V. Greenwood (eds.): *Long-term Management of Patients after Myocardial Infarction.* 1988   ISBN 0–89838–352–8
85. W.H. Gaasch and H.J. Levine (eds.): *Chronic Aortic Regurgitation.* 1988
                                                                        ISBN 0–89838–364–1
86. P.K. Singal (ed.): *Oxygen Radicals in the Pathophysiology of Heart Disease.* 1988
                                                                        ISBN 0–89838–375–7
87. J.H.C. Reiber and P.W. Serruys (eds.): *New Developments in Quantitative Coronary Arteriography.* 1988   ISBN 0–89838–377–3
88. J. Morganroth and E.N. Moore (eds.): *Silent Myocardial Ischemia.* Proceedings of the 8th Annual Symposium on New Drugs and Devices (1987). 1988
                                                                        ISBN 0–89838–380–3
89. H.E.D.J. ter Keurs and M.I.M. Noble (eds.): *Starling's Law of the Heart Revisted.* 1988   ISBN 0–89838–382–X
90. N. Sperelakis (ed.): *Physiology and Pathophysiology of the Heart.* (Rev. ed.) 1988
                                                                        ISBN 0–89838–388–9
91. J.W. de Jong (ed.): *Myocardial Energy Metabolism.* 1988   ISBN 0–89838–394–3
92. V. Hombach, H.H. Hilger and H.L. Kennedy (eds.): *Electrocardiography and Cardiac Drug Therapy.* Proceedings of an International Symposium, held in Cologne, F.R.G. (1987). 1988   ISBN 0–89838–395–1
93. H. Iwata, J.B. Lombardini and T. Segawa (eds.): *Taurine and the Heart.* 1988
                                                                        ISBN 0–89838–396–X
94. M.R. Rosen and Y. Palti (eds.): *Lethal Arrhythmias Resulting from Myocardial Ischemia and Infarction.* Proceedings of the 2nd Rappaport Symposium, held in Haifa, Israel (1988). 1988   ISBN 0–89838–401–X
95. M. Iwase and I. Sotobata: *Clinical Echocardiography.* With a Foreword by M.P. Spencer. 1989   ISBN 0–7923–0004–1
96. I. Cikes (ed.): *Echocardiography in Cardiac Interventions.* 1989
                                                                        ISBN 0–7923–0088–2
97. E. Rapaport (ed.): *Early Interventions in Acute Myocardial Infarction.* 1989
                                                                        ISBN 0–7923–0175–7
98. M.E. Safar and F. Fouad-Tarazi (eds.): *The Heart in Hypertension.* A Tribute to Robert C. Tarazi (1925–1986). 1989   ISBN 0–7923–0197–8
99. S. Meerbaum and R. Meltzer (eds.): *Myocardial Contrast Two-dimensional Echocardiography.* 1989   ISBN 0–7923–0205–2

Developments in Cardiovascular Medicine